Evidence-Based Practice:
Toward Optimizing Clini

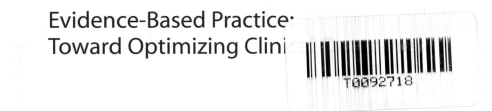

T0092718

Francesco Chiappelli (Editor)

Xenia Maria Caldeira Brant
Negoita Neagos
Oluwadayo O. Oluwadara
Manisha Harish Ramchandani (Co-Editors)

Evidence-Based Practice: Toward Optimizing Clinical Outcomes

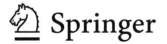 Springer

Prof. Dr. Francesco Chiappelli
ADA Champion, Evidence-Based Dentistry
Divisions of Oral Biology and Medicine
and Associated Clinical Specialties (Joint)
University of California, Los Angeles
School of Dentistry
Divisions of Oral Biology and Medicine
Los Angeles, CA 90095-1668
USA
fchiappelli@dentistry.ucla.edu

Prof. Dr. Xenia Maria Caldeira Brant
Rua Aimorés 2480/609
Belo Horizonte-MG
Brazil
xenia.brant@gmail.com

Dr. Negoita Neagos
University of California, Los Angeles
School of Dentistry
Divisions of Oral Biology and Medicine
Los Angeles, CA 90095-1668
USA
nneagos@yahoo.com

Dr. Oluwadayo O. Oluwadara
University of California, Los Angeles
School of Dentistry
Divisions of Oral Biology and Medicine
Los Angeles, CA 90095-1668
USA
oluwadara@yahoo.com

Dr. Manisha Harish Ramchandani
University of California, Los Angeles
School of Dentistry
Divisions of Oral Biology and Medicine
Los Angeles, CA 90095-1668
USA
rmanisha@ucla.edu

ISBN: 978-3-642-05024-4   e-ISBN: 978-3-642-05025-1

DOI: 10.1007/978-3-642-05025-1

Springer Heidelberg Dordrecht London New York

Library of Congress Control Number: 2010923771

Cover design: eStudio Calamar, Figueres/Berlin

Printed on acid-free paper

Springer is part of Springer Science+Business Media (www.springer.com)

Foreword

Evidence-Based Decision-Making in Health Care: Implications and Directions for the Future

In the current political climate, health care is in crisis with no conceivable, long-term solution. Its future portends a shortage of primary care physicians with an estimated 50 million new patients needing basic health care [1]. It is expected that in the next decade 40,000 medical providers must be added to the existing 100,000 or the system for health care response to expected need will be overwhelmed. While the agenda for universal health care and reform has become a major stimulus for political action, dentistry has provided concrete advances in knowledge, technology, and mechanisms toward credible and practical responses to this crisis.

These advances come in the form of new knowledge and research into oral biomarkers in screening for systemic diseases with mechanisms to systematically review published information for best evidence, and practical models to implement this best evidence for service providers and their patients. This implementation is integrated into the shared decision-making, patient assessment, evaluation, and treatment planning encounter occurring within real timeframes and without disturbing practice routines. The effort of dentistry to provide these workable solutions is particularly profound in that the knowledge, mechanisms, and models offered attempt to maximize effective, efficacious, and cost containment treatment options for patients with best health care evidence for all within the dynamics of change in knowledge and treatments.

Thus, there is a paradigm shift occurring in the concept of health care practice in general and dental practice in particular. The approach to patient-centered care is envisioning dental practice as part of primary care, creating a concept in which dental practice has expanded to become a center for dental medicine and oral health wellness. Evidence of this paradigm shift is the work being done by David Wong in salivary diagnostics. Malamud [2] extols this new approach as *"point-of-care (POC)"* diagnostics that will revolutionize the way a limited amount of resources may be used to handle increased patient loads, providing the ability to diagnose disease conditions: reciprocal and inclusive of those performed in diagnostic medicine. Here, a *"noninvasive, well-tolerated"* oral sampling may be used to identify biomarkers in diagnosing disease at initial or periodic dental maintenance visits.

As part of primary care, dental providers become part of the interdisciplinary team whose responsibility is to manage health care, including dental services, for shared patients. This health care management and service delivery may occur in hospital, nursing home, or private practices and clinics. For dentists, or any health care provider, this requires a knowledge base for interpretation of data and translation of its information into service or treatment options. EBR and translational evidence mechanisms are needed to provide trusted best evidence to perform within the dynamics of this new concept of dental practice.

There are two major categories within which EBR has provided to meet changes in future health care practices. One has been in the reasoning of evidence and the other in application of this reasoning to improving patient decision-making in the presence of uncertainty about health care options, their value to individuals, and cost trade-offs.

Evidence-based advances in reasoning have expanded knowledge or data to include the value and application of best evidence to patients and society. Current mechanisms include comparative effectiveness research (CER) and EBR. CER may be independent or synergistic with EBR. CER both conducts studies and uses systematic review analyses to compare similar treatments or procedures in maximizing the choice of the most effective cost/benefit option within the context of new evidence [3]. EBR uses similar analyses; however, the result is to determine best evidence in maximizing best outcomes not costs. Clinicians use these advances to promote shared understanding and decision-making in providing informed consent as well as oral health services and their maintenance along with disease control in individuals, their patients [5].

While CER and EBD in health care assist in reasoning individual health and treatment choices during shared-decision making with dentists, translational evidence mechanisms explain the development of data, its transformation into best evidence, clinical relevance, and meaning in practice. These mechanisms, which rely on human information technology (HIT) systems, propose to understand, define, and characterize the underlying process involved in clinical decision-making for CER and EBD. For health care in the twenty-first Century, the triad of CER-EBD-HIT defines the compact between researcher (research synthesis), clinician (clinical expertise, local long-term monitoring and implementation of evidence), patients (patient choice and compliance) in providing the essential components of the biological, behavioral, and social interventions involved in clinical decision-making related to health care delivery, and coverage of costs by third-party providers [4].

The future of these advances is profound for patients because dentists and physicians are known for providing services, treatments, and therapies in the nongovernmental, private business sector that responds to market forces in maximizing effective, efficacious, and cost containment for oral health care and service delivery. Dentistry and medicine, as well as nursing and allied health care professions, function as part of the primary care – interdisciplinary team systems approach. This is a reality today, which will subsist in coming decades.

Therefore, the contributions contained within this book explain the advances made in evidence-based and CER for decision-making in health care. This literature provides the background and knowledge of the development, validation, and implementation of research methodologies and mechanisms in providing relevant and practical solutions for physicians, dentists, nurses, and patients. These advances are timely in their promotion of best evidence used in informed consent and assisting the choices and trade-offs patients often are required to make when uncertainties in health care choices and options arise. The benefit of these developments toward resolving the current crisis in health care delivery nationally and internationally is critical and timely as it proffers practical models for translating the best available research evidence to patients and society for improvement in health care and well-being of the patient populations we serve.

Janet G. Bauer, DDS, MSEd, MSPH, MBA
Associate Professor and Director
June and Paul Ehrlich Endowed Program
in Geriatric Dentistry
UCLA School of Dentistry
23-088E CHS, 10833 Le Conte Avenue
Los Angeles, CA 90095-1668, USA

References

1. Associated press: 50 million new patients? Expect doc shortages. Revamped health care system could swamp primary care physicians. [article online] cited 14 September 2009. Available from: http://www.msnbc.msn.com/id/32829974
2. Malamud D (2006) Salivary diagnostics: the future is now. J Am Dent Ass 137:284–286
3. A new analysis released by the RAND Corporation (8 September 2009) suggests that while there are benefits to having better information for health care providers, third-party providers (e.g., insurance companies), and patients about what works best in treating different health problems short-term, it is uncertain that comparative effectiveness research will lead to reductions in spending and waste or improvements in patient health…. "there is not enough evidence at this point to predict exactly what the result might be for the cost of the nation's health care system.." Elizabeth McGlynn, codirector of COMPARE, RAND Corporation http://www.randcompare.org/publications/summary/comparative_effectiveness_research_may_not_lead_to_lower_health_costs_or_improve_health_analysis_finds
4. Chiappelli F, Cajulis O, Newman M. Comparative Effectiveness Research in Evidence-Based Dental Practice. J Evid Based Dent Pract 2009 9:57–8
5. Chiappelli F, Cajulis OS. The logic model in evidence-based clinical decision-making in dental practice. J Evid Based Dent Pract 2009 9:206–10

Preface

Just over 10 years ago, the American Dental Association produced its original policy statement on evidence-based dentistry (February, 1999). Later that year, a colleague at UCLA School of Dentistry, Professor Lindemann, told me "Francesco, you really should look into this evidence-based dentistry." His suggestion changed my research direction, and, I suppose, that moment was the true genesis of this book.

Of course, the movement toward evidence-based practice in dentistry had been ushered in a few years earlier by medicine (evidence-based medicine). The notion had spread fast both nationally and internationally and across fields, and, within a few years, one could find common references to evidence-based nursing, evidence-based specialties across the branches of health care, and even evidence-based law, economics, and the like. As I began to explore the field, I was fortunate to develop colleagues interested in evidence-based research (EBR) and decision-making in the health sciences in general, and in dentistry in particular, across the globe.

Students and post-docs in my research group became increasingly actively engaged in this new and cutting edge field, and we soon published a carefully crafted definition of the meta-construct of evidence-based dentistry [1], and of salient issues in this emerging field [2]. In 2003, the *Brazilian Journal of Oral Sciences* invited me to be the guest editor of a special issue dedicated to evidence-based dentistry – to my knowledge, the first ever peer-reviewed journal dedicating a special issue to evidence-based dentistry. By 2006, when the *California Dental Association Journal* invited me to do the same, evidence-based dentistry was fast becoming established in the national and international dental literature. Working on both these issues was transforming, that is, it gave me a broad awareness of the depth of the field, its potentials, impediments, hurdles, and benefits.

It was during that time that my students, coresearchers, and I realized the methodological void that still remained to be addressed in the field. We developed the Wong scale [3] to assess and to quantify the quality of the research methodology, design, and data analysis based on commonly accepted criteria, and soon revised it and improved its validity and reliability [4]. We refined our skills in research synthesis, and in our ability to generate the best available evidence, be it in dentistry, medicine, alternative and complementary medicine, or any domain of the health sciences [5]. We realized that, whereas our research group was well versed in obtaining a consensus of the best available evidence, we had done little in terms of utilizing the evidence-based paradigm to optimize clinical outcomes. We were aware of the need to fill the gap between clinical practice based on the evidence, patient-oriented evidence that matters (POEM), and research synthesis (or, specifically for the field of dentistry: research evaluation and appraisal in dentistry [READ]) [6], and endeavored to do more in that domain. Hence this book.

Upon this fertile ground, an idea burgeoned, which we shared with Stephanie Benko at Springer, and the proposal for this comprehensive book addressing cutting edge issues about utilizing evidence-based concepts in clinical practice in order to optimize clinical outcomes was in the making. Soon, Irmela Bohn (Springer) stepped in the project, and we were most fortunate because, without Irmela's expertise, patience, and guidance, the project would have remained just that: an idea – a good idea perhaps, but just an idea. I will never be able to thank Irmela enough for her dedication, encouragement, and superlative hard work along the way.

It was mainly because of her, and through her consistent support that the project really took a life of its own. And soon I was discussing it with selected colleagues in various countries – from Brazil to Nigeria, from Romenia to the US - inviting them to be on the editorial team. Together, we carefully chose the "rose" of experts in the field to invite to contribute chapters. Therefore, of course, I must thank profusely my friends and colleagues – Drs. Brant, Neagos, and Oluwadara – who worked long and arduous hours on this project as coeditors. Without them, the final product would never have achieved the level of perfection and excellence it has.

My profound thanks, which I know are shared as well by the coeditors, go to the authors of the chapters in this work. They wrote assiduously, edited and perfected their chapters patiently responding to each and every one of Irmela's and my and the coeditors' requests for timeliness, precision, format, and all the possible details one could imagine. It is their expertise and their dedication to this project that makes this book the superb *ouvrage* and the timely and critical anthology of evidence-based decision (EBD)-making in health care the high quality product that it is.

Los Angeles, California, USA   Francesco Chiappelli

References

1. Chiappelli F, Prolo P (2001) The meta-construct of evidence based dentistry: Part I. J Evid Based Dental Pract 1:159–165
2. Chiappelli F, Prolo P, Newman M, Cruz M, Sunga E, Concepcion E, Edgerton M (2003) Evidence-based dentistry: benefit or hindrance. J Dental Res 82:6–7
3. Wong J, Prolo P, Chiappelli F (2003) Extending evidence-based dentistry beyond clinical trials: implications for materials research in endodontics. Braz J Oral Sci 2:227–231
4. Chiappelli F, Prolo P, Rosenblum M, Edgeron M, Cajulis OS (2006) Evidence-based research in complementary and alternative medicine II: the process of evidence-based research. Evid Based Complement Altern Med 3:3–12
5. Chiappelli F (2008) The science of research synthesis: a manual of evidence-based research for the health sciences – implications and applications in dentistry. NY, NovaScience, pp 1–327
6. Chiappelli F, Cajulis OS (2008) Transitioning toward evidence-based research in the health sciences for the XXI century. Evid Based Complement Altern Med 5:123–128

Acknowledgements

This work would not have been possible without the arduous and serious dedication of the many predental students who, in the past several years, have contributed to our research groups. Most of them have found over the years a most deserved acceptance into dental school, some jointly with a Master's degree or even a PhD degree. To name only a few, I wish to commend Dr. Jason Wong for his original work on the Wong scale, and Dr. Jason Kung for his original work on the revision of the AMSTAR. I also want to mention particularly Ms. Audrey Navarro (dental student and PhD candidate), Mr. David Moradi (dental student and Master's candidate); and Ms. Raisa Avezova, Mr. George Kossan, Mr. Cesar Perez, Ms. Linda Phi, and Ms. Nancy Shagian, predental students, for their current contribution to our research progress in EBD-making. By their assiduous dedication to forwarding the field of research synthesis for EBD-making and for comparative effectiveness analysis, they enact the beautiful words uttered not so long ago by the French writer Antoine de Saint-Exupéry (29 June 1900 – 31 July 1944): "*Fais de ta vie un rêve et de tes rêves la réalité...*"

I thank colleagues at UCLA and beyond for their precious intellectual contributions, especially Drs. Janet Bauer, Carl Maida, and Jeanne Nervina, and the Evidence-Based Dentistry Center at the American Dental Association.

I thank the UCLA Senate for funding in support of this and other research endeavors by my group.

And most of all, I, on behalf as well of the coeditors of this work, profusely thank Ms. Irmela Bohn of Springer (Heidelberg, Germany) for her kind support, patience, and guidance in making this anthology of EBD-making the high-quality product that it is.

I dedicate this and all of my academic endeavors to Olivia, to Aymerica and to Fredi, and to honor *...la gloria di Colui che tutto move/per l'universo penetra e risplende/in una parte più e meno altrove...*(Dante Alighieri, 1265–1321; La Divina Commedia, Paradiso, I 1–3).

Contents

The Science of Research Synthesis in Clinical Decision-Making

Introduction: Research Synthesis in Evidence-Based Clinical Decision-Making

1

Francesco Chiappelli, Xenia M. C. Brant, Oluwadayo O. Oluwadara, Negoita Neagos, and Manisha Harish Ramchandani

Core Message

> It is important and timely to facilitate evidence-based decision making that results in better patient outcomes, enhanced research planning, better products, and improved policy development. This book is a compilation of the writings of several experts in the field, and their collaborators. Each chapter examines specific facets of the process of evidence-based clinical decision making in the principal domains of health care, which is subsumed briefly here as dentistry, medicine, and nursing.

F. Chiappelli (✉)
Divisions of Oral Biology and Medicine, and Associated Clinical Specialties (Joint), University of California at Los Angeles, School of Dentistry, CHS 63-090, Los Angeles, CA 90095-1668, USA
e-mail: fchiappelli@dentistry.ucla.edu

X.M.C. Brant
Rua Aimorés 2480/609, Belo Horizonte-MG, Brazil
e-mail: xenia.brant@gmail.com

O.O. Oluwadara
N. Neagos
M.H. Ramchandani
University of California, Los Angeles, School of Dentistry, Divisions of Oral Biology and Medicine, Los Angeles, CA 90095-1668, USA
e-mail: oluwadara@yahoo.com
e-mail: nneagos@yahoo.com
e-mail: rmanisha@ucla.edu

1.1 Introduction: Evidence-Based Health Care

1.1.1 The Example of Dentistry

Health care and treatment modalities continue to evolve from its earliest introduction in the Western society. In dentistry, for example, the concept of oral pathology and dental intervention as a field in its own right was first articulated by Dr. Pierre Fauchard (1678–1622 March 1761) [18]. In the last three centuries, three periods have characterized the evolution of clinical dentistry; the first 200 years, followed by a period of five decades or so, leading to the last decade. The first "drill and fix" reparative mode focused upon the repair of damaged or decayed dental structures, and most often the performance of extractions. The second great period of dental care emerged as the "prevention" model, and integrated specific benchmark measures that included the patient dental exam and history, and the dentist's expertise and training, in addition to utility indices, such as cost, risk, overall benefits, and, as insurance coverage grew, cost modalities, and most importantly novel research evidence. Emerging "magic bullets," drugs, materials, and medicaments were developed, tested in vitro, in animal models, with control human subjects, and eventually in full-scale clinical trials. Evidence mounted in support of this or that intervention, and was integrated in the decision making of treatment. It was not long before some prided themselves to follow this new model of dental care as "dentistry based on the evidence" [3, 4, 7, 35].

The sheer amount of new research evidence called for articulated guidelines by which the new information could be identified, evaluated, and synthesized into some form of a consensus of the totality of the *best available* evidence for the purpose of elaborating revised clinical practice guidelines (rCPGs). Dental care emerged in the late 1990s into its third and current period of "evidence-based dentistry (EBD)[1]" [3, 4, 19, 22, 27, 39, 43, 44, 54].

In brief, EBD is now conceptualized as consisting of two principal, intertwined, and cross-feeding features:

- Identification of the best available research evidence
- Integration of the best available evidence into treatment intervention

The process by which the available evidence is gathered in response to a given clinical question, and rigorously evaluated, following the stringent protocols of research synthesis (RS) [33], for obtaining the best available evidence is sometimes referred to as evidence-based research (EBR); and the process by which this best available evidence is incorporated into clinical practice pertains to evidence-based practice (EBPr) (Fig. 1.1).

The best available evidence that is gathered through EBR is meant to complement, not replace the set of elements that the clinician utilizes in decision-making. EBD is simply intended to formulate recommendations (cf., note 1) for decision making, and not to

dictate what practitioners should or should not do."... *Rather, the EBD process is based on integrating the scientific basis for clinical care, using thorough, unbiased reviews and the best available scientific evidence at any 1 time, with clinical and patient factors to make the best possible decision(s) about appropriate health care for specific clinical circumstances. EBD relies on the role of individual professional judgment in this process...*" (ADA Positions and Statements).

Undoubtedly, certain interventions in dentistry need not, or cannot be subjected to the evidence-based paradigm. Take, for example, a superficial cavity in the enamel compartment of a molar: here an aggressive restoration involving a root canal, a crown, or an implant is most likely uncalled for. By contrast, carious lesions that project proximal to the pulp chamber, will, in all likelihood require aggressive restoration. In this particular case, evidence-based dental care is most probably not needed. EBD, and evidence-based medicine (EBM) and evidence-based nursing (EBN), fundamentally incorporates into clinical decisions for treatment interventions and for updating policies a plethora of well-articulated information about:

- The patient:
  - Dental and medical history
  - Wants and needs
  - Exam results, symptoms, X-rays, laboratory tests
- The health care provider:
  - Training, expertise
  - Clinical judgment, experience
  - Recommendations
- Utility concerns:
  - Risk/benefit ratio
  - Cost/benefit ratio
  - Insurance coverage/private payment

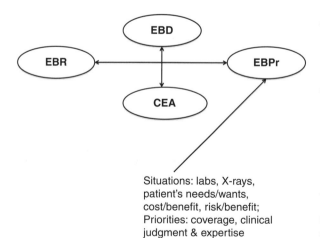

Situations: labs, X-rays, patient's needs/wants, cost/benefit, risk/benefit; Priorities: coverage, clinical judgment & expertise

Fig. 1.1 Evidence-based dentistry (EBD), and similarly EBM (evidence-based medicine) and EBN (evidence-based nursing), is composed of two fundamental and intertwined processes: evidence-based research (EBR) that seeks to obtain the best available evidence, and evidence-based practice (EBPr) that incorporates the best available evidence into clinical intervention, and related to cost-effectiveness research analysis (CER, aka CEA)

[1]The American Dental Association (ADA) Board of Trustees examined this new approach to clinical practice and dental care, and adopted resolution (B-18-1999) in February 1999 as: "...*an approach to treatment planning and subsequent dental therapy that requires the judicious melding of systematic assessments of scientific evidence relating to the patient's medical condition and history, the dentist's clinical experience, training and judgment and the patient's treatment needs and preferences.*" The ADA further states that "...*evidence-based clinical recommendations are intended to provide guidance, and are not a standard of care, requirement or regulation...(they serve as) a resource for dentists...*"

- Best available research evidence:
  - Consensus of the best available research evidence following systematic reviews (SRs) and meta-analyses (RS process)
  - rCPGs

EBD requires the synthesis of the available research in a process that involves:

- Framing the clinical problem as patient-intervention-comparison-outcome (PICO) question, which permits timely retrieval and critical evaluation of the available research literature, and the evaluation of validity of the integrated information.
- The rigor of process of research integration and synthesis (i.e., inclusion and exclusion criteria; level and quality evidence[2]) [3, 4, 33].
- The data from separate reports are pooled, when appropriate, for meta-analysis, meta-regression, Individual Patient Data analyzes, and acceptable sampling statistics [2, 3, 13, 33, 40].
- The data are interpreted from the perspective of Bayesian modeling in order to obtain statistical significance, infer clinical relevance and effectiveness, and extract Markov estimates (e.g., Markov model[3]).

A recent superbly articulated guide to evidence-based decision making for dental professionals presented a step-by-step process for making evidence-based decisions in dental practice [19]. The model consists of five distinct levels of mastery:

- Formulating patient-centered questions – i.e., the PICO question described above
- Searching for the appropriate evidence – i.e., the initial step of RS
- Critically appraising the evidence – i.e., the core of RS
- Applying the evidence to practice – i.e., EBPr and care
- Evaluating the process – i.e., evaluating outcomes and policies

Whereas this discussion took dentistry and EBD as a model example, it is self-evident that it applies to EBM and EBN as well. In evidence-based health care in general, the presentation and evaluation of the findings of RS in a summative evaluation model is often referred to as a systematic review [33], because of the emphasis on the systematic gathering of all of the available

research evidence, and the systematic analysis of the level [45] and quality of the evidence [2, 9, 11, 14, 34, 38], based on established criteria of research methodology, design, and statistical analysis [2, 3, 33] (cf., note 2). A well-conducted systematic review produces a clear, concise, and precise consensus of the best available research evidence in direct response to the PICO question. The consensus statement permits statements of rCPGs, which in turn lead to evidence-based treatment (EBT) interventions, and evidence-based policies (EBPo) [4, 5, 7, 12] (Fig. 1.2).

In brief, evidence-based health care rests on the consensus of the best available evidence to revise clinical practice guidelines, treatment protocols, and policies. Because the instruments and the process utilized to reach that consensus must be scrutinized, evaluated, and standardized, it is imperative that SRs be of high quality and follow a rigorous, detailed, and tested RS protocol, including that for the acceptable sampling and meta-analytical processing of the data [2, 33]. Therefore, it is important to develop and to validate standards for the evaluation of the quality and reliability of SRs and meta-analysis[4].

As the EBD/M/N literature grows, multiple SRs are produced in response to any given clinical PICO question. In some instances, multiple SRs are concordant in the generated consensus statements; in other instances, discordant SRs may arise. In either instance, it is becoming increasingly important to refine RS

---

[2] cf., Criteria for the level of evidence, and the "strength of recommendation taxonomy grading (SORT) guidelines" offered in the forward of the Journal of Evidence-Based Dental Practice.

[3] This is usually achieved by means of the Markov model-based decision tree. This approach permits to model events that may occur in the future as a direct effect of treatment or as a side effect. The model produces a decision tree that cycles over fixed intervals in time, and incorporates probabilities of occurrence. Even if the difference between the two treatment strategies appears quantitatively small, the Markov model outcome reflects the optimal clinical decision, because it is based on the best possible values for probabilities and utilities incorporated in the tree. The outcome produced by the Markov decision analysis results from the sensitivity analysis to test the stability over a range probability estimates, and thus reflects the most rational treatment choice [55, 59].

[4] e.g., Quality of reporting of meta-analysis, QUOROM – The QUOROM criteria were recently revised as the preferred reporting items for systematic reviews and meta-analysis (PRISMA) (cf., [32]).

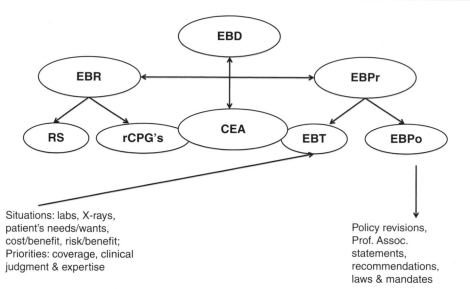

Situations: labs, X-rays,
patient's needs/wants,
cost/benefit, risk/benefit;
Priorities: coverage, clinical
judgment & expertise

Policy revisions,
Prof. Assoc.
statements,
recommendations,
laws & mandates

Fig. 1.2 EBR in dentistry/medicine/nursing is conducted as a process of research synthesis (RS), whose product, the systematic review generates a consensus of the best available evidence, evaluated for the level and the quality of the evidence, and analyzed by means of acceptable sampling and meta-analysis statistics. The consensus revised clinical practice guidelines (rCPGs) are incorporated into evidence-based treatment (EBT), which is duly evaluated for efficacy and effectiveness before it becomes new and improved evidence-based policy (EBPo). CEA is interdependent with rCPGs and EBT, and shown on the figure as partially overlapping

tools to evaluate the overall evidence across multiple SRs (e.g., assessment of multiple SRs, AMSTAR; [49, 50]) for the generation of what has been termed either "complex systematic" reviews [56] or "meta-SRs" [3, 7].

1.2 Probabilistic Models for Clinical Decision Making

Clinical decisions rest on a complex admixture of facts and values. They can be made on the basis of experience in situations in which the presenting condition and patient characteristics are consistent with the findings that are associated with predictable outcomes. In this case, the dentist's expertise helps to recognize these types of clinical situations triggered by key elements that are rapidly integrated into a mental model of diagnostic categories and an overall concept of treatment modalities. Here, treatment options derive most directly from clinical experience and judgment. They aim to meet accepted standards of care, but are rarely altered by consensus statements of the best available evidence.

By contrast, analytical decision making applies to those presenting conditions and patient characteristics that are less certain, and that require recommending treatment modalities whose benefits and harms are variable or unknown. In this context, clinical experience and judgment is insufficient in meeting accepted standards of care, and clinical decisions must be carefully pondered. Decision aids, such as the Markov tree are useful, as are quite often, recommendations that arise from the best available evidence [1].

In brief[5], clinical decision-making problems often involve multiple transitions between health states. The probabilities of state transitions, or related utility values, require complex computations over time. Neither decision trees nor traditional influence diagrams offer as practical a solution as state of transition models (i.e., Markov models). Markov models represent cyclical, recursive events, whether short-term processes, and therefore are best used to model prognostic clinical cases and associated follow-up. Markov models are often used to calculate a wide variety of outcomes, including average life expectancy, expected utility, long-term costs of care, survival rate, or number of recurrences.

---

[5]For in depth discussion, see 2.

Discrete Markov models enumerate a finite set of mutually exclusive possible states so that, in any given time interval (called a cycle or stage), an individual member of the Markov cohort can be in only one of the states. In order to determine a value for the entire process (e.g., a net cost or life expectancy), a value (an incremental cost or utility) is assigned to each interval spent in a particular state. The assignment of value in a Markov model is called a reward, regardless of whether it refers to a cost, utility, or other attribute. A state reward refers to a value that is assigned to the members of the cohort in a particular state during a given stage. The actual values used for state rewards depend on the attribute being calculated in the model (e.g., cost, utility, or life expectancy). A simple set of initial probabilities is used to specify the distribution of model subjects among the possible state rewards at the start of the process. The resulting matrix of transition probabilities is used to specify the transitions that are possible for the members of each Markov reward state at the end of each successive stage.

Two methods are commonly used to calculate the value of a discrete Markov model: a) cohort (expected value) calculations, and b) Monte Carlo trials. In a cohort analysis, which corresponds more realistically to a clinical situation, the expected values of the process are computed by multiplying the percentage of the cohort in a reward state by the incremental value (i.e., cost or utility) assigned to that state. The outcomes are added across all state rewards and all stages. In the more theoretical Monte Carlo simulation trial, the incremental values of the series of reward states traversed by the individual are summed.

The Markov model is most often represented in a graphical form known as a cycle tree. Since it is based on a node and branch framework, it is easily integrated into standard decision tree structures and can be appended to paths in a Markov decision tree. The root node of the Markov cycle tree is called a Markov node. Each of the possible health states is listed on the branches emanating from the Markov node, with one branch for each state. Possible state transitions are graphically displayed on branches to the right. A state from which transitions are not possible, such as the Dead state, is called an absorbing state. No state rewards are given for being in the Dead state, and zero values are assigned to the state rewards of all absorbing states. In this fashion, the Markov process integrates a termination condition, or stopping rule, specified at the Markov node to determine whether a cohort analysis is complete. This rule is the termination condition at the beginning of each stage. When the termination condition is verified, the Markov process ends and the net reward(s) are reported. The termination condition can include multiple conditions, which may be cumulative or alternative.

The Markov model generates an expected value analysis that is performed at, or to the left of each Markov node in cohort analysis. The expected value analysis can generate additional information about the Markov cohort calculations. For example, in a model designed to measure the time spent in the diseased state diagnosed as dementia of the Alzheimer's type, the expected value will generate the average life expectancy for a patient in the cohort. Additional calculated values will include the amount of time spent, on average, in each of the specified states of Alzheimer's dementia. The percentage of the cohort in each state will be computed at the end of the process. When the termination condition has been set to continue the process until most of the cohort is absorbed into the Dead state, the final probability of patients in the Dead state will approach 1.0. In brief, one of the strongest assets of the Markov model is its capacity to yield both an extensive numerical description of the process under study, as well as a detailed graphical representation and associated costs.

From this viewpoint, cost-effectiveness analysis (CEA)[6] can be performed either on the basis of expected value calculations or using Monte Carlo simulation. This is particularly important in the case of complex state transition models, because in order to evaluate individual outcomes – as distinguished from cohort analysis – Markov models must be calculated using Monte Carlo simulation.

CEA is a collection of methods for the evaluation of decisions based on two criteria using different outcome scales. It is of particular interest in situations where resource limitations require balancing the desire to maximize effectiveness and the need to contain costs.

CEA can simultaneously compare the expected costs and the expected effectiveness values of the options at a decision node. CEA generates a cost-effectiveness graph, which is interpreted as the best available evidence in support of fundamental CEA tools, calculations, results, and findings, including

---

[6]cf., [6, 52].

incremental values and the existence of dominance[7] or extended dominance[8].

The remainder of this discussion pertains to the circumstance of analytical decision making in health care.

Analytical decisions, generally speaking, refer to the behavioral and the cognitive processes of making rational human choices, from the logical and rational evaluation of alternatives, the probability of consequences, and the assessment and comparison of the accuracy and efficiency of each of these sets of consequences. Decision-making principles are designed to guide the decision-maker in choosing among alternatives in light of their possible consequences [1].

Decision theory has emerged principally from two schools of thought: first, the probability theory recognizes that decisions may involve conditions of certainty, risk, and uncertainty. In this model, the probability of occurrence for each consequence (i.e., utility) is quantifiable, and alternatives of occurrence are associated with a probability distribution. The correctness of decisions can be measured as the adequacy of achieving the desired objective, and by the efficiency with which the result was obtained [3, 15, 51].

The process of making a decision driven by a probabilistic estimation of either the "prospects" or the "utility" of its outcome is in effect the informed choice among the possible, probable, and predicted occurrence. Whereas decisions are most often made without advance knowledge of their consequences, three fundamental rules guide probabilistic decision making:

- The multidimensional nature of the prospect/utility associated with the decision.
- The subjectively expected maximization of the benefit in the outcome.
- The analytical process (usually Baysian in nature) that incorporates previous experience with current knowledge and evidence [1, 2].

The prospect theory [30] rests on empirical evidence, and seeks to describe how individuals evaluate potential losses and gains, and make choices in situations where they have to decide between alternatives that involve a known or anticipated risk.

The prospect-based decision-making process involves two stages:

- In the initial editing stage, possible outcomes of the decision are estimated, ranked, and evaluated heuristically.
- In the final evaluation phase, decisions are estimated if their outcome could be quantified and computed, based on potential outcomes, gains and losses, and their respective probabilities, evaluation.

The aim of prospect-based decisions is to yield a choosing and deciding heuristic that establishes the more likely outcome in terms of having the more profitable utility. The utility perspective on decision making follows from the prospect-theoretical framework, and finds its roots in Antiquity [3] to our contemporary Peter Singer (6 July 1946), presently holding an academic appointment both at Princeton University and at University of Melbourne.

In the context of decision research, the term utility refers to a measure of perceived or real benefit, relative satisfaction from, or desirability of – such as, for example, "increase in quality of life" – a direct consequence of the utilization of goods or services, and health care intervention. It follows that certain interventions, or modifications thereof may contribute to increasing or decreasing such benefits, and therefore the utility of the said goods or services. For this specific reason, utility-based decision making rests largely on a rationale centered upon utility-maximizing behavior, rather than strictly economic constraints. That is to say, good dentistry should be driven by the intent of benefitting the patient, and of providing the best possible care at the lowest possible cost (cf., CEA), and are expressed as cost-to-benefit ratios.

---

[7]In the context of CEA, one alternative is said to be dominant if offers the more effective and less costly alternative. When this is the case, the dominated alternative normally may be removed from consideration. The use of relative position to infer dominance can be inferred from the analysis of the cost-effectiveness graph: effectiveness increases from left to right, and cost increases from bottom to top. The crossing point of the axes represents one alternative. Its comparators can then be placed on the graph: more costly alternatives above, and more effective alternatives to the right. An alternative is said to be "dominated" if it lies both above and to the left of another alternative.

[8]When making certain population-wide policy decisions, two strategies may be used together as a sort of "blended" policy, instead of assigning a single treatment strategy to all patients. Hence, we speak of "extended dominance." Blending strategies only becomes relevant when the most effective strategy is too costly to prescribe for the entire population.

The fundamental assumptions of the utility theory of decision making state that:

- Utilities and probabilities of one alternative (or set of alternatives) should not influence another alternative.
- Alternatives are "transitive," and are subject to ordering based on preferences.
- By the very nature of the process, creativity and any form of cognitive input is excluded, as it strictly rests on probabilistic rules.

As we discussed elsewhere [3], utility theory proposes to generate two types of measurable outcomes:

- Cardinal utility, the magnitude of utility differences, as an ethically or behaviorally relevant and quantifiable measure.
- Ordinal utility, that is utility rankings, which do not quantify the strength of preferences or benefits.

As such, utility is often described by an indifference curve, which plots the combination of commodities that an individual or a society would accept to maintain a given level of satisfaction. In that respect, individual utility (or societal utility) is expressed as the dependent variable of functions of, for instance, production or commodity[9] [3].

Probability-based decision making can be driven by, and carried out for the purpose of altering utility outcomes. Nevertheless, the latter point can be particularly problematic since cognitive dissonance does arise between the outcome of the purely probabilistic process, and the clinician's knowledge, information processing, beliefs, preferences, expertise, whether or not in the context of newly rCPGs resulting from SRs.

Cognitive and social psychologists correctly argue, however, that individuals in a social group – such as dentists, doctors, physician assistants, nurses and nurse practitioners, and patients – often have different value systems upon which to establish the utility of a given intervention. Consequently, it is unclear how cardinal and ordinal utility can be reconciled across these different perspectives. Neither does the utility theory of decision making nor its alternative that is concerned with the prospect of risk and benefits (hence, prospect theory of decision making) permit adequate normative and summative evaluation of outcome and success.

Alternate decision-making theories may actually be prone to be more useful than utility or prospect theory in the context of evidence-based health care.

1.3 Logic Evidence-Based Decisions in Clinical Practice

Rather than relying on probabilistic conditions, the decision-making process may rest on cognitions and reasoning, such as either rationality or logic. In that respect, the cognition-based approach to decision making would become akin to the so-called *intelligence cycle*, which originated as the processing of information in the context of a civilian or military intelligence agency or in law enforcement as a closed path consisting of repeating nodes, and the closely logically related target-centric approach [3, 10]. This process of decision making is critical to the analysis of gathered intelligence, and may be summarized in certain fundamental steps, or phases, which exemplify the process of evidence-based cognitive decision making, whether it be a rational model or a logic model (*vide infra*):

1. In the *directive phase,* the specific "intelligence question" is posed – in the preceding chapter, we indicated that the directive phase of the evidence-based process is the statement of the PICO question.
2. In the *collection phase,* the data, information, processed intelligence, and corporate "wisdom" resides – in the context of evidence-based decision making, we stressed the need to integrate expertise and experience with the entire body of available evidence.
3. In the *analysis phase,* the collected information is collated, analyzed, and evaluated. This is identical to the step we described above where the best evidence is obtained from the entire body of available evidence, based on the level and the quality of the evidence, followed by acceptable sampling and meta-analysis.
4. In the *dissemination phase,* the processed information, data and intelligence is presented in a form that is useful, relevant, in context, and most importantly, timely. This step corresponds, for all intents and purposes, to the systematic review format of reporting the evidence-based process.

---

[9]cf., Pareto's efficiency curve.

5. In the *reflection phase*, the newly discovered information is incorporated into corporate wisdom, from which flows new and improved questions and tasks. The evidence-based paradigm here speaks of the dissemination of the consensus of revised guidelines.

The traditional intelligence cycle, and the rational and the logic cognition-based models of decision making, distinguish "collectors," "processors," and "analysts." In a remarkable parallel, so does the evidence-based paradigm separate those who perform RS and EBR to produce the consensus for rCPGs, from those who integrate consensus statements into evidence-based treatment intervention (EBT) and practice (EBPr), and from the policy makers, who integrate normative and summative evaluations into new and improved EBPo for the benefit of the stakeholders (cf. Fig. 1.2). The remainder of this writing compares and contrasts the rational vs. the logic model of clinical decision making, and argues in support of the latter in the context of evidence-based health care.

A fundamental difference exists between rationality and logic. A *sine qua non* of a rational argument is that it be logically valid, but rationality per se is broader than logic because it can include uncertain but sensible arguments based on probability expectations and personal experience. Logic can concern itself only with directly provable facts and consequential valid relations among them. To be grounded in logic, an argument must rest on elements that are consistent, sound, and complete. The argument may follow from given premises, and be deductive in nature; or it may reliably derive a generalization from observations, and be inductive. Platonian informal logic concerns itself with natural language arguments, whereas the Aristotelian formal logic is concerned with inferences of both formal and explicit content [3].

Rational decisions can be taken *ad hominen*[10], rather than logic, and *ad hominem* decisions may be both logically unsound but fully rational, sensible, and practical. Case in point, the simple example below:

I am hungry – I don't want to be hungry.
If I cook myself a sausage, I will not be hungry.
Therefore, I will cook myself a sausage.

A decision is said to be rational, when it is based on guesses (heuristic, trial-error), intuition, beliefs, or knowledge and previous experience. Rational choice theory argues that patterns of behavior in societies reflect the choices made by individuals as they seek to maximize benefits and minimize costs. In this light, decision making depends primarily and rationally from comparing costs and benefits of different courses of action, and patterns of individual and social behavior develop and become established solely as a result of those choices [3, 5].

Several models of rational choice exist, but all converge on the fundamental tenet that individuals choose and decide upon the best action according to, and based upon the set of preferences, psycho-cognitive functions, and socio-environmental constraints facing them. Models then differ for the additional assumptions they propose, although it is widely recognized that none provide a full and complete description of reality: they simply allow the generation of testable working hypotheses, which must then undergo empirical tests.

Indeed, Weber's social decision model[11] could appear attractive in the context of EBD/M/N, and suggests that Weber's *Zweckrational* mode[12] might be optimally integrated in a rational model of evidence-based clinical decision making. But, this view has encountered serious debate by contemporary social psychologists, including Ezioni, who reframed the decision-making process and proposed that purposive/instrumental rationality is actually subordinated by normative ideas on how people "ought" to behave and effective considerations of how people "wish" to behave [17]. As we discussed elsewhere [3], Weber's theoretical paradigm is severely challenged for the prohibitive limitations in empirical outputs and quantifiable measures that this rational choice theory can

---

[10]Arguments are *ad hominem* when they use factual claims or propositions by attacking or appealing to a characteristic or a belief of the source or origin of the proposition or claim (i.e., the person – argument *to the person*, Latin: "*ad hominem*"), rather than by addressing the substance of the argument itself, and producing evidence for or against it following the rules of logic. These arguments may be logically *valid*, but they also can be logically unsound, because not based on the rules of logic. Therefore, rational decisions may at times appear "illogical."

[11]cf., [3].

[12]Purposeful and instrumental type of behaviors that characterize the expectations of the behaviors of others in a social context, and that lead to pondered "rationally pursued and calculated social decisions."

generate, particularly in the domain of political and social science [23, 46].

The logic model is characterized as a mode of "evaluability assessment" [57, 58], and is designed as a general framework for describing the fundamental, rational, and logic process of decision making that an individual, a group, or an organization may follow. In its simplest form, the logic model presents decision making as a process that consists of four distinct, intertwined, and logically flowing categories [3, 5, 36], which actually mirror the evidence-based process (cf. Fig. 1.3):

1. *Inputs*, the identified available research evidence that becomes additive to the decision-maker's experience, expertise, and skills. Inputs incorporate, and rest upon

needs/wants, situations, priorities based on clinical diagnosis, expertise, coverage, etc.

2. *Activities*, the process of sifting through the available research evidence in order to single out the best available evidence on the basis of widely accepted criteria of research methodology, research design, and research data analysis: what needs to be done, what is *de facto* done as a clinical intervention.

3. *Outputs*, the conclusive steps of the evidence-based process that yield a consensus of the best available evidence by means of acceptable sampling and meta-analysis [2], and that produce a set of revised criteria for practice decision making based on these results: measurable clinical outcomes.

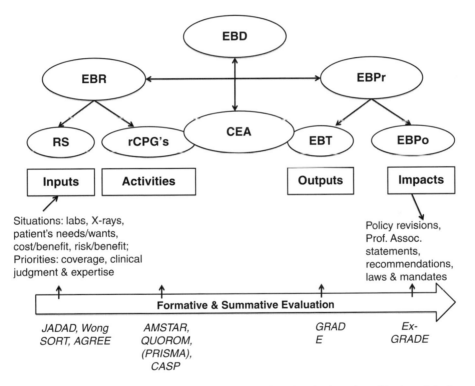

Fig. 1.3 EBD/medicine/nursing, which is intertwined with comparative effectiveness analysis, is positioned at the center of the logic model of clinical decision making for optimizing treatment outcomes. The model incorporates the situation of the patient, the priorities set by the health care provider, with the input of the best available evidence generated by the process of RS. Quantifiable formative evaluation of these elements is permitted by the model at this stage. Taken together, these elements yield rCPGs with direct application and implications to the patient condition, from which the PICO originated. As noted, the model incorporates a formative evaluation step to verify the clinical relevance of these recommendations. The evidence-based paradigm then leads to the utilization of the best available evidence in EBT intervention, which the logic model considers the outputs of the clinical decision-making process. Formative evaluation of the efficacy and the effectiveness of EBTs is an integral part of the logic model. When deemed clinically satisfactory and relevant, these new and improved EBT intervention can be articulated into policies, recommendations, mandates, and laws, and can have long-lasting impact. Formative evaluation of the logic model output at this stage is critical, and often involves national and international professional associations. The overall process is also subject to quantifiable overall summative evaluation (adapted from [5])

4. *Impacts*, the logical flow from this step-wise progression from short-term, to intermediate, to long-term impacts and consequences of delivering services, and include normative and summative evaluations of outcome quality, validity, and reliability, as well as stockholder's satisfaction.

The strength of the logic model lies in the fact that it represents the most probable view of reality[13]. As such, it permits the flexibility that several models do not have to be circular, spiral-shaped, or to consist of series of feedback loops that enhance or dampen each other. For any given decision-making process, working hypotheses can be clearly stated in the context of the logic model at each step, tested and verified by means of quantifiable, reliable, and valid performance measures (Fig. 1.3).

Needs evaluation is primordial in establishing the situation, priorities, and inputs. Process evaluation quantifies the progression, the activities, and output stages. Outcomes evaluation ranks the validity and the reliability of the short-term and intermediate products of the process. Intermediate and long-term summative impacts can also be evaluated [29].

Figure 1.3 shows that formative and summative evaluation [25] are obtained at key capstone time-points in order to ensure steady progress toward obtaining anticipated outputs, and desired outcomes, and, in the final analysis, providing justification for testing the model experimentally in any given situation in the first place. At the RS stage of EBR, the available evidence is evaluated following established criteria and standards of research design[14], methodology, and data analysis [2, 33] (cf. note 3). Validated instruments for this purpose include the Jadad scale [28] and the Wong-revised scale [2, 9]. This initial process results in SRs and meta-analyses, which must be evaluated as well along established standards (cf., note 4) and with validated tools (e.g., AMSTAR), and its revision [3]. In a similar fashion, EBPr calls for standards and instruments of evaluation. One such approach is provided by GRADE[15], a validated approach for going from research evidence to clinical intervention, and for assessing the quality of evidence for diagnostic recommendations [5, 21, 24, 47]. GRADE addresses issues of concern to patients, clinicians, and, to some extent, policy makers. GRADE provides a sound evaluative assessment of EBT in terms of the quality of evidence for each outcome, the relative importance of outcomes, the overall quality of evidence, the balance of benefits, harms, and costs, and considers the strength of recommendation and the overall value of implementation [3, 5].

As we introduced elsewhere [3, 5, 9], the final stage of EBPr that concerns EBPo still requires the validation of an evaluative instrument that may extend and expand GRADE to include assessment of policies, because a key feature of an EBPr environment is that it must support and promote the use of best evidence by requiring clinical practice policies and procedures to be evidence-based [41]. The expanded version of GRADE (Ex-GRADE), which we, at present, are endeavoring in validating[16], includes the fundamental elements of policy evaluation that have been in health care practice for the last decade [20], and which we outlined elsewhere as follows [5]:

- What is the extent of relevance to practice?
- Are the condition and interventions specific?
- Is the target population well-defined?
- How good is the policy's evidence?
- What biases does the policy reflect?
- Is the policy ready to implement?
  - By assembling a team and building consensus
  - By documenting all clinical processes
  - By modifying the policy for local use
  - By communicating changes in processes
  - By establishing modalities to evaluate the policy
  - By testing possible changes or interventions
  - By adopting the revised clinical policy
  - By evaluating the new policy

The promise of the logic model in evidence-based decision making lies in its ability to formulate in quantifiable terms the emerging situation, the required action-response, and the concrete results. It provides quantifiable, normative, and summative evaluation of the evidence, and describes the relationships between

---

[13]As discussed elsewhere [3], views and perceptions of reality differ. This discordance pertains to a separate and distinct, yet related and pertinent domain of cognitive psychology termed "person-environment fit." For the implications of this model in the context of evidence-based decision-making in medicine and dentistry, please see: Chiappelli et al. [8].

[14]e.g., The consolidated standards of clinical trials, CONSORT.

---

[15]Another noteworthy assessment guideline in the EBR-EBPr spectrum is the "appraisal of guidelines, research and evaluation – Europe" (AGREE) instrument [11].

[16]Chiappelli et al., in progress.

investments/inputs, activities, and results. It yields a concrete approach for integrating planning, implementation, evaluation, and reporting.

1.4 Conclusions

Clinical problems in must be reliably diagnosed and treated as per practice guidelines approved by the professional body, and uniquely required for the case and recommended by the specialty in whose domain the case falls. But, not all domains of clinical dentistry can be handled in an evidence-based paradigm [1, 5, 19, 37].

Evidence-based decision making in medicine, dentistry, and nursing is based upon the application of the scientific method for the conscientious, explicit, and judicious use of current best evidence, evaluated by a systematic process of the level *and* the quality of the research evidence. SRs provide a tool to apply stringent scientific strategies to quantify the quality of the accumulated research evidence, and limit bias. They utilize and integrate both acceptable analysis and meta-analysis to establish the level of overall significance of the gathered evidence, and are vastly different in purpose and format from narrative reviews and health technology assessments [4, 5, 34].

The consensus of the total best available evidence is obtained and utilized cogently in making clinical decisions that pertain to the health care of each individual patient. But, one fundamental question remains: how do we "translate" the evidence derived from group data, as commonly obtained in research studies and synthesized in SRs and meta-analyses, to have any degree of pertinence and direct applicability to the individual patient.

In its simplest elaboration, as in its most complex iteration, the logic model of decision making has fundamental strengths that set it apart from other models. From the perspective of the initial consideration of the task, it permits to forge a master plan that "sees" the end, does more than simply considering inputs or tasks, and visualizes and focuses upon the ultimate outcomes and the results to be gained. The logic model is a proactive approach to identify the optimal procedural steps to achieve the desired results, and to prove the working hypothesis under study. It permits focus on accountability for investment based on long-term outcomes [3, 5, 16].

Furthermore, the logic model, which need not be linear, provides sound indicators of finality, in terms of output and outcome measures of performance (i.e., work-hours, manpower), as well as success. Short-term, intermediate, as well as long-term outcomes are clearly identifiable, which permits to set criteria for immediate and for mission success far in the future. In these cases, intermediate or shorter-term outcomes that provide an indication of progress toward the ultimate long-term outcome may be identified. Therefore, and most importantly, the logic model, with intertwined, formative, and summative evaluative protocols that can be integrated at every step, is being increasingly imparted to the students of the field[17]. In summary, it may be argued that the logic model is a timely response to the call by Spring [53] for "...*a good theory of integrative, collaborative health decision-making...*" [53].

In brief, this dichotomy of evidence-based decision making – i.e., probabilistic vs. logic-grounded, might in reality be better viewed as a spectrum of possibilities, depending largely upon the clinical circumstances (e.g., the PICO question). In fact, it is likely that the field of evidence-based decision making in health care will soon find itself converging toward, and finding much conceptual richness in the parallel academic science of knowledge management[18].

---

[17]Note: the critical appraisal skills program (CASP) was developed by Oxford Regional Health, in association with the Evidence Based Medicine Working Group, a group of clinicians at McMaster university, Hamilton, Canada, to promote the skills necessary for critical appraisal of the evidence, and decision-making grounded on the best available evidence (cf., [42]).

[18]For example, "...*organizational knowledge that constitutes "core-competency" is more than "know-what" explicit knowledge which may be shared by several. A core competency requires the more elusive "know-how" – the particular ability to put know-what into practice...*" [48], contrasting to "...*Knowledge exists on a spectrum. At one extreme, it is almost completely tacit, that is semiconscious and unconscious knowledge held in peoples' heads and bodies. At the other end of the spectrum, knowledge is almost completely explicit or codified, structured, and accessible to people other than the individuals originating it. Most knowledge of course exists between the extremes. Explicit elements are objective, rational, and created in the "then and there," while the tacit elements are subjective experiential and created in the "here and now..."* [31]. Hence, the distinction between what people know and can articulate, quantify, or document in conscious cognitive act (knowing what) – considered by some as "hard" knowledge, vs. what people know to know, which can be articulated or quantified, a subconscious knowing how, an innate or acquired quality of knowing by inference, reason and logic, rather than by quantifiable measures – spuriously called "soft" knowledge [26].

The purpose of this book is to explore the field outlined above in greater depth in order to grasp a better understanding of evidence-based health care and how to optimize clinical outcomes in health care. This endeavor is a rather wide-casting net, which should be relevant and applicable to the breadth of the health sciences, while focused to the domain of the process of evidence-based clinical decision making toward improving benefits for the patients. In order to articulate the complexities of the field, this work consists of four sections.

- *Part I* addresses the science of RS, and its place and role in clinical decision making. Following this brief introductory chapter by the editors (Chap. 1), Dr. Bartolucci provides, in Chap. 2, some historical context, the key definitions, elements, and output of meta-analytic methods, and reviews them with illustrative examples. Understanding these allows one to appreciate better the advantages and limitations of this approach to interpreting results from the literature. In Chap. 3, Dr. Susin further provides an overview of the methods used to combine the results of several studies, and discusses the application and interpretation of meta-analytic methods.
- *Part II* of this book explores the process of making evidence-based decisions in the clinical domain. It opens with Chap. 4 by Dr. Cajulis who discusses the extent to which the translation of EBPr in nursing has been difficult and challenging, but has a promising future in the next decade. Dr. Faggion discusses in Chap. 5 the strengths and the weakness of a model for implementing evidence-based decisions in dental practice. In brief, these authors discuss the use of three checklists (CASP, QUOROM, and AMSTAR) to assess the methodological quality of two SRs of randomized controlled trials (RCTs), regarded as the strongest form of evidence using the treatment of peri-implantitis as an example to illustrate the process. In Chap. 6, Dr. Arimie discusses the complexities associated with evidence-based decisions in HIV/AIDS. High number of infected persons, difficulty of treatment, and other comorbidity factors might increase the risk of cardiovascular diseases. Dr. *Rastogi* (Chap. 7) expands the frontiers of the field to evidence-based complementary and alternative health care intervention. In brief, the specific focus of this chapter is the correct use and appropriate utilization

of Prakriti (Constitution) analysis in Ayurveda, – from the realm of empirical research to evidence-based clinical decisions. In Chap. 8, Dr. *Akadiri* evaluates evidence-based clinical decisions in oral surgery.

- In *Part III* of this work, the authors specifically discuss the applications and implications of EBPr toward improving clinical outcomes by examining selected ways and means by which the evidence-based paradigm can be optimized for the benefit of the patient. Continuing in the field of evidence-based decisions in oral surgery, Dr. Akadiri continues, in Chap. 9, an elegant discussion of the spectrum of evidence-based issues in maxillofacial trauma. Chap. 10, authored by Dr. Nocini further examines the strengths and weaknesses of the evidence-based movement specifically in the context of improving clinical outcomes in dentistry and oral surgery. Dr. Foschi, in Chap. 11, discusses the role of evidence-based decisions in the pharmacological management of alcohol dependence and alcoholic liver disease. Chapter 12 by Dr. Bessa concludes this selective anthology of evidence-based decisions and comparative effectiveness research with a discussion of the efficacy of TMD/TMJ therapy from the viewpoint of an evidence-based approach to analysis. This section is concluded by Dr. Esposito and colleagues at the Cochrane Organization (Chap. 13), who present a prototype of Cochrane systematic review for assessing the efficacy of dental implants in the specific context of the efficacy of horizontal and vertical bone augmentation procedures. This chapter, both in its format and approach, represents an example of the current most highly recommended process in the field. The Cochrane Group (Cochrane.org) is unquestionably the leader in the domains of EBR, the structure and depth of SRs, and the generation of consensus of the best available evidence that is required and utilized in evidence-based decision making.
- This work concludes with *Part IV*, in which Dr. Frustaci tackles, in Chap. 14, the arduous question of the clinical relevance of EBM in general, and in oncological care in particular, and present an elegant consideration of the forthcoming issues. *In finis*, the editor's *postscriptum* (Chap. 15) traces, in broad strokes, the most likely avenues of future research in the field for the next decade.

References

1. Bauer JG, Spackman S, Chiappelli F, Prolo P, Stevenson RG (2006) Making clinical decisions using a clinical practice guideline. Calif Dent Assoc J 34:519–528
2. Chiappelli F (2008) The science of research synthesis: a manual of evidence-based research for the health sciences – implications and applications in dentistry. NovaScience, Hauppauge, NY
3. Chiappelli F (2009) Sustainable evidence-based decision-making. Monograph. NovaScience, Suffolk, USA
4. Chiappelli F, Cajulis OS (2008) Transitioning toward evidence-based research in the health sciences for the XXI century. Evid Based Compl Alt Med 5:123–128
5. Chiappelli F, Cajulis OS (2009) The logic model in evidence-based clinical decision-making in dental practice. J Evid Based Dent Pract 9(4):206–210
6. Chiappelli F, Cajulis O, Newman M (2009) Comparative effectiveness research in evidence based dental practice. J Evid Based Dent Pract 9:57–58
7. Chiappelli F, Cajulis OC, Oluwadara O, Ramchandani MH (2009) Evidence-based based decision making – implications for dental care. In: Columbus F (ed) Dental care: diagnostic, preventive, and restorative services. NovaScience, Hauppauge, NY
8. Chiappelli F, Manfrini E, Edgerton M, Rosenblum M, Cajulis KD, KD PP (2006) Clinical evidence and evidence-based dental treatment of special populations: patients with Alzheimer's disease. Calif Dent Assoc J 34:439–447
9. Chiappelli F, Navarro AM, Moradi DR, Manfrini E, Prolo P (2006) Evidence-based research in complementary and alternative medicine III: treatment of patients with Alzheimer's disease. Evid Based Compl Alt Med 3:411–424
10. Clark RM (2003) Intelligence analysis: a target-centric approach. CQ, Washington, DC
11. Cluzeau FA, Burgers JS, Brouwers M, Collaboration AGREE (2003) Development and validation of an international appraisal instrument for assessing the quality of clinical practice guidelines: the AGREE project. Qual Saf Health Care 12:18–23
12. Cook DJ, Greengold NL, Ellrodt AG, Weingarten SR (1997) The relation between systematic research and practice guidelines. Acad Clin 127:210–216
13. CRD – Critical Review Dissemination (2009) Systematic reviews. York University, York GB
14. Deeks J (2001) Systematic reviews of evaluations of diagnostic and screening tests. In: Egger M, Davey Smith G, Altman D (eds) Systematic reviews in health care: meta-analysis in context. BMJ, London
15. Edwards W, Fasolo B (2001) Decision technology. Annu Rev Psychol 52:581–606
16. Engel-Cox J, Van Houten B, Phelps J, Rose S (2009) Conceptual model of comprehensive research metrics for improved human health and environment. Cien Saude Colet 14:519–531
17. Etzioni A (1988) Normative-affective factors: towards a new decision-making model. J Economic Psychol 9:125–150
18. Fauchard P (1728) Le chirurgien dentiste (The Surgeon Dentist). Paris
19. Forrest JL, Miller SA, Overman PR, Newman MG (eds) (2008) Evidence-based decision making: a translational guide for dental professionals. Lippincott, Williams & Wilkins, Philadelphia, PA
20. Gilbert TT, Taylor JS (1999) How to evaluate and implement clinical policies. Fam Pract Manag 6:28–33
21. GRADE Working Group (2004) Grading quality of evidence and strength of recommendation. BMJ 328:1–8
22. Gray MJ (ed) (1967) Evidence-based health care. Churchill-Livingstone, London
23. Green DP, Shapiro I (1994) Pathologies of rational choice theory: a critique of applications in political science. Yale University, New Haven
24. Guyatt GH, Oxman AD, Kunz R, Falck-Ytter Y, Vist GE, Liberati A, Schünemann HJ, GRADE Working Group (2008) Going from evidence to recommendations. BMJ 336:1049–1051
25. Hastings BS, Madaus G (1971) Handbook of formative and summative evaluation of student learning. McGraw-Hill, New York, NY
26. Hildreth PM. Kimble C (2002) The duality of knowledge. Information Research, 2002 8 (October), # 142; http://InformationR.net/ir/8-1/paper142.html
27. Ismail A, Bader J (2004) Evidence-based dentistry in clinical practice. JADA 135:78–83
28. Jadad AR, Cook DJ, Browman GP (1997) A guide to interpreting discordant systematic reviews. Can Med Assoc J 156:1411–1416
29. Julian DA (1997) The utilization of the logic model as a system level planning and evaluation device. Eval Program Plann 20:251–257
30. Kahneman D, Tversky A (1979) Prospect theory: an analysis of decision under risk. Econometrica XLVII:263–291
31. Leonard D, Sensiper S (1998) The role of tacit knowledge in group innovation. Calif Manag Rev 40:112–132
32. Liberati A, Altman DG, Tezlaff J, Murlow C, Getzsche PC, Ionnidis JPA, Clarke M, Devereaux PJ, Kleijnen J, Moher D. PLoS 2009 6 e1000:100
33. Littell JH, Corcoran J, Pillai V (2008) Systematic reviews and meta-analysis. Oxford Univeristy, New York, NY
34. Manchikanti L (2008) Evidence-based medicine, systematic reviews, and guidelines in interventional pain management, part I: introduction and general considerations. Pain Phys 11:161–186
35. Martin JA (2004) From repair to prevention: the wellness model of care. Int J Periodontics Restorative Dent 24:411
36. Mayeske GW, Lambur MT (2001) How to design better programs: a staff centered stakeholder approach to program logic modeling. The Program Design Institute, Crofton, MD
37. Merijohn GK (2006) Implementing evidence-based decision making in the private practice setting: the 4-step process. J Evid Base Dent Pract 6:253–257
38. Moher D, Schultz KF, Altman DG (2001) The CONSORT statement: revised recommendations for improving the quality of reports of parallel-group randomized trials. Ann Int Med 134:657–662
39. Newman M, Baudendistel CL (2001) Editorial. J Evid Based Dent Pract 1:1–2
40. Nieri M, Clauser C, Pagliaro U, PiniPrato G (2003) Individual patient data: a criterion in grading articles dealing with therapy outcomes. J Evid Base Dent 3:122–126

41. Oman KS, Duran C, Fink R (2008) Evidence-based policy and procedures: an algorithm for success. J Nurs Adm 38:47–51

42. Oxman AD, Sackett DL, Guyatt G (1993) Users' guides to the medical literature. I. How to get started. The Evidence-Based Medicine Working Group. JAMA 270: 2093–2095

43. Reeves A, Chiappelli F, Cajulis OS (2006) Evidence-based recommendations for the use of sealants. Calif Dent Assoc J 34:540–546

44. Robbins JW (1998) Evidence-based dentistry: what is it, and what does it have to do with practice? Quintessence Int 29:796–799

45. Sackett DL, Rosenberg WMD, Gray JAM, Haynes RB, Richardson WS (1996) Evidence-based medicine: what it is and what it isn't. BMJ 312:71–72

46. Schram SF, Caterino B (eds) (2006) Making political science matter: debating knowledge, research, and method. New York University, New York

47. Schünemann HJ, Oxman AD, Brozek J, Glasziou P, Bossuyt P, Chang S, Muti P, Jaeschke R, Guyatt GH (2008) GRADE: assessing the quality of evidence for diagnostic recommendations. Evid Based Med 13:162–163

48. Seely Brown J, Duguid P (1998) Organizing knowledge. Calif Manag Rev 40:90–111

49. Shea BJ, Bouter LM, Peterson J, Boers M, Andersson N, Ortiz Z, Ramsay T, Bai A, Shukla VK, Grimshaw JM (2007) External validation of a measurement tool to assess systematic reviews (AMSTAR). PLoS ONE 2:e1350

50. Shea BJ, Grimshaw JM, Wells GA, Boers M, Andersson N, Hamel C, Porter AC, Tugwell P, Moher D, Bouter LM (2007) Development of AMSTAR: a measurement tool to assess the methodological quality of systematic reviews. BMC Med Res Methodol 7:10

51. Simon HA (1982) Models of bounded rationality. MIT, Cambridge, MA

52. Simon HA (1947) Doctoral dissertation: administrative behavior: a study of decision-making processes in administrative organizations

53. Spring B (2008) Health decision making: lynchpin of evidence-based practice. Med Decis Making 28:866–874

54. Steele DC (2000) Evidence-based care: a new formula for an old problem? J Indiana Dent Assoc 79:76

55. Sugar CA, James GM, Lenert LA, Rosenheck RA (2004) Discrete state analysis for interpretation of data from clinical trials. Med Care 42:183–196

56. Whitlock EP, Lin JS, Chou R, Shekelle P, Robinson KA (2008) Using existing systematic reviews in complex systematic reviews. Ann Intern Med 148:776–782

57. Wholey JS (1979) Evaluation: promise and performance. Urban Institute, Washington, DC

58. Wholey JS (1987) Evaluability assessment: developing program theory. In: Bickman L (ed) Using program theory in evaluation. New Directions for Program Evaluation. No. 33. Jossey-Bass, San Francisco, CA

59. Yu F, Morgenstern H, Hurwitz E, Berlin TR (2003) Use of a Markov transition model to analyse longitudinal low-back pain data. Stat Methods Med Res 12:321–331

Overview, Strengths, and Limitations of Systematic Reviews and Meta-Analyses

2

Alfred A. Bartolucci and William B. Hillegass

Core Message

> It is important and timely to provide some historical context, the key definitions, elements, and output of meta-analytic methods, and to review them with illustrative examples. Understanding these allows one to better appreciate the advantages and limitations of this approach to interpreting results from the literature.

2.1 Introduction

The support of medical decisions comes from several sources. These include individual physician experience, pathophysiological constructs, pivotal clinical trials, qualitative reviews of the literature, and, increasingly, meta-analyses. Historically, the first of these four sources of knowledge largely informed medical and dental decision makers. Meta-analysis came on the scene around the 1970s and has received much attention. What is meta-analysis? It is the process of combining the quantitative results of separate (but similar) studies by means of formal statistical methods. Statistically, the purpose is to increase the precision with which the treatment effect of an intervention can be estimated. Stated in another way, one can say that

meta-analysis combines the results of several studies with the purpose of addressing a set of related research hypotheses. The underlying studies can come in the form of published literature, raw data from individual clinical studies, or summary statistics in reports or abstracts.

More broadly, a meta-analysis arises from a systematic review. There are three major components to a systematic review and meta-analysis. The systematic review starts with the formulation of the research question and hypotheses. Clinical or substantive insight about the particular domain of research often identifies not only the unmet investigative needs, but helps prepare for the systematic review by defining the necessary initial parameters. These include the hypotheses, endpoints, important covariates, and exposures or treatments of interest. Like any basic or clinical research endeavor, a prospectively defined and clear study plan enhances the expected utility and applicability of the final results for ultimately influencing practice or policy.

After this foundational preparation, the second component, a systematic review, commences. The systematic review proceeds with an explicit and reproducible protocol to locate and evaluate the available data. The collection, abstraction, and compilation of the data follow a more rigorous and prospectively defined objective process. The definitions, structure, and methodologies of the underlying studies must be critically appraised. Hence, both "the content" and "the infrastructure" of the underlying data are analyzed, evaluated, and systematically recorded. Unlike an informal review of the literature, this systematic disciplined approach is intended to reduce the potential for subjectivity or bias in the subsequent findings.

Typically, a literature search of an online database is the starting point for gathering the data. The most common sources are MEDLINE (United States Library of

A.A. Bartolucci (✉)
W.B. Hillegass
Department of Biostatistics, School of Public Health,
University of Alabama at Birmingham, 1665 University
Boulevard, Birmingham, AL 35294-0022, USA
e-mail: abartolucci@ms.soph.uab.edu

F. Chiappelli et al. (eds.), *Evidence-Based Practice: Toward Optimizing Clinical Outcomes,*
DOI: 10.1007/978-3-642-05025-1_2, © Springer-Verlag Berlin Heidelberg 2010

Medicine database), EMBASE (medical and pharmacologic database by Elsevier publishing), CINAHL (cumulative index to nursing and allied health literature), CANCERLIT (cancer literature research database), and the Cochrane Collaborative [9]. These online resources have increased the likelihood that investigators will have ready access to all the available results from research directed at a common endpoint.

The third aspect is the actual meta-analysis. Meta-analysis is the statistical synthesis of the results of the studies included in the systematic review. Meta-analysis is the process of combining the quantitative results of separate (but similar) studies by means of formal statistical methods in order to increase the precision of the estimated treatment effect. It is generally used when individual trials yield inconclusive or conflicting results. It may also be used when several trials asking similar questions have been conducted and an overall conclusion is needed.

While the main focus of this chapter will be meta-analysis, it cannot be completely isolated from several prerequisites assessed in the systematic review. For example, the studies must address a common question. The eligibility criteria of the underlying studies must be well established. Evaluation techniques for endpoints must be reasonably consistent across the studies. In the clinical setting, when making comparisons between a treatment and control, the underlying studies must be properly randomized. Exploratory meta-analyses and meta-regressions may examine the associations between interventions, covariates, and secondary events [1].

After providing some historical context, the key definitions, elements, and output of meta-analytic methods will be reviewed with illustrative examples. Understanding these allows one to appreciate better the advantages and limitations of this approach to interpreting results from the literature.

2.1.1 Background

This idea of combining results from several studies is not new. Karl Pearson in 1904 established the first identifiable formal technique for data pooling [16]. He examined the correlation coefficients between typhoid and mortality by inoculation status among soldiers in various parts of the British Empire. As a summary measure, Pearson calculated the arithmetic mean of the correlation coefficients across five two-by-two contingency tables. In 1931, Tippett described a method for evaluating the likelihood of a significant effect from the ordered p-values observed across studies [22]. Subsequently in 1932, Fisher established a procedure for combining p-values from various studies asking a similar question [10]. In the hope of making a definitive statement about a treatment effect, he examined the null hypothesis of no treatment effect over all the studies vs. the alternative research hypothesis of a pooled treatment effect. A fairly straight forward statistical procedure, Fisher's method is still used to combine the study results. If we assume that there are $k > 1$ studies being examined for the superiority of some form of intervention, call it A vs. not having A, then each of these studies has a p-value associated with it. Call them $p_1, p_2, \ldots, p_k$. Fisher established that the statistic, $2\Sigma i =_{1,k} \log(p_i)$, has a chi square distribution with $2k$ degrees of freedom (df). Fisher computed Y and compared that value to the tabled chi square value on $2k$ df for an alpha level of 0.05. If Y was greater than that tabled value, then the null hypothesis would be rejected at the 0.05 level. Hence, the intervention, A, would be declared effective or superior to not having A. As an example of Fisher's method, suppose there were five studies comparing some form of intervention, A, to a control, and the p-values for the five studies were $p_1 = 0.07$, $p_2 = 0.06$, $p_3 = 0.045$, $p_4 = 0.035$, and $p_5 = 0.05$, Y would have the value 29.843 which is greater than the tabled value of 18.31 on $2 \times 5 = 10$ df. Thus A is effective overall from the five studies at the alpha $= 0.05$ level. Extensions of Fisher's methods with weighted p-values were subsequently developed.

As the statistical methods for pooling data across studies evolved, the concept of combining the treatment effects has largely replaced combining the p-values. Further, the influence of each trial in the combined estimate of treatment effect is now typically weighted. Most commonly, each study's contribution to the overall treatment effect is weighted by the inverse of the variance of the estimated treatment effect for that particular study. Since variance is largely a function of sample size, studies with large sample size will have smaller variance (and larger inverse variance.) Hence, larger studies will generally have a greater influence on the overall estimated treatment effect across studies.

The term "meta-analysis" was coined by Glass in 1976 who stated that, "Meta-analysis refers to the analysis of analyses...the statistical analysis of a large collection of analysis results from individual studies for the purpose of integrating the findings" [11]. Meta-analytic techniques have continued to evolve and be refined with seminal advances such as DerSimonian and Laird's development of the random-effects model and the advancement of meta-regression methods to explain across study heterogeneity [6]. The application of meta-analysis to enhance clinical decision making, craft guidelines, and inform policy has rapidly flourished and been widely embraced.

Every clinician in training knows the old saw, "For every study cited, an equal and opposite study can be found." When studies address a similar question and the results do not agree, the role of meta-analysis is to hopefully put all the results together and reach a definitive conclusion about the positive, negative, or inconclusive impact of an intervention. Whether gathering aggregate data from the literature or pooling raw individual patient data (IPD) from multiple studies, the motivation is to reach a definitive conclusion about a therapy when several studies involving that intervention have been conducted. Tamoxifen treatment of early stage breast cancer provides a classic example [7]. Most of the individual separate studies had a favorable but statistically insignificant treatment effect. Several had unfavorable results albeit statistically insignificant. The beneficial mortality effect of tamoxifen therapy could not be definitively established until the patient-level data was combined from all the trials in a meta-analysis.

"Real world" limitations such as funding, available patients, access to testing and follow-up resources, and logistical limitations often inherently preclude adequately powered mega-trials to answer many investigative questions. Hence, methods to properly combine studies to obtain more precise results have understandable utility and appeal. Most disciplines, whether oncology, cardiovascular health, or dental interventions, tend to employ similar endpoints within their respective fields. Mean effects, response rates, odds ratios, time to events (survival, disease-free survival), correlations, etc. are common measures. As stated above, most meta-analyses are performed from data gathered in the literature or from pooled raw data. One has to understand that studies contributing to a meta-analysis are all asking a similar question, but all are not necessarily asking the same question. For example, if one wanted to examine whether receiving a statin after the

first myocardial infarction reduces the chance of death within 5 years, several studies have addressed this issue. One may involve one type of statin vs. a placebo control, while another may be a different statin vs. a fibrate. They do not involve the same active treatment or the same control. However, they are asking a similar question in that does receiving a statin in some form vs. not receiving a statin reduce the risk of death over a certain period of time.

When one pools data from various trials it enhances the power. Small or moderate, but potentially meaningful differences can be detected that individual trials could not definitively establish. A clinical trial may be inconclusive in that it did not demonstrate statistical superiority of a treatment or intervention. Sometimes, one refers to this as a "negative" trial. However, that may not be a proper term. One learns something from all trials. One may prefer the term "inconclusive" for a study demonstrating neither clear benefit nor harm. Studies not having sufficient sample size or long-enough follow-up to attain statistical significance to reach a definitive endpoint is commonplace because of resource limitations. Obviously, inconclusive results in a clinical trial do not necessarily mean the treatment is ineffective. Unfortunately, dismissal of an inconclusive trial as "negative" may contribute to publication bias. Since "positive" trials are more apt to receive prompt well-placed publication than the inconclusive trials, overly optimistic impressions of the treatment effect may arise from this publication bias. Diligent search for and location of both unpublished trials and those in less prominent journals is warranted. The meta-analyst must carefully evaluate this less formal data. This additional information gathered from more studies or subjects may lead to more accurate estimation of the treatment effect. Also, several studies may have a more heterogeneous sample than a single study. The result from this more diverse population may have more generalizability to unselected populations. Thus hopefully, one gathers a more global solution to a question or hypothesis based on most, if not all, existing evidence from all relevant studies.

This is particularly true in oncology where treatment effects are often small and contradictory results are likely to occur. The advantages of a meta-analysis of the pooled raw data from studies, if it can be obtained, are that, one can have more descriptive capabilities and apply covariate adjustment as well as have a rich database for future analysis as longer follow-up is accrued

[17]. Most meta-analyses, however, are done using summary data from published articles, abstracts, or reports. The advantages are that data is easily gathered in statistical summary form and there are statistical techniques available for accurately combining the results. It may be necessary to summarize the results from older studies, where the data is lost, inaccessible, or too expensive to retrieve. A meta-analysis of the aggregate data from several trials may be the first step in motivating the commitment of effort and resources in pursuing the raw data for more detailed analyses. Methods have been developed and validated for mixed models combining IPD from some trials with aggregate data from other trials when the IPD is unavailable [19]. Granted there are limitations such as inadequate details in the publications, protocol violations, undocumented patient compliance rates, and insufficient follow-up in longitudinal trials. Fortunately, in recent times, publications for the most part receive a good statistical review and the results are generally reliable.

2.1.2 Overview of Statistical Terms and Approaches

An appreciation of the terms and methods of meta-analysis assures deeper understanding of the ultimate results and their proper interpretation and limitations. Our strategy in this section is to present two meta-analyses, the first involving continuous data in Sect. 2.1.1 and the second involving categorical data in Sect. 2.1.2. We introduce the terms and analysis approaches with some attention to the limitations of which the readers may wish to be aware.

Meta-analyses deal with common endpoints which are well defined, easily measurable, and have been measured in a consistent way over all studies over time. Rather than combining p-values like Fisher, each individual study's result is translated into an effect size (ES). ESs may be the differences in the mean effect of treatment or intervention, A, vs. the mean effect of treatment or intervention, B. Other ES examples are response rates (proportion of successes on A vs. proportion of successes on B) and time to event endpoints such as survival, time to progression, time to second myocardial infarct (MI), etc. ES can also be expressed in terms of odds ratios (OR), relative risk (RR), or hazard ratios (HR). The methodology of meta-analysis

is to examine the ES from each study and then to statistically combine these ES to determine a common overall ES from all the studies and test the statistical significance of this combined statistic, ES.

2.1.2.1 Continuous Data

In the first example, meta-analysis examines continuous endpoint data such as LDL cholesterol level. In general terms, we wish to know if the mean reduction in LDL cholesterol is greater with treatment A than with treatment B. There are seven studies ($k=7$) in this example, where A is the treatment of interest and its comparison group is represented by B. The standardized ES δ_i in each individual study in this application is:

$$\delta_i = (\mu_{Ai} - \mu_{Bi})/\sigma_i. \qquad 2.1$$

This difference in the population means μ_{Ai} and μ_{Bi} with treatment A compared to treatment B in the ith study is then standardized by dividing it by the population standard deviation σ_i in the ith study. This standard ES may vary depending on how the standard deviation is defined. For example, it can be the standard deviation of group A or group B (the reference or control group) or the pooled standard deviation of the two populations [12]. We will assume the pooled estimate for our example. The population ES δ_i as defined by the population parameters μ_{Ai}, μ_{Bi}, and σi is of course estimated by the realizations of these parameters in the observed data of the ith study.

$$ES_i = (Y_{Ai} - Y_{Bi})/S_i, \qquad 2.2$$

In our case, each study will have an estimate of the ES, where Y_A minus Y_B is the difference in mean observed LDL cholesterol levels between treatment A and B in the particular study divided by the pooled standard deviation of the cholesterol levels in both A and B groups. The standardized ES becomes unitless or "scale free." The pooled ES will be calculated from these 7 ES from the seven studies (see Table 2.1). The values, n_A and n_B, in the first column of Table 2.1 are the number of subjects on each treatment from A and B, respectively. The middle column of Table 2.1 is the ES from each of the seven studies. One can see that in studies 1, 2, 3, 6, and 7, the ES is negative indicating a treatment effect in favor of A. This is not true for studies 4 and 5.

Table 2.1 Effects sizes and p-values for the seven LDL studies

Study name(n_A, n_B)	Effect size $=(Y_A-Y_B)/S$	p-value
1(32, 26)	−0.160	0.545
2(26, 33)	−0.717	0.008
3(32, 43)	−0.261	0.266
4(37, 41)	0.324	0.156
5(37, 38)	0.432	0.064
6(35, 40)	−0.112	0.629
7(48, 38)	−0.627	0.005
Overall	−0.143	0.114

The last column gives the p-value for testing the ES = 0 in each study. Only studies 2 and 7 have a significant effect in favor of A. The overall ES in the last row is −0.143 showing a greater mean reduction in cholesterol on A. However, the overall p-value is 0.114 in the last column indicating no significant effect overall.

There is some discussion as to the accuracy of equation (2) in estimating the true population ES represented by equation (2.1) [12]. When the combined sample size of A and B within a single study is less than 50, the ES of (2) may overestimate the true population ES. Some authors [12] have suggested a correction factor (CF) with theoretical justification of CF = (1−3/(4N-9)) multiplied by ES of (2.2) or CFxES to more closely approximate the true population ES where N is the sum of the sample sizes of the two groups, A and B, within a study ($N=n_A + n_B$). Clearly, as N becomes large this CF approximates one. This CF adjustment was made to the middle column of Table 2.1, although it was hardly necessary as all our sample sizes are fairly large.

The individual and overall study data from such meta-analyses is typically displayed in a Forest Plot as shown in Fig. 2.1. The Forest plot is a graphical summary of the meta-analytic statistics. The title, "std diff in means and 95% CI" is the ES with the 95% confidence intervals for each study. The dark rectangles represent the ES of each study found in the middle column of Table 2.1. Note that the larger the area of the rectangle the larger the sample size. Also, the horizontal lines of the boxes represent the 95% confidence interval of the ES. The rectangles to the left of the null line (treatment difference between A and B equals 0)

favor treatment A. Those to the right of the null line favor treatment B. The horizontal lines that overlap the 0 vertical line indicate statistical nonsignificance at the 0.05 level for that particular study. This is consistent with the last column of Table 2.1. The diamond at the bottom of the Forest plot is the overall ES of the seven studies. The vertical points of the diamond overlap or are equal to the value, −0.143, favoring treatment, A, and the horizontal points are the lower and upper limits of the 95% confidence interval. The 95% confidence interval for the overall population ES is (−0.320, 0.034), which includes 0 and thus overlaps the null line in the Forest Plot. Hence, the overall combined results are not statistically significant. The actual p-value = 0.114.

2.1.2.1.1 Heterogeneity

Now, having understood the contents of Table 2.1 and Fig. 2.1, we can discuss and demonstrate one of the issues in meta-analysis called heterogeneity. When doing a meta-analysis, the issue of heterogeneity across the studies may affect the study results. This is simply the variation among the studies. In terms of a statistical hypothesis, we can write the null hypothesis: H_0: no heterogeneity or that the treatment effect is the same in all k (in our case $k=7$) studies. The alternative hypothesis is: H_1: the treatment effect varies over the k studies included in the meta-analysis, thus giving

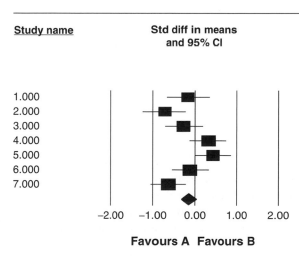

Study name

Std diff in means and 95% CI

Meta Analysis

Fig. 2.1 Forrest plot of the seven LDL studies

heterogeneity. All we are doing here is testing for consistency among the ESs across the studies. If we reject H_0, then we have heterogeneity. This is important because heterogeneity implies that there is some underlying difference or differences among the included studies. We often want to know what this difference is. We would like to be able to understand the cause and explain this heterogeneity or variance. Note in Table 2.1 that 5 of the ES are negative or favor treatment A and 2 of the ES are positive or favor treatment B. Note also in Fig. 2.1 that 5 of the rectangles are to the left of the vertical 0 line and 2 are to the right. We want to know if statistically, this is a sufficient enough discrepancy to cause us to be concerned about heterogeneity.

So, the next task is to formally test for significant heterogeneity among the studies at some prespecified level of significance, typically $\alpha = 0.05$ or 0.10. So, in addition to some visual indication of heterogeneity in the Forest Plot, we have a formal test statistic called the Q statistic. The Q statistic is used to determine the degree of heterogeneity across studies. The benchmark we use is that if Q is close to 0 then there is no heterogeneity. The formula for calculating Q involves calculating a function of the difference between each study ES and the overall mean ES of all studies combined [13]. If the ES from each study is close to the overall mean ES, showing little or no difference among the ES, then the Q statistic will be close to zero indicating little or no difference among the ESs. The Q has a chi square distribution [13] on k-1 df or the number of studies minus one. Like other statistics we calculate, the Q statistic is compared to a critical value for the chi square distribution. The null hypothesis is that there is no heterogeneity in the combined analysis or H_0: $Q = 0$ vs. the alternative hypothesis, H_1: $Q \neq 0$ implying that there is significant heterogeneity. The critical value of the k studies for a chi square distribution on $71 = 6$ df at an alpha level of 0.05 is 12.59. The calculated value of Q from our data is 19.76. Clearly, the calculated Q is much greater than the critical value. Therefore, we reject the null hypothesis and determine that there is significant heterogeneity among our studies. As a matter of fact, the exact p-value is 0.003.

This does not change our conclusion that there is no significant treatment effect due to A. However, it does alert us that we should try to determine the source of the heterogeneity. Some possible sources of heterogeneity may be the clinical differences among the studies such as patient selection, baseline disease

severity, differences in the treatment applied, management of intercurrent outcomes (toxicity), patient characteristics, time point or conditions of measurements, or others. One may also investigate the methodological differences between the studies such as the mechanism of randomization, extent of withdrawals, and follow-up failure in longitudinal studies. One should also note that heterogeneity can still be due to chance alone and the source not easily detected. Quantifying heterogeneity can be one of the most troublesome aspects of meta-analysis. It is important, because it can affect the decision about the statistical model to be selected (fixed or random effects described below). If significant heterogeneity is found, then potential moderator variables can be found to explain this variability. It may require concentrating the meta–analysis on a subset of studies that are homogeneous within themselves.

Another statistic used to quantify heterogeneity is the I^2 index which quantifies the extent of heterogeneity from a collection of ESs by comparing the Q statistic to its expected value assuming homogeneity, that is to its degrees of freedom, $(df = k-1)$. When the Q statistic is smaller than its df, then I^2 is truncated to 0. The I^2 index can easily be interpreted as the percentage of heterogeneity in the system or the amount of the total variation accounted for by the between studies variance. For example, a meta-analysis with $I^2 = 0$ means that all variability in ES estimates is due to sampling error within studies. On the other hand, a meta-analysis with $I^2 = 60$ means that 60% of the total variability among ESs is caused not by sampling error, but by true heterogeneity among studies. In our seven-study case, $I^2 = 68.63$ or 68.6% of the variability among them is due to heterogeneity across the underlying studies.

2.1.2.1.2 Meta-Regression

If one finds significant heterogeneity with a significant Q statistic and fairly large I^2, say greater than 0.55, one may use what is referred to as a "meta-regression" to determine significant variants or causes of among study variability [15]. Such sources of variability are given in the previous paragraphs (for example, patient characteristics, baseline disease severity, management of inter current outcomes or toxicity, etc.), and are sometimes referred to as covariates. The meta-regression approaches model the heterogeneity among study treatment effects. Simply stated, the dependent variable is the ES, such as OR's, RR, standardized mean differences, etc. from each study and is regressed on the covariates of interest. The suspected covariates and their strength of association with the differences in ES is determined with usual regression statistics such as the estimated regression coefficients or the β-values, the p-values, and the R-squares. Those covariates which are determined to have a statistically significant association with the dependent variable, ES, are assumed to be the major causes of heterogeneity. The assumption in using a meta-regression is that all the variables of interest suspected of being the sources of heterogeneity are available in all publications so they can be included in the meta-regression. Absence of data about important covariate variables in the literature can be a major limitation in assessing heterogeneity in meta-analyses with meta-regression. For example, in one study or publication, one may know the average age of individuals on each treatment or intervention, while in another study, only age groupings are given, and those groupings may be so restrictive as to not permit extrapolation of a meaningful average across treatment groups.

Other issues with meta-regression have been noted as well [21]. That is to say, the associations derived from meta-regressions are observational, and have a less rigorous interpretation than the causal relationships derived from randomized comparisons. This applies particularly to our example above when averages of patient characteristics in each study are used as covariates in the regression. Data dredging is the term used to describe the main shortcoming in reaching reliable conclusions from meta-regression. It can be avoided only in the strict statistical sense by prespecifying the covariates that will be investigated as potential sources of heterogeneity. However, in practice, this is not always easy to achieve as one has no guarantee that this information will be available in a reasonable form for coding before undertaking the literature search or systematic review. Only in the case of doing a meta-analysis of the raw patient-level data, if available, may this be possible.

Further statistical issues of meta-regression are also at hand. In a meta-analysis, the unit of analysis is the study, so the regression performance is determined by the number of studies in the meta-analysis. Thus the power of the regression is limited, and in most cases, as in the meta-regression from the literature, one could not expect much power depending on the number of covariates one considers in the model. Also with a restricted sample size, investigations of confounding interactions could be a challenge. One could derive weights for a weighted regression by study size. However, the usual inverse variance technique used for weighted regression would be difficult. Also, in the case of a meta-regression, most of the regressions performed use linear regression with no attempt to check the underlying assumptions of linearity or normality. Despite all these challenges, if one is determined to get a handle on the sources of heterogeneity, meta-regression is the tool of choice particularly with prespecified covariates. Again, the clinician's or investigator's substantive insight into the domain of the research can significantly enhance methodological planning for the systematic review and subsequent meta-analysis.

2.1.2.1.3 Funnel Plots to Measure Bias

Another useful diagnostic tool in examining meta-analyses is the funnel plot. The underlying studies' effect estimates are plotted on the horizontal axis against sample size in ascending order on the vertical axis. These may be useful in assessing the validity of meta-analyses. This is often referred to as "publication bias." The funnel plot is based on the fact that precision in estimating the underlying treatment effect will increase as the sample size of the included studies increases. Results from small studies will scatter widely at the bottom of the graph. The spread should narrow at the top of the graph among studies with larger sample sizes. In the absence of bias, the plot will resemble a symmetrical inverted funnel. Conversely, if there is bias, funnel plots will often be skewed and asymmetrical. Funnel plots are usually constructed as plotting the ES vs. the sample size or the ES vs. the standard error.

In meta-analysis, we can use a linear regression approach [8] to measure funnel plot asymmetry on the ES. The ES is regressed against the estimate's precision, the latter being defined as the inverse of the standard error. The regression equation is: $ES = a + b*$ precision, where a is the intercept and b is the slope. If the regression line passes through the origin, the intercept $a = 0$, then the funnel plot is symmetric. The null hypothesis is Ho: $a = 0$ which assumes symmetry of the effects about the null value of 0 in the case of continuous data. Since precision depends largely on sample size, small trials will be close to zero on the horizontal axis and vice versa for larger trials. If the null hypothesis is rejected, the intercept of the regression line is different from 0 indicating bias in the relationship between precision and ES. We demonstrate this concept for our seven studies in which the funnel plot is not really very informative. Although symmetrical (see Fig. 2.2 which is the standard error on the vertical axis and the ES or "std diff in means" on the horizontal), it is rather flat because there are few studies with approximately the same sample size. However, the symmetry is preserved as shown by the plot and the regression results. The test of the null hypothesis that the intercept is equal to zero is not significant at the 0.05 alpha level indicating that the line goes through the origin. See the vertical mid line on Fig. 2.2. The actual p-value is 0.5194 indicating that there is not any bias in the relationship between ESs and precisions. Thus there is no publication bias. However, a limitation of this test is that it may not be accurate for small sample sizes, i.e., small number of studies in the meta-analysis. Figure 2.3 is a funnel plot of 14 studies addressing the same issue as our seven study plot, and one can see that with enough studies, the plot does take a nice funnel shape indicating no bias. Detailed discussions of funnel plots and test of symmetry can be found throughout the literature [3, 8] pertaining to meta-analyses.

2.1.2.2 Categorical Data

We next consider a second type of meta-analyses i.e., when data are categorical. This can involve statistics such as ORs, proportion of response, or relative risk ratios. In Table 2.2 are the results from six clinical studies comparing an intervention A with a control group B noted by the subscripts. O represents the observed number of responses in the treated, A group, and the control, B group. N represents the total sample size in each group, A and B. The odds ratio ($OR = [O_A/(N_A - O_A)]/[O_B/(N_B - O_B)]$) or the odds of response vs. no response in group A vs. group B is noted in the sixth column. For example, in study 1, one interpretation could be that the odds of a responses vs. a nonresponse is 1.3 times more likely in group A than in group B showing superiority of intervention A to control B. We see that in studies 1, 2, 3, and 6, there is superiority of A to B with respect to achieving a higher odds of response and the opposite is true in studies 4 and 5. The p-values for each study is seen in the last column and the overall p-value using the Mantel–Haenszel statistic is 0.001, showing superiority of A over B with respect to the endpoint. Recall that the null hypothesis being tested in this context is that the $OR = 1$ vs. the alternative hypothesis where the $OR \neq 1$. The overall $OR = 1.223$ with 95% confidence limits (1.094, 1.366). The p-value = 0.001. Figure 2.4 is the Forest plot with 95% confidence intervals on the ORs. Notice the larger rectangle for study 6 indicating a larger sample size than the other studies.

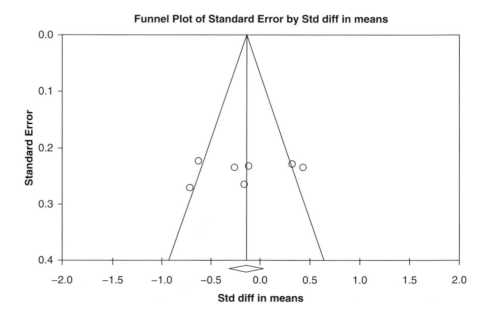

Fig. 2.2 Funnel plot of the 7 LDL studies

Fig. 2.3 Funnel plot of 14 studies showing symmetry

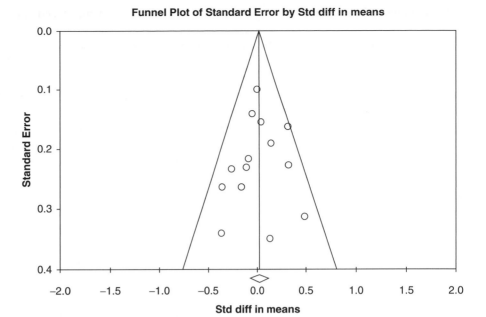

Table 2.2 Six clinical studies involving categorical data

Study	O_A	N_A	O_B	N_B	OR	p-value
1	392	512	358	498	1.277	0.090
2	286	483	249	482	1.358	0.018
3	164	427	297	848	1.157	0.235
4	34	152	36	137	0.808	0.439
5	36	154	51	172	0.724	0.202
6	334	1107	274	1116	1.328	0.003
Overall	–	–	–	–	1.223	0.001

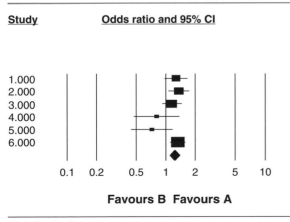

Meta Analysis

Fig. 2.4 Forest plot of the six studies of Table 2.2

Just as in the previous case, not only do we have the treatment comparison effects, but also we can generate the other statistics testing for heterogeneity and publication bias. The Q statistic is 8.249 with a p-value $= 0.143$ indicating no heterogeneity. The I^2 statistic is 38.389 indicating that about 38% of the variance in heterogeneity is due to the between studies variation. The funnel plot is not shown here. However, Egger's test for symmetry yields a p-value $= 0.019$ indicating possible publication bias. Examining the statistics (not shown here) indicates that the larger studies 1, 2, 3, and 6 do in fact have smaller standard errors than do the smaller studies, 4 and 5. Thus this test of symmetry may not be very informative in this case as we mentioned above, as the sample size (number of studies) is rather small.

2.1.2.3 Time to Event Data

Figure 2.5 is a survival plot comparing two interventions, A and B. The vertical axis is the probability of remaining free of the event or failure and the horizontal axis is the time. Often, data from survival studies, generally known as the time to event analyses, are presented as survival curves as pictured in this figure. One can see in this study that the curve for intervention, A, is above the curve for B indicating a slower rate of failure over time for A as compared to B. In order to do a meta-analysis on aggregate data such as this, one has to know the hazard ratio (HR) or the log(HR), where HR is the ratio of hazards. The hazard function is a function associated with a survival curve or experience. The hazard function is basically the failure (death) rate over time. It can be thought of as the odds of failure over time. It is the chance of failure at any point in time. Just as the hazard function is a failure rate on a particular treatment, the HR is a measure of relative treatment effect. For example, suppose we have two groups (A or B), H_A is the hazard associated with A and H_B is the hazard associated with B. In Fig. 2.5, we wish to compare their survivals. Our null hypothesis is that the two survivals are not different or the hazard ratio, HR = 1 i.e.,

H_0: HR = H_A/H_B = 1 (null hypothesis)
H_1: HR = H_A/H_B ≠ 1 (alternative hypothesis)

Thus the HR = [Failure rate (new treatment)/Failure rate (control group)].

If the HR < 1, then the outcome favors treatment A. This indicates that A has smaller hazard or chance of failure over time as compared to B. If HR > 1 then the outcome favors treatment B. Thus HR = 1 implies no difference between treatment and control groups. Meta-analysis combining several time-to-event studies determines whether treatment A is superior to its comparison group. If we do not have the raw patient data, an aggregate data approach may be required for some or all included studies. With meta-analysis of randomized controlled trials with time-to-event outcomes, the challenge is that there may be variation in the reporting of survival analyses [23]. Often, no single method for extracting the log(HR) estimate will suffice. Methods have been described for estimating the log(HR) from survival curves [23]. These methods extend to life-tables. In the situation where the treatment effect varies over time and the trials in the meta-analysis have different lengths of follow-up, heterogeneity may be evident. In order to assess whether the hazard ratio changes with time, several tests have been proposed and compared [23]. All issues discussed above for the OR applies to the hazard ratio. One can test for treatment effect, heterogeneity, and publication bias. As mentioned, one of the greatest sources of heterogeneity would be the differing length of follow-up across the studies included in the meta-analysis.

2.1.3 Other Tests in Meta-Analysis

In Sect. 2.0 above, we have discussed the background and the major tests for determining the overall treatment effect and its significance as well as heterogeneity in meta-analysis. There are other topics that one can pursue which are informative and will point out precautions that one must take in discussing meta-analyses.

2.1.3.1 Test for Interaction

One possible test is that of interaction. This involves grouping studies according to some characteristic of the study; for example, is the treatment effect homogeneous over the groups such as age categories, modalities, etc.? Let us suppose for the six studies of Table 2.2, that we believe the treatment effect to be nonhomogeneous over the age groups in our studies. In particular, we might suspect that the treatments may perform

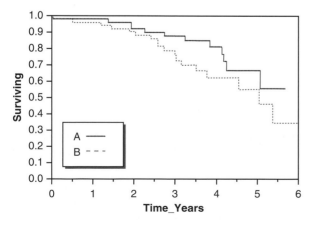

Fig. 2.5 Survival comparison of A vs. B for time to event data

Table 2.3 Test of age by treatment interaction for the combined six studies of Table 2.2

Age category	Range	OR
1	20–30	1.23
2	31–40	1.04
3	41–50	1.09
4	51+	0.82
Interaction	–	p = 0.02

differently in the older than younger age groups. Assuming that we have the information to stratify the individual study results by age, we calculate OR comparing treatment A to treatment B in four age categories (Table 2.3). Note that overall, the results for Table 2.2 indicated superiority of A over B at $p = 0.001$. When the data was combined from all six studies in Table 2.3 and broken into age categories, we see that A is superior to B in ages 20–50 as the OR are all greater than one. Note that for age 50 or more, the OR is less than one, indicating superiority of B over A in the oldest group. In the last row of Table 2.3, we list the p-value for testing significant interaction of treatment with age which is $p = 0.02$ indicating significant interaction. This identifies a limitation of doing a meta-analysis on aggregate data. Unless one had the raw data from the six studies, or information on age categories and response was available in all 6 published articles, one would not be able to detect this potentially meaningful interaction. Hence, one might not discover that the overall result of the meta-analysis may not be true in a clinically important subgroup.

2.1.3.2 Test for Trend

Another important test to examine meta-analytic results is testing for a trend in the treatment effect. The technique is to split the data of each study according to some ordinal characteristic of the subjects which is suspected to influence the treatment effect; e.g., age, nodal status, disease stage, or severity, etc. Is there a systematic tendency of the treatment effect to increase/decrease with the severity of disease? Again, unless one has the raw data, or the ordinal categorization is obvious from the aggregate or published results, this may be impossible to do.

A meta-analysis was done on several studies to compare two interventions A and B. Was there a significant trend in response based on disease severity? We assume that we can group the data results from a number of studies by three classes of disease severity: low, medium, and high. When analyzing the data, we note that the OR of A vs. B (OR > 1) with respect to achieving a response overall was statistically significant, $p \leq 0.05$. When combining all the studies, we note a trend in the OR as 3.65, 1.72, and 1.05 for low, medium, and high disease severity respectively. Note the decreasing effect of A as the severity increases. A test for trend was significant at $p = 0.01$ indicating a statistically significant trend in the effect of A, with greater effect in less severe cases.

2.1.3.3 Sensitivity Analysis and "File-Drawer Effect"

One of the challenges in a meta-analysis is finding all of the studies on the subject. A critical issue in meta-analysis is what has been dubbed "the file-drawer effect." That is, a study is conducted without a significant result, and it is not published. The time, effort, and resources necessary to publish the study are not expended particularly because it may be difficult to receive publication in a respected journal. It is very tempting for someone with inconclusive, nonsignificant data to quietly put it in a file drawer, intending to write it up when one gets some free time. Other more promising projects take priority.

The reason why publication bias is so important to a meta-analysis is that even if there is no real treatment effect, 5% of studies will show a significant positive result at the $p < 0.05$ level. That is, there is a 5% probability of getting a significant result if the null hypothesis is actually true. Counterbalancing inconclusive studies which would contribute to a more accurate overall ES estimate may be absent. Suppose one in fact performs a meta-analysis and achieves a significant effect, to evaluate the sensitivity of the result to publication bias, an estimate of how many unpublished, nonsignificant studies would reduce the overall effect to nonsignificance can provide some intuitive sense of the robustness of the result. Obviously, if the number of studies required to negate the observed effect is very large, you can be more confident that your meta-analysis's significant treatment effect is not arising from the "file-drawer effect." For example, in Table 2.2, at least 10 more studies with a sample size of at most 200 with nonstatistically significant results would be required to reduce the observed result to nonsignificance. Hence, we can be pretty confident that the results are not highly sensitive to publication bias. Sensitivity analysis, therefore, helps determine the robustness of the meta-analytic result.

Another form of sensitivity analysis is to reexamine the result when one or more studies are excluded. The reasons for doing this may include suspicion that one or more of the studies has undue influence on the overall result. Therefore, the question may arise as to the effect of certain studies in the meta-analysis that one believes may be over influencing the result, and if they were removed, would the effect be diminished? For example, in a meta-analysis of a longitudinal or time to event outcome, omit those studies with less follow-up than others to determine if the results still hold. Additionally, one may wish to perform a sensitivity analysis where studies judged to be of lower quality are excluded. Strategies have been employed to weight the studies by the presence of prespecified characteristics generally associated with optimal study design and conduct [5].

2.1.4 Statistical Techniques to Account for Study Size and Quality

In medicine and dentistry, one needs to properly weight all the evidence available to make sound principled decisions. Similarly, the studies in a meta-analysis can and should be weighted by study size (inverse variance) and perhaps other factors such as study quality.

2.1.4.1 Weighing of Evidence

Now that we have discussed what a meta-analysis does and some of the issues involved, we are keenly aware of the fact that not all studies will behave in the same way. That is, they are of different sizes, perhaps different precision of the estimates of the effects across the studies and differing amounts of information such as subject characteristics from study to study. The ultimate goal of the meta-analysis is to calculate a "weighted average" of the effects of interest such as OR, risk ratio, hazard ratio, or standardized mean effect across the studies.

While there are various potential measures of ES, the overall goals are the same:

- Calculating a "weighted average" measure of effect
- Performing a test to see if this estimated overall effect is different from the null hypothesis of no effect.

The general concept is simple: determine the average effect across studies and assess its significance with a p-value. The mathematics is also straightforward.

The main challenge is to choose the type of weights to assign. By far, the most common approach is to weight the studies by the "precision" of the estimates. Precision is largely driven by the sample size and reflected by the widths of the 95% confidence limits about the study-specific estimates. Another way of considering precision is the variance of the effect within the study. The larger the variance, the less precise the estimate of the effect (i.e., OR, risk ratio, hazard ratio, or standardized mean effect). The smaller the variance, the more precise the estimate of the effect. The precision is defined in several ways, but has the same impact. The precision is sometimes defined as the inverse of the variance, inverse of the standard deviation, or inverse of the standard error of the mean. In any case, the smaller the variance, standard error, standard deviation, etc. usually as a result of a larger sample size within a study, the greater the precision.

When weights are assigned by the precision of the estimates, they are proportionate (1/(variance of the study)). This is the "statistician's" approach. A possible problem, however, is that it could assign a bigger weight to the large and poorly-done study than it does to the small and well-done study. A meta-analysis that includes one or two large studies is largely a report of just those studies. However, for the most part, this is a reasonable assignment of weights. So, if we assume that we have chosen our studies well, we want the larger study to impact more on the meta-analysis than a smaller study. Some authors have assigned weights to studies based on the study quality or the amount of information provided about the study design, analysis, and study presentation. This is a scoring method and the studies with the most detail receive a higher score which is factored into the weighting [5]. The most widely used is the Jadad scale (Oxford quality scoring system) that assigns a score of 0–5 based on the study characteristics of randomization, blinding, and withdrawals/dropouts [14].

2.1.4.2 Random Effects

In Sect. 2.1.2, we discussed the Q statistic as a measure of the heterogeneity across studies in a meta-analysis. Heterogeneity in the underlying studies can be a challenge when interpreting the results of a meta-analysis. The diverse nature of the patient populations, designs, and overall methods employed in the underlying studies can lead one to question the applicability of the results to a specific individual or group of patients. Also, the confidence interval surrounding the estimated overall effect, if derived from just the variance within each study, is too small when heterogeneity is present across the studies. Because of the varying sample sizes and underlying patient populations, it has been pointed out [6] that each study has a different sampling error associated with it. The inverse variance weights defined above account for the within study variance but do not account for the between studies variation. With these fixed-effects methods of meta-analysis, one of the assumptions is that there is no variation between studies. However, if all the studies are not sampling from the same parent population, there may well be additional variance between the studies. In other words, one possible explanation for the heterogeneity of ESs among the studies is that each individual study in a meta-analysis may be sampling from a different parent distribution.

To allow for the randomness between the studies, we want to account for both the within and between study variation. Unlike fixed-effects models, random effects meta-analysis methodologies account for both within and between study variations. This allows one to adjust for the heterogeneity among the studies and gives a more accurate interpretation of the results when integrating studies. Several authors [6] have done an excellent job of describing this process and constructing what is known as a random effects model. The convenience of the random effects model is that we need not worry about heterogeneity and discussion of the Q statistic and I^2 with regard to the estimation of the confidence interval around the overall ES. The additional

between study variance has been adjusted for in the calculations of the confidence interval surrounding the treatment effect. The estimate of the between study variance is calculated in the τ statistic. The square of this statistic is added to the variance of each individual study variance before calculating the inverse variance $[1/(s_i^2 + \tau^2)]$.

This is not necessarily reassuring to some investigators who wish to know the degree of heterogeneity even before the random model is invoked. This does not necessarily prevent one from computing the Q and I^2 statistic as described above in Sect. 2.1.2. Hence, many investigators will compute the results of the meta-analysis with a fixed-effects approach to explicitly and formally examine heterogeneity. If heterogeneity is found, typically a random effects model will then be invoked as the more sound estimate of the summary treatment effect and the surrounding confidence interval.

While there is a convenience to the random effects model, it generates wider 95% confidence intervals. This is true because the 95% confidence interval on the summary ES takes into account two sources of variation, the between study as well as the within study sampling variation. To demonstrate this, note from the seven-study example in Sect. 2.1.2 and Table 2.1 and Fig. 2.1, that the ES = −0.143 and the 95% confidence interval for the overall population ES is (−0.320, 0.034). For the random effects model, the ES = −0.154 and the 95% confidence interval for the overall population ES is (−0.476, 0.169). The results are the same in that there is no significant treatment effect, $p = 0.350$. However, the confidence interval in the random context is almost twice as large (1.8 times) as that for the fixed effects confidence interval. As another example, note the results of Sect. 2.1.2 for the categorical data in Table 2.2. The overall OR = 1.223 with 95% confidence limits (1.094, 1.366) for the fixed effects analysis. For the random effects analyses, the OR is 1.187 with 95% confidence interval, (1.019, 1.382). The results remain statistically significant ($p = 0.028$), but the confidence interval width in the random context is 1.33 times that for the fixed effects confidence interval. Given this, if no significant heterogeneity is detected between the ESs of the underlying studies, a fixed effects model may be appropriate. When a fixed effects assumption is appropriate, there is greater power to detect a significant overall treatment effect than with the random effects model.

2.1.4.3 Random Effects vs. Fixed Effects

The question naturally arises as to which is the better approach – a random effects model or a fixed effects model? One might determine that the more conservative approach is to consider the random effects since the confidence intervals are wider. However, an excellent discussion of this approach and its controversy has been put forth by several authors. [18]. They point out that "conservative" in this context is generally taken to mean that random-effects approaches tend to have higher estimated variances than fixed effects models due to the inclusion or addition of the between study variation, which results, as we saw above, in wider confidence intervals. They point out that, when random-effects summaries are conservative in this context, they need not be conservative in other, equally important considerations. Specifically, random-effects ES can be farther from the null value and can have smaller p values, so they can appear more strongly supportive of causation or prevention than fixed-effects statistics or ES. The presence of this condition depends on the situation. For example, let us consider our two data examples in Sects. 2.2.1 and 2.1.2. Note that in Sect. 2.1.1, when considering the case of the continuous data summarized also in the previous paragraph, the confidence interval for the fixed effects is narrower than the confidence interval for the random effects. Also the ES of −0.154 for the random model is farther from the null value of 0 than is −0.143 for the fixed effects model. The p-value for the fixed effects is 0.114 and for the random model is 0.350. Here, the p-value of the random model is not smaller than the fixed effects model or more supportive of causation despite the larger estimated ES with the random model. Also in Sect. 2.1.2 for the OR example, the ES for the fixed effects is 1.223 with a p-value = 0.001 and the ES for the random effects is 1.187 which is closer to the null value of 1 and a p-value = 0.028. All this indicates is that the random effects model is not always more conservative than the fixed effects model when one not only focuses on the confidence intervals and p-values, but also examines the magnitude of the ESs [18].

Usually, the presence of heterogeneity among studies motivates employing the random effects design. While the random effects approach is a good mathematical way of accounting for the variation across studies, the researcher should still be aware of and investigate the potential sources of heterogeneity. It may not always be possible to determine or explain the heterogeneity, but every attempt should be made to examine it, explain it, and determine if proceeding with the meta-analysis is appropriate. An assumption is that the characteristics of the studies that generated the results allow those results to be combined [18]. Some may question that assumption and after examining those characteristics decide that it may not be reasonable scientifically or clinically to combine those results. Hence, rather than being mutually exclusive, examining fixed effects, random effects, and tests of heterogeneity are all a part of the total reporting of a sound meta-analysis.

Another possible way of examining the data accounting for the randomness among the studies is by conducting a Bayesian meta-analysis.

2.1.5 Bayesian Meta-Analysis

There are times when one has a prior belief about the performance of therapies before the trial or study begins. Thus it is assumed that their performance on an average is random. This is also the case before proceeding with a systematic review to gather studies for a meta-analysis. Just as meta-analysis is the technique used to combine the information from similar trials into a formal summary, Bayesian analysis takes it one step further and combines prior information or prior beliefs with the meta-analysis. These beliefs are called the prior distribution. The term "Bayesian" comes from Bayes Theorem which is a simple mathematical formula for computing conditional probabilities. Thomas Bayes was an 18th century English clergyman [4].

For example, in our data in Table 2.2 from Sect. 2.1.2, one may believe before starting the study that the gains in odds of response on A is 20% better than that on B and that this is a random component with a reasonable probability distribution. The evidence from the trial or data from the literature is described as the sampling distribution of results. Combining the prior belief and the evidence in the data gives the posterior distribution of beliefs. This gives an estimate of the actual OR or what is termed the posterior OR. Differences from the analysis done in Sect. 2.1.2 or classical analyses include the incorporation of prior beliefs and the absence of p-values. The posterior estimate of the effect or OR is via a credibility interval which is analogous to a

Table 2.4 Posterior estimates of odds ratios for the data in Table 2.2

Study	Posterior OR	Lower (2.5%)	Upper (97.5%)
1	1.235	1.011	1.533
2	1.272	1.054	1.573
3	1.185	0.976	1.409
4	1.109	0.714	1.424
5	1.048	0.620	1.372
6	1.269	1.088	1.498
Overall	1.195	0.9724	1.413

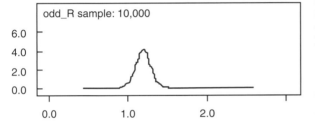

Fig. 2.6 Posterior density of the composite odds ratio for the Bayesian analysis

classical point estimate of the OR and its associated confidence interval, but has a direct interpretation in terms of belief. As many people interpret a confidence interval as the region in which the effect probably lies, they are essentially acting as Bayesians.

Table 2.4 and Fig. 2.6 give the results of the Bayesian application to the data in Table 2.2. The prior belief incorporated into the analysis was that the prior odds of A in favor of B is random with a probability distribution and ranged from 0.9 to 1.26. We omit the details of the underlying distribution as it is not necessary for us to proceed with the overview of the procedure. Combined with the data in Table 2.2 from the columns titled, O_A, N_A, O_B, N_B, we derive the posterior OR in Table 2.4 for each of the 6 studies. That is, the OR column of Table 2.2 updates the prior information to yield the "Posterior OR" column in Table 2.4. The columns titled Lower (2.5%) and Upper (97.5%) for studies 1–6 are the lower and upper limits respectively for the 95% posterior credible regions of the posterior OR from each of the studies. Note that in Table 2.4, studies 3, 4, and 5 have a lower limit below 1 indicating possibly no difference in the two treatments. Studies 1, 2,

and 6 have a lower limit above the value 1 indicating superiority of A to B. The last row of Table 2.4 is the overall Bayesian meta-analytic posterior OR with the 95% credible regions. Note that the posterior OR = 1.195 with a lower limit equal to 0.972 or very close to one. This indicates possible evidence from the combined six studies for no difference between the two treatments. However, note Fig. 2.6, which is the posterior density of the OR from the combined studies. We note that the bulk of the density is above 1, favoring treatment A. The feature of the Bayesian approach is that now the parameters of interest, such as the ESs, are random and have a distribution which allow us to determine the credibility of certain values of that parameter with some probability. No p-value is generated confining us to a region of 0.05 or less. The interpretation is based on the credible interval or region and the posterior density distribution.

Also in Fig. 2.6, the label odd R stands for posterior OR from the meta-analysis and the number 10,000 is a feature of the software we used indicating the number of high speed iterations used to converge to our solutions [20]. We used much more than actually needed for this particular application. We note that the Bayesian computations can be computer intensive, but the availability of the software to perform these calculations makes it routine in most cases [20].

Another feature of the Bayesian analysis is that one can derive a predictive distribution. That is, if a new study were to be done comparing A and B, then based on our results, we can predict what the OR would be and it's credible region. For our data, the predictive value of the OR is 1.227 with a credible region of (0.762, 1.761) indicating some evidence in favor of no treatment effect.

The Bayesian analysis is very attractive in that one can incorporate prior information into the meta-analysis and update this information with the new sample data from studies gathered. Also, should more articles addressing a similar question be published in the future, one can then use the posterior distribution from the present meta-analysis as the new prior distribution for the next meta-analysis. For example from Table 2.4, the new prior density region for the OR for the next meta-analysis could be in the range of 0.972–1.41. There are no statistical multiplicity issues involved in terms of p-value adjustment for repeated significance testing since there are no p-values to consider. The major criticism of the Bayesian approach is that one has to specify a prior distribution and that it may be too subjective. Such need not be the case as one can always use previous data from previous studies or the literature to empirically construct a prior distribution.

2.2 Discussion

There are many advantages to doing a meta-analysis. They include, but are not limited to the following:

1. One is able to detect small but clinically relevant effects of an intervention.
2. Considering the heterogeneous nature of subjects across studies, the more diverse groups of subjects across studies hopefully permits a more global solution to a question or hypothesis. The conclusion has the potential advantage of being based on most, if not all, existing evidence from relevant studies.
3. One can avoid the time and expense of doing a larger confirmatory study if the evidence from many studies is available, properly handled statistically, and the meta-analysis provides a sufficiently conclusive result.
4. Although most meta-analyses are done from published results, the more powerful results are garnered from actual subject data. However, for many studies the data are too old, too expensive to retrieve, or cannot be retrieved. A meta-analysis of aggregate data may be all that is possible.
5. The statistical tools are such that most sources of bias and heterogeneity can be statistically examined. Sensitivity of statistically significant results can be measured.
6. The statistical techniques to analyze results from meta-analyses are generally not new and many standard techniques apply.
7. The resources to help accomplish a systematic review of studies to be included in the meta-analysis are available.
8. The statistical software to perform meta-analyses are available, but should not be used without appropriate understanding of the underlying methods and limitations.

Some of the more prominent issues facing meta-analyses include:

1. The assumption that the evaluation techniques are consistent across studies.

2. It still may be difficult to locate all the articles necessary for a meta-analysis or data sources, although resources are available. This can still lead to the "file-drawer" effect.
3. Some statistics such as ESs for continuous data may be biased and must be adjusted accordingly.
4. Inconsistent coding of variables across studies limiting their utilization for detecting heterogeneity.
5. Although one can detect the presence and severity of heterogeneity, the exact sources of heterogeneity may not be detectable from the literature even with meta-regression.
6. Because the study is the unit of analysis, the adequacy of statistical power of any meta-analysis may be in question.
7. Unless the data is available and consistent across studies, detection of interaction and trends can be difficult.
8. When combining studies for analysis, appropriate weights and scoring must be considered.
9. The underlying statistical assumptions of meta-regression and random effects are sometimes ignored and must be validated.
10. Although the Bayesian approach involves a broader inclusion of prior knowledge to a meta-analysis, some are reluctant to specify a prior distribution unless it can be empirically justified.
11. The statistical computations of the Bayesian approach are complex and should be performed by those experienced in that skill.

All of these latter issues are addressed statistically and certainly do not preclude one performing meta-analyses. One should certainly be aware of these issues. The attempt has been made here to demonstrate most of the strengths and limitations of meta-analyses by way of definition and application.

2.2.1 Conclusion and Resources

Meta-analysis is controversial. However, every attempt is made to guard against bias through proper systematic review, examination of heterogeneity, and publication bias. Heterogeneity should be exposed, explored, and explained if feasible. Limitations obviously result from selection of studies, choice of relevant outcome, methods of analysis, interpretation of heterogeneity, and generalization and application of results. Typically, the statistical tools at hand are certainly adequate for addressing these issues. There are good online sources which provide guidelines for conducting a meta-analysis. These include CONSORT, QUORUM, and MOOSE. These can be entered as key words to locate the resource. The Cochrane Collaborative mentioned above in section 1.0 provides excellent guidelines as well. A good source for arranging onsite training for nonstatistically oriented investigators with an overview for understanding and conducting meta-analyses can be found by contacting QuantitativeAppl@aol.com. However, one should keep in mind that meta-analyses should neither be a replacement for well-designed large-scale randomized studies [2] nor a justification for conducting small underpowered studies. It is a tool which, when properly utilized, helps one to arrive at a reasonable and defensible decision from the scientific information already presented.

References

1. Baldessarini RJ, Hegarty JD, Bird ED, Benes FM (1997) Meta-analysis of postmortem studies of Alzheimer's disease-like neuropathology in schizophrenia. Am J Psychiatry 154:861–863
2. Bartolucci AA (1999) The significance of clinical trials and the role of meta-analysis. J Surg Oncol 72(3):121–123
3. Bartolucci AA, Howard G (2006) Meta-analysis of data from the six primary prevention trials of cardiovascular events using aspirin. Am J Cardiol 10:746–750
4. Carlin JB (1992) Meta-analysis for 2 × 2 tables: a Bayesian approach. Stat Med 11:141–58
5. Chalmers TC, Smith H Jr, Blackburn B, Silverman B, Schroeder B, Reitman D, Ambroz A (1981) A method for assessing the quality of a randomized clinical trial. Control Clin Trials 2:31–49
6. DerSimonian R, Laird N (1986) Meta-analysis in clinical trials. Control Clin Trials 7:177–188
7. Early Breast Cancer Trialists Collaborative Group (1988) Effects of adjuvant tamoxifen and cytotoxic therapy on mortality in early breast cancer: an overview of 61 trials in 28, 896 women. N Eng J Med 319:1681–1692
8. Egger M, Davey G, Schneider M, Minder C (1997) Bias in meta-analysis detected by a simple graphical test. BMJ 315:629–634
9. Egger M, Davey Smith G, Altman D (eds) (2001) Systematic Reviews in Health Care: Meta-Analysis in Context. 2nd edition. London, British Medical Journal 323:101–105
10. Fisher RA (1932) Statistical methods for research workers, 4th edition. Oliver and Boyd, London
11. Glass R (1976) Primary, secondary, and meta-analysis of research. Edu Res 5:3–8
12. Hedges LV, Olkin O (1985) Statistical methods for meta-analysis. Chapter 6, pp 107–118 Academic Press, San Diego
13. Higgins JPT, Thompson SG (2002) Quantifying heterogeneity in meta-analysis. Stat Med 21:1539–1558
14. Jadad AR, Moor RA, Carroll D, Jenkinson C, Reynolds DJM, Gavaghan DJ, McQuay HJ (1996) Assessing the quality of reports of randomized clinical trials: is blinding necessary? Control Clin Trials 17(1):1–12
15. Morton SC, Adams JL, Suttorp MJ, Shekelle PG (2004) Meta-regression Approaches: What, Why, When, and How? Technical Review 8 (Prepared by Southern California–RAND Evidence-based Practice Center, under Contract No 290-97-0001). AHRQ Publication No. 04-0033. Rockville, MD: Agency for Healthcare Research and Quality
16. Pearson K (1904) Report on certain enteric fever inoculation statistics. BMJ 3:1243–1246
17. Peto R (1986) Five years of Tamoxifen, or more? National Cancer Inst 88(24):1791–1793
18. Poole C, Greenland S (1999) Random-effects meta-analysis are not always conservative. Am J Epidemiol 150(5): 469–475
19. Riley RD, Lambert PC, Staessen JA, Wang J, Gueyffier F, Thijs L, Boutitie F (2007) Meta-analysis of continuous outcomes combining individual patient data and aggregate data. Stat Med 27:1870–1893
20. Spiegelhalter D, Thomas A, Best N, Lunn D (2003) WinBugs User Manual. Version 1.4, Cambridge, UK. http://www.mrc-bsu.cam.ac.uk/bugs
21. Thompson SG, Higgins JPT (2002) How should meta-regression analyses be undertaken and interpreted? Stat Med 21:1559–1573
22. Tippett LHC (1931) The method of statistics. Williams and Norgate, London
23. Williamson PR, Smith CT, Hutton JL, Marson AG (2002) Aggregate meta analysis with time to event outcomes. 2002. Stat Med 21(22):3337–3351

Understanding and Interpreting Systematic Review and Meta-Analysis Results

3

Cristiano Susin, Alex Nogueira Haas, and Cassiano Kuchenbecker Rösing

Core Message

> Here, we provide an overview of the methods used to combine the results of several studies. Specifically, we discuss the application and interpretation of meta-analytic methods.

3.1 Introduction

Systematic reviews and meta-analysis have become the *de facto* gold standard in evidence-based health care. Nevertheless, most health care providers do not have a clear understanding of how systematic reviews and meta-analyses are conducted and how to interpret their results. This fact greatly hinders the application and dissemination of evidence that could have an important impact on the population health. Frequently,

evidence from systematic reviews reaches mainstream health care only when they are adopted or endorsed by professional associations/societies and governmental bodies. In an evidence-based era, it is interesting to note that some of the journals with higher impact in medicine and dentistry are still based on narrative reviews written by invited authorities. This underlines the fact that most health care providers have trouble understanding one of the most important sources of evidence. In this context, the aim of the present chapter is to provide an overview of the methods used to combine the results of several studies. We will focus on the application and interpretation of meta-analytic methods.

First, we would like to acknowledge that systematic reviews and meta-analyses are not easy topics for most readers. This is especially true for health care providers who focused most of their efforts on learning biology-related subjects instead of mathematical concepts. As a consequence, most researchers do not like statistics-related topics, most professionals do not use it in their appraisal of the medical literature, and majority of the students are not willing to learn it. This is an unfortunate truth with known causes and consequences. Our approach to try to explain these concepts will be as intuitive as possible and we will try to avoid the classic mathematical approach whenever possible.

It is beyond the scope of this chapter to review all steps of a systematic review. Thus, we will assume that the necessary steps to carry out a systematic review have been fulfilled (identification of the need for the review, preparation of a review protocol, identification and selection of the studies, quality assessment and data collection, etc.), and we will focus on the analysis and presentation of the results.

C. Susin (✉)
Laboratory for Applied Periodontal and Craniofacial Regeneration, Department of Periodontics and Oral Biology, Medical College of Georgia School of Dentistry, 1459, Laney Walker Blrd, Augusta, GA 30912, USA
e-mail: csusin@mcg.edu/csusin@me.com

A.N Haas
C.K Rösing
School of Dentistry, Federal University of Rio Grande do Sul, Rua Ramiro Barcelos, 2492, 90035-003, Porto Alegre, RS, Brazil
e-mail: alexnhaas@gmail.com
e-mail: ckrosing@hotmail.com

F. Chiappelli et al. (eds.), *Evidence-Based Practice: Toward Optimizing Clinical Outcomes*,
DOI: 10.1007/978-3-642-05025-1_3, © Springer-Verlag Berlin Heidelberg 2010

3.1.1 Example: Studies Characteristics and Descriptive Results

To illustrate this chapter, let us imagine that we are conducting a systematic review about the effect of a new antiviral therapy for recurrent herpes labialis. For simplicity, our main outcome will be reduction in the number of days with pain, i.e., a continuous outcome. Also for simplicity, let us assume that all studies used placebo as the control group.

Most systematic reviews use tables to present the methodological characteristics and outcomes of the selected studies. For example, the success of secondary root canal treatment was investigated in a systematic review published by Ng et al. [7]. The search strategy identified 40 studies, of which 17 were included in the analyses. Table 3.1 describes the methodological characteristics and outcomes of the 17 included studies. The methodological characteristics of the studies facilitate the reader interpretation of the meta-analysis results. Other study characteristics frequently reported are sample characteristics, randomization method, blindness of patients, therapists and examiner, follow-up time, and dropout rate.

In addition to the methodological characteristics, most systematic reviews present the original results in descriptive forms using tables and graphs. Table 3.2 combines study characteristics and results for our systematic review describing 12 studies that tested the effect of our new antiviral therapy. The table presents the year of publication, total sample size, source of funding, sample size in each experimental group (n), estimate of the intervention effect (mean), an estimate of the intervention variability (standard deviation – SD), and the p-value.

The overall trend of the studies is used to suggest if a given intervention is better than the standard treatment or no intervention when only descriptive tables are used to present results. This approach is very intuitive and does not need any statistical expertise to be conducted. However, as you will later see in this chapter, it can be misleading for several reasons. An overall assessment of Table 3.2 indicates that between 1997 and 2002, mostly small studies were conducted, with large studies being published only in the last 4 years. This finding is consistent with most new therapy studies since large, costly, time-consuming studies are only conducted after some evidence of positive effect and safety is available. A closer look at the results of the studies shows that within small studies the results are very inconsistent, with few studies showing large positive or negative effects for the therapy when compared to placebo. In contrast, large studies do not show major differences between experimental groups. As expected, variability is larger in smaller studies due to the sample size effect on standard deviation estimates. Only the first two studies reached statistical significance, and in three other studies somewhat borderline results were found ($p \sim 0.10$).

3.2 Main Results: Overall Estimates of Effect

The treatment effect could be estimated by calculating an overall mean of the results simply by summing up the individual results dividing by the number of studies. This approach, although very intuitive, would not take into consideration the studies characteristics, with studies contributing equally to the overall estimate. Looking at the estimates in Table 3.2, it is obvious that some studies have more precise estimates than others. Factors that may affect the precision of the estimates are various, including sample characteristics, sample size, measurement precision, and reliability. In the meta-analysis framework, sample size is often the most important factor to be taken into consideration. Thus, overall estimates should take into account the sample size with larger studies contributing more than small studies. Mathematically, this can be accomplished by multiplying each study estimate by the sample size or, in other words, by weighting the estimates according to sample size. The sum of the estimates can then be divided by the total sample size. Table 3.3 shows the weight of each study of our example according to sample size. Using this approach, the mean reduction in days with pain would be 2.8 days for the treatment group and 3.1 days for the control group. Thus, the placebo treatment reduced in approximately 0.3 days patients' symptoms.

In essence, this is what is done in a meta-analysis to take into consideration the contribution of each study. A similar strategy can be used to account not only for the sample size, but also for the variability in the estimates of the original studies. The overall weighted estimate is calculated multiplying each study estimate by the inverse of the square of the standard error (inverse-variance weighting method), which is highly associated with the sample size of the study. Using this

Table 3.1 Methodological characteristics and outcomes of included studies by Ng et al. [7]

Study authors	Operator	Design	Recall rate (%)	Sample size	Unit of measure	Assessment of success	Radiographic criteria success	≥4 years after treatment	Calibration	Reliability test	Statistical analysis
Grahnen	UG	R	64	502	Ro	C&R	S	✓	–	–	–
Engstrom	UG	R	72	153	T	C&R	L	✓	–	–	X^2
Selden	Sp	R	20	52	T	C&R	L	–	–	–	X^2
Bergneholtz	UG	R	66	556	Ro	C&R	S	–	–	✓	–
Pekruhn	Sp	R	81	36	T	C&R	S	–	–	–	X^2
Molven	UG	R	50	226	Ro	Ra	S	✓	✓	✓	X^2
Allen	–	R	53	315	T	C&R	S	–	✓	–	X^2
Sjogren	UG	R	46	267	Ro	C&R	S	✓	✓	✓	LR
Van Nieuwenhuysen	–	R	–	612	Ro	C&R	S	–	✓	✓	X^2
Friedman	Sp	C	78	128	T	C&R	S	–	–	–	X^2
Danin	Sp	RCT	100	18	T	Ra	L	–	✓	✓	X^2
Sundqvist	UG	C	93	50	T	C&R	S	✓	–	–	X^2
Chugal	PG	R	75	85	Ro	Ra	S	✓	–	–	LR
Hoskinson	Sp	R	78	76	Ro	C&R	S	✓	✓	✓	GEE
Farzaneh	Sp	C	22	103	T	C&R	S	–	✓	✓	LR
Gorni	PG	C	94	452	T	C&R	S	✓	✓	✓	M–W
Çaliskan	Sp	R	96	86	T	C&R	S	–	✓	✓	X^2

"–" missing information; *UG* undergraduate students; *PG* postgraduate students; *Sp* specialist endodontists; *R* retrospective study; *C* prospective cohort study; *RCT* randomized controlled trial; *T* teeth; *Ro* root; *C&R* combined clinical and radiographic examination; *Ra* radiographic examination only; *S* strict criteria; *L* loose criteria; *LR* single level logistic regression; *GEE* generalized estimating equations; *X²* chi-square test; *M-W* Mann–whitney U-test

Table 3.2 Description of study characteristics and original results

Year of publication	Sample size	Source of funding	Treatment			Control			*p*-value
			n	Mean	SD	*n*	Mean	SD	
1997	42	Private	21	2.0	1.7	21	3.9	2.1	0.003
1998	31	Private	16	1.8	2.4	15	3.8	2.7	0.04
1998	44	Private	22	2.1	2.6	22	3.5	2.8	0.09
1999	33	Public	18	3.3	2.7	15	1.8	2.4	0.11
2001	30	Private	14	3	3.2	16	2.1	2.9	0.43
2001	29	Private	13	2.1	2.9	16	3.2	3.2	0.35
2002	27	Public	13	2.9	2.9	14	2.5	2.5	0.70
2002	31	Private	15	2.5	2.5	16	3	2.9	0.61
2005	190	Public	96	2.9	2.1	94	3.1	2.5	0.55
2007	80	Public	39	3.5	2.6	41	3.1	2.2	0.46
2007	145	Public	73	3.2	2.4	72	2.9	1.9	0.41
2008	394	Public	198	2.8	1.7	196	3.1	1.8	0.09

Table 3.3 Study weights according to sample size and inverse-variance methods

Year of publication	Weight based on sample size (%)	Weight based on inverse-variance method (%)
1997	3.9	4.6
1998	2.9	1.9
1998	4.1	2.4
1999	3.1	2.0
2001	2.8	1.3
2001	2.7	1.2
2002	2.5	1.5
2002	2.9	1.7
2005	17.7	14.2
2007	7.4	5.5
2007	13.5	12.4
2008	36.6	51.3
Total	100	100

the greatest precision (smaller standard deviations and confidence intervals). Studies with lower variability receive greater weight and therefore have greater influence in the estimate.

Tables and graphs are popular ways of presenting the results of a meta-analysis. Table 3.4 presents the WMD and the 95% confidence interval for each study. The weighted mean provides an estimate and direction of the effect, and the confidence interval provides an assessment of the variability of the estimates. Confidence intervals also indicate the significance of the results and when it does not include zero (or 1 when the results are presented in odds ratio), the weighted mean is statistically significant.

3.3 Forest Plots

Figure 3.1 is a Forest plot of the results and has essentially the same information presented in Table 3.4. Studies are identified by their year of publication and sample size on the left side of the graph. The WMDs are presented in a graphical form with point estimates being presented as dots or short vertical lines and confidence intervals as horizontal lines. The size of the plotting symbol for the estimate is proportional to the weight of each study in the meta-analysis. The actual estimates are also presented on the right side together with the weight of the study. The overall estimate and

approach, the weighted mean difference (WMD) between treatments is 0.26 mm in favor of the new antiviral therapy. Table 3.3 also shows the weight attributed to each study according to the inverse-variance method. It is clear that the study published in 2008 dominates the overall estimate not only because it has the largest sample size, but also because it has

Table 3.4 Meta-analysis result using the inverse-variance method

Year	Sample size	Weighted mean difference	95% CI		Weight (%)
			Lower	Upper	
1997	42	−1.9	−3.056	−0.744	4.6
1998	31	−2	−3.803	−0.197	1.89
1999	44	−1.4	−2.997	0.197	2.41
1998	33	1.5	−0.241	3.241	2.03
2001	30	0.9	−1.297	3.097	1.27
2001	29	−1.1	−3.323	1.123	1.24
2002	27	0.4	−1.649	2.449	1.46
2002	31	−0.5	−2.403	1.403	1.7
2005	190	−0.2	−0.857	0.457	14.21
2008	80	0.4	−0.658	1.458	5.48
2006	145	0.3	−0.404	1.004	12.38
2007	394	−0.3	−0.646	0.046	51.33
Pooled weighted mean difference		−0.257	−0.504	−0.009	100
Significance test of weighted mean difference$=0$		$p=0.042$			

confidence interval are marked by a diamond. A dotted vertical line is used to present the overall estimate.

Since Table 3.4 and Fig. 3.1 have the same information, most publications present only the Forest plot. Looking at Fig. 3.1, it is easier to observe that the first two studies had a significant large effect in favor of the new therapy since both estimates are on the left side and the confidence interval does not include zero. No clear tendency is seen in the next six studies with half of them favoring therapy and the other half favoring control. It is important to note that the confidence intervals include zero for all studies. The overall WMD estimate is clearly dominated by the last study.

The last information in Fig. 3.1 is the I-square (I^2) statistic. The I^2 statistic represents the percentage of heterogeneity that can be attributed to variability between studies. The I^2 statistic varies between 0 and 100% and can be interpreted as follows: low heterogeneity for <50%, moderate heterogeneity for ≥50−<75%, and high heterogeneity for ≥75%. In this example, the I^2 statistic is approximately 53%, which indicates moderate heterogeneity. This finding can be explained by the inconsistent results of the small studies published between 1997 and 2002. The I^2 statistic is statistically significant with a p-value of 0.016, further indicating that there is heterogeneity in the results. The only

information that the Forest plot does not present is the p-value for the overall estimate ($p=0.042$).

3.4 Exploring Heterogeneity

To further explore heterogeneity, let us try to look into the sample size effect. We stratified the studies into small and large sample sizes. Figure 3.2 presents the Forest plot with estimates for each stratum. Small studies showed a significant effect in favor of the therapy with antiviral treatment reducing the number of days in pain in 0.8 days ($p=0.01$). In contrast, no significant effect was observed in large studies since the confidence interval includes zero ($p=0.29$). An overall test for heterogeneity between small and large studies is significant ($p=0.05$). It is interesting to notice that the I^2 statistic for the small sample size shows moderate heterogeneity (56.8%, $p=0.02$) indicating that other factors may further explain these results. We will address this finding later on.

Let us try to explore the heterogeneity of the data even more. Figure 3.3 is the Forest plot using a fixed-effect model stratified by funding source: public or private. For public-funded studies, the WMD is 0.10

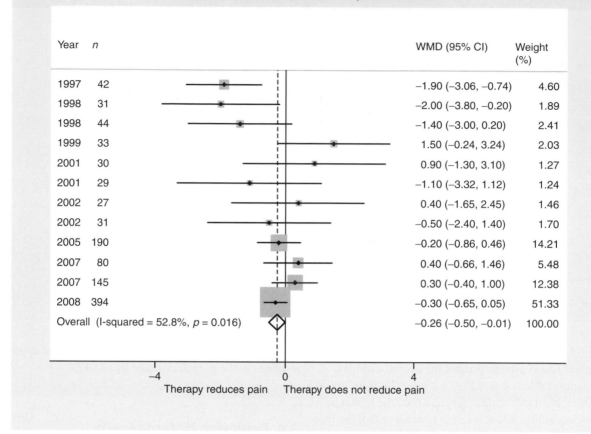

Fig. 3.1 Forest plot showing effect estimates and confidence intervals for individual studies and meta-analysis (fixed-effect model)

($p=0.46$, not reported in the Forest plot) in favor of the antiviral therapy, whereas for private-funded studies the antiviral therapy reduces pain, in average, in 1.29 days ($p<0.001$, not reported in the Forest plot). The heterogeneity test between groups is highly significant, also indicating that funding is an important source of variability.

3.5 Fixed-Effects vs. Random-Effects

So far we have found two possible sources of heterogeneity indicating that these studies may have different characteristics. We have used what is called a fixed-effect model to combine studies in a meta-analysis. When heterogeneity between studies exists, a different approach called random-effects model should be used. The fixed-effect model assumes that the meta-analysis

overall estimate represents the same underlying effect and that differences between studies are due to sampling error, i.e., individual studies have the same single effect. The random-effects model includes an estimate of between-study variability assuming that the meta-analysis overall estimate is the mean effect around which individual studies have a normal distribution. In other words, random-effects models assume that the intervention is not the only explanation for the overall estimate allowing for other factors (such as study design, sample characteristics, and treatment differences) to partly explain the results.

In practice, random-effects models yield more conservative estimates with lower p-values and larger confidence intervals than fixed-effect models. Disparities in the overall WMD between treatments can also be seen due to the fact that random-effects models give greater weight to smaller studies than fixed-effect

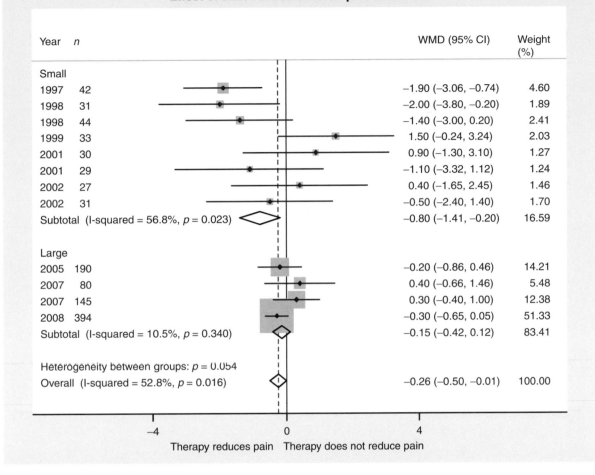

Fig. 3.2 Forest plot showing effect estimates and confidence intervals for individual studies and meta-analysis stratified by study sample size (fixed-effect model)

models (Table 3.5). As can be seen in Fig. 3.4, the overall WMD using the random-effects model is slightly different than the estimate using the fixed-effect model (0.30 vs. 0.26). However, the major difference can be seen in the confidence interval that now includes zero, and therefore, is associated with a non-significant p-value ($p=0.22$). In other words, when the heterogeneity is taken into consideration in the calculation of the estimates, no overall significant differences were observed between treatments with regard to pain reduction. This is in contrast to the conclusion that could be drawn from the fixed-effect model.

Sometimes researchers present the Forest plot of the fixed-effect model and include the random-effects estimate for comparison (Fig. 3.5). This may be confusing

for the inexperienced reader because different models may have opposite results. As a rule of thumb, if the I^2 statistic is moderate or high (>50%) and the p-value is significant ($p<0.05$), a random-effects model should be used. In our example, a random-effects model is warranted.

3.6 Meta-Regression

Stratified analysis is an important tool for detecting heterogeneity, but has the same drawbacks of subgroup analysis in clinical trials. A better approach to evaluate between-group difference is to use a meta-regression

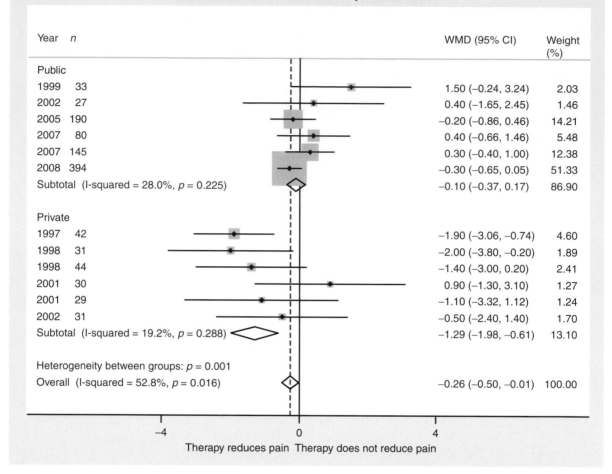

Fig. 3.3 Forest plot showing effect estimates and confidence intervals for individual studies and meta-analysis stratified by source of funding (fixed-effect model)

or meta-analysis regression. For those familiar with regression analysis, a meta-regression could be thought as a regression analysis performed at the study-level, i.e., using study-level data instead of individual-level data. Table 3.6 shows the result of the random-effects meta-regression using sample size and source of funding as explanatory variables. As observed before in the stratified analysis, both factors were significant sources of heterogeneity and funding seems to have the biggest impact on the effect estimates.

Similarly, Pavia et al. [8] conducted a meta-analysis of observational studies about the contribution of fruit and vegetable intakes to the occurrence of oral cancer. They included 16 studies and found that each portion of fruit consumed per day significantly reduced the

risk of oral cancer by 49% (pooled odds ratio 0.51 95%CI 0.40–0.65). They found a significant heterogeneity across studies. To additionally explore heterogeneity, a meta-regression analysis was performed. This meta-regression analysis examined the effect of certain variables, such as quality score, type of cancers included, citrus fruit and green vegetable consumption, population studied (men, women, or both), and time interval for dietary recall, on the role of fruit or vegetable consumption in the risk of oral cancer. Table 3.7 shows the results for the meta-regression analysis, demonstrating that the lower risk of oral cancer associated with fruit consumption was significantly influenced by the type of fruit consumed and by the time interval of dietary recall.

Table 3.5 Study weights according to fixed- and random-effects methods

Year of publication	Fixed-effect model (%)	Random-effects model
1997	4.6	9.24
1998	1.9	5.16
1998	2.4	6.15
1999	2.0	5.43
2001	1.3	3.78
2001	1.2	3.71
2002	1.5	4.23
2002	1.7	4.75
2005	14.2	14.73
2007	5.5	10.14
2007	12.4	14.13
2008	51.3	18.54

3.7   Funnel Plots and Publication Bias

Another important issue in meta-analysis is publication bias. Publication bias arises from the fact that studies with statistically significant results are more likely to be reported by authors and accepted for publication. Consequently, there is a risk that meta-analysis estimates are positively biased. It should be remembered that some publication bias might be diminished during the search strategy, looking for grey literature (unpublished data). Graphical and statistical methods have been developed to assist in the identification of publication bias. The Funnel plot is the most commonly used graphic to investigate bias in meta-analysis. Funnel plots are scatterplots of each study treatment effect (i.e., WMD) by a measure of the study precision (i.e., standard error of the treatment effect). Figure 3.6 shows the Funnel plot of the present data. The WMD is plotted in the horizontal axis (x-axis) and the standard error

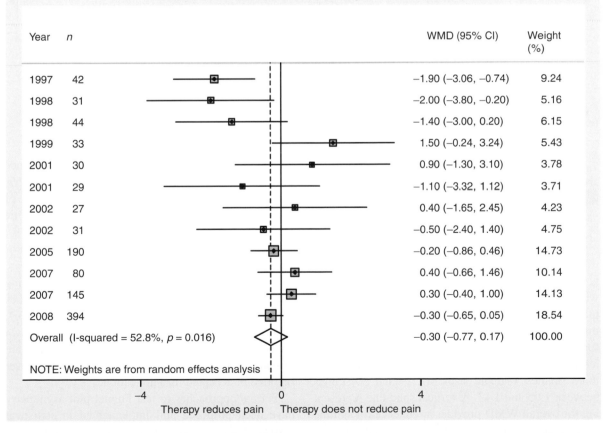

Fig. 3.4 Forest plot showing effect estimates and confidence intervals for individual studies and meta-analysis stratified using a random-effects model

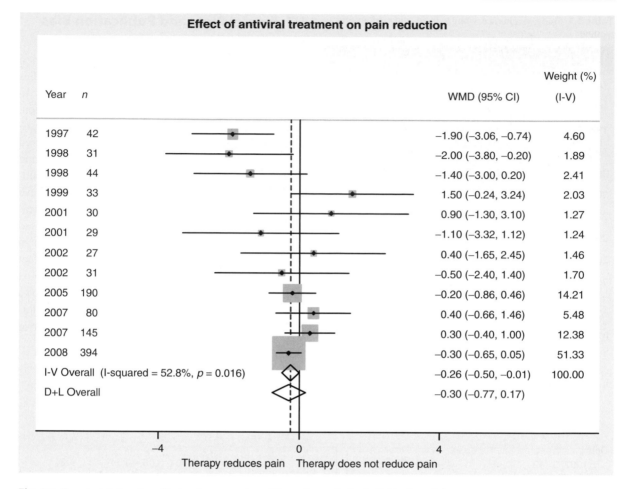

Fig. 3.5 Forest plot showing effect estimates and confidence intervals for individual studies and meta-analysis stratified using a fixed-effect and random-effects model

Table 3.6 Meta-regression analysis using study sample size and source of funding as explanatory variables

Variable	Coefficient	SE	p-value
Sample size	−0.66	0.28	0.04
Funding	−2.06	0.52	0.003

is plotted in the vertical axis (y-axis). Larger studies will often concentrate in the upper part of the Funnel plot because their standard error is generally smaller than smaller studies. For instance, the standard error for the three largest studies (sample sizes: 145, 190 and 394) ranged between 0.18 and 0.36, whereas that for three smallest (sample sizes: 27, 29 and 30) ranged between 1.05 and 1.13. A vertical solid line representing the overall WMD provides a reference for symmetry. A similar number of studies should be on both sides of this line. In our example, the same number of studies

is plotted on the left and right sides of this reference line. The two doted diagonal lines represent the 95% confidence limits for the Funnel plot. In the absence of bias and heterogeneity, 95% of the studies should lie within the confidence limits lines. Two out of 12 (17%) studies are outside the confidence limits, further providing evidence of heterogeneity and perhaps bias.

A clear example of asymmetric Funnel plot using our data could be created by removing four studies with effects favoring the control treatment. In Fig. 3.7, it can be easily seen that small studies (generally shown on the bottom part of the plot) with negative results are missing, which may indicate that they were never reported or accepted for publication.

Formal approaches to test Funnel plot asymmetry have been proposed and implemented in statistical softwares. The Egger test uses a linear regression to draw a straight-line relationship between the WMD

Table 3.7 Meta-regression conducted by Pavia et al. [8]

Variable	Regression coefficient	SE	p
Fruit			
Only citrus fruit (no=0; yes=1)	−1.53	0.56	0.006
Dietary recall (lifelong= 0, 2 years=1, 1 year=2)	0.63	0.3	0.04
Population studied			
Men and women=0	0	–	–
Only women=1	−1.06	1.07	0.33
Only men=2	0.01	0.56	0.99
Study quality score (low=0, high=1)	−0.32	0.54	0.56
Vegetables			
Only green vegetables	−0.23	0.43	0.59
Dietary recall (lifelong=0, 2 years=1, 1 year=2)	−0.03	0.21	0.88
Population studied			
Men and women−0	0	–	–
Only women=1	1.14	0.73	0.12
Only men=2	0.25	0.64	0.69
Study quality score (low=0, high=1)	0.23	0.47	0.63

and standard errors. When this regression line is plotted in the Funnel plot, it will appear as a vertical line as can be seen in Fig. 3.8. If asymmetry is present, the regression line will be plotted away from the vertical and the slope of the line will indicate the direction of bias (Fig. 3.9). The Egger's bias coefficient provides a measure of the asymmetry. The Egger's bias coefficient and its p-value for Fig. 3.7 are small (coefficient: −0.18, SE: 0.75, $p=0.81$), indicating small chance of bias. On the other hand, the bias coefficient for Fig. 3.8 is larger with a p-value approaching significance (coefficient: −1.42, SE: 0.81, $p=0.13$), indicating some evidence of bias. A negative bias coefficient indicates that the effect estimated from the smaller studies is smaller than the effect estimated from the larger studies. This may be interpreted as evidence that small sample size studies with nonsignificant results were not included in the meta-analysis. In general, bias tests for Funnel plots have lower power; thus, lower p-values should be carefully considered especially when less than ten studies are included in the analysis.

Even though we have focused on publication bias, Funnel plot asymmetry can be explained by other reasons such as poor study quality, true study heterogeneity, and chance. As discussed before, study quality can be addressed during study selection, and quality assessment and heterogeneity can be evaluated by stratified analysis and meta-regression.

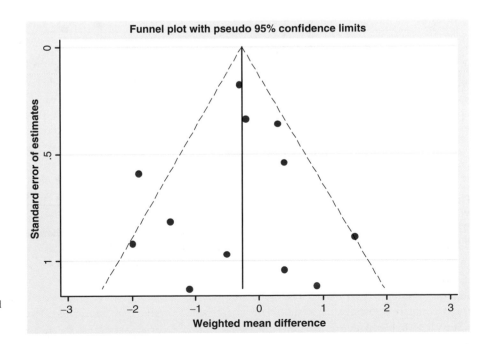

Fig. 3.6 Funnel plot of the weighted mean difference (WMD) against its standard error showing a symmetric distribution of studies

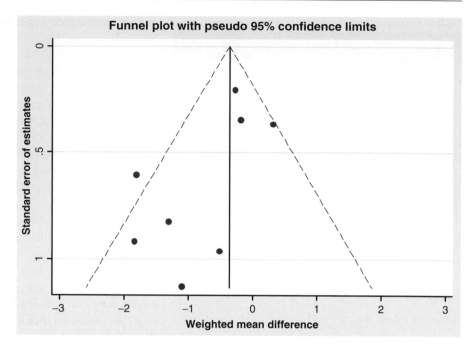

Fig. 3.7 Funnel plot of the WMD against its standard error showing an asymmetric distribution of studies (four studies with effects favoring the control treatment were removed)

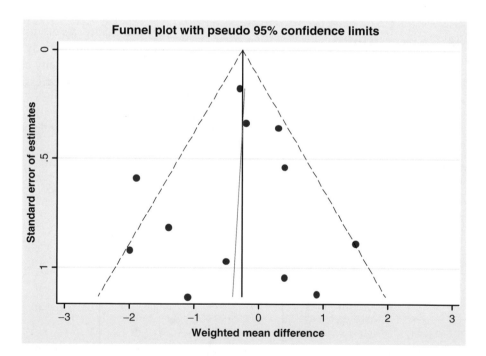

Fig. 3.8 Funnel plot of the WMD against its standard error and Egger regression line

Fig. 3.9 Funnel plot of the WMD against its standard error and Egger regression line. (four studies with effects favoring the control treatment were removed)

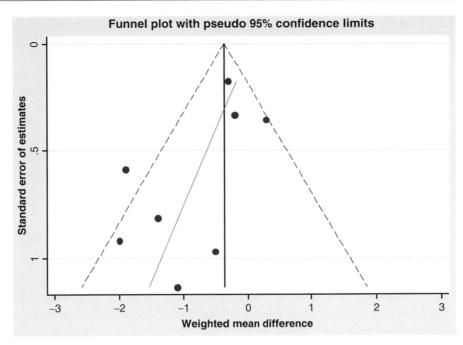

3.8 Exploring Influential Studies

Sometimes a single study has a great impact in the estimates. Table 3.8 shows the WMD and 95% confidence intervals for the meta-analysis when one study is omitted at a time. Among the studies that showed large positive effect for the antiviral therapy, the first study published in 1997 has the greatest impact in the WMD. Omitting this study from the meta-analysis would change the WMD from −0.26 days to −0.18 days. A similar but contrary effect would be observed if the 2006 study was omitted. In this case, the WMD would change from −0.26 days to −0.34 days. The impact of a single study in the overall estimate is dependent upon the effect size and sample size. The study with largest influence on the confidence intervals (i.e., precision of the estimate) is the study published in 2007 due to its large sample size. The exclusion of this study would widen the confidence interval in approximately 40%. The search for very influential studies should be done with caution and more attention should be paid to influential small studies.

Table 3.8 Meta-analysis results after omitting one study at a time

Omitted study		Weighted mean difference	95% CI	
Year	Sample size		Lower	Upper
1997	42	−0.18	−0.43	0.08
1998	31	−0.22	−0.47	0.03
1999	44	−0.23	−0.48	0.02
1998	33	−0.29	−0.54	−0.04
2001	30	−0.27	−0.52	−0.02
2001	29	−0.25	−0.50	0.00
2002	27	−0.27	−0.52	−0.02
2002	31	−0.25	−0.50	0.00
2005	190	−0.27	−0.53	0.00
2008	80	−0.29	−0.55	−0.04
2006	145	−0.34	−0.60	−0.07
2007	394	−0.21	−0.57	0.14
Pooled weighted mean difference when all studies are included		−0.26	−0.50	−0.01

3.9 The Cochrane Collaboration Forest Plot

We have used Stata [9] to perform this meta-analysis due to personal preferences, but there are other software and statistical packages that can be used with minor differences in the results. The Cochrane Collaboration has the software Review Manager [5] for preparing systematic reviews and meta-analysis. The Forest plot generated by this software is presented in Fig. 3.10, which is very similar to Fig. 3.1.

3.10 Standardized Mean Differences

We have focused in this chapter on WMDs because it is more intuitive and easy to understand. With respect to continuous outcomes, the standardized mean difference can be used instead of the WMD. The standardized mean difference can be used when studies have measured the outcomes in different units. However, standardized mean differences are usually difficult to interpret because these measures are not directly related to everyday outcomes. In this case, the reader should look for the interpretation given to the results by the authors. Usually, standardized mean differences can be presented as the proportion of patients benefiting from the intervention, or a measure of the minimal important difference can be provided to assist the reader. As a rule of thumb, standardized mean differences ≥0.7 may be

considered large effects. For our data, the standard mean difference would be −0.11 (95% confidence interval: −0.23 to 0.01, $p=0.07$) using a fixed-effect model, and −0.12 (95% confidence interval: −0.32 to 0.08, $p=0.24$) using a random-effects model (Table 3.9). These results indicate a small effect of the antiviral therapy, but the interpretation of the results is difficult to translate in practical terms. Several methods to calculate the standardized mean difference have been proposed such as the Glass method, Cohen method, and Hedges method.

3.11 Dichotomous Outcomes

Similar meta-analysis methods can be used for dichotomous (odds ratios and risk ratios), ordinal (indices and scales), counts and rates (number of events), and time-to-event data (survival). We will briefly present below some differences with regard to dichotomous outcomes because they are frequently reported in the medical and dental fields. In addition to the inverse-variance method already discussed for continuous data, three other methods are available for meta-analysis of dichotomous outcomes: Mantel–Haenszel and Peto methods for fixed-effect models and DerSimonian and Laird method for random-effects models. The Mantel–Haenszel is frequently used for fixed-effect models and is the standard method for several statistical programs. The Forest plot is also used to present the results with minor differences. Odds ratios and risk

Study or Subgroup	Therapy Mean	SD	Total	Control Mean	SD	Total	Weight	Mean difference IV, Fixed, 95% CI	Mean difference IV, Fixed, 95% CI
1997 42	2	1.7	21	3.9	2.1	21	4.6%	−1.90 (−3.06, −0.74)	
1998 31	1.8	2.4	16	3.8	2.7	15	1.9%	−2.00 (−3.80, −0.20)	
1998 44	2.1	2.6	22	3.5	2.8	22	2.4%	−1.40 (−3.00, 0.20)	
1999 33	3.3	2.7	18	1.8	2.4	15	2.0%	1.50 (−0.24, 3.24)	
2001 29	2.1	2.9	13	3.2	3.2	16	1.2%	−1.10 (−3.32, 1.12)	
2001 30	3	3.2	14	2.1	2.9	16	1.3%	0.90 (−1.30, 3.10)	
2002 27	2.9	2.9	13	2.5	2.5	14	1.5%	0.40 (−1.65, 2.45)	
2002 31	2.5	2.5	15	3	2.9	16	1.7%	−0.50 (−2.40, 1.40)	
2005 190	2.9	2.1	96	3.1	2.5	94	14.2%	−0.20 (−0.86, 0.46)	
2007 145	3.2	2.4	73	2.9	1.9	72	12.4%	0.30 (−0.40, 1.00)	
2007 80	3.5	2.6	39	3.1	2.2	41	5.5%	0.40 (−0.66, 1.46)	
2008 394	2.8	1.7	198	3.1	1.8	196	51.3%	−0.30 (−0.65, 0.05)	
Total (95% CI)			**538**			**538**	**100.0%**	**−0.26 (−0.50, −0.01)**	

Heterogeneity: Chi² = 23.29, df = 11 ($p = 0.02$); $I^2 = 53\%$
Test for overall effect: Z = 2.03 ($p = 0.04$)

−4   −2   0   2   4
Favors experimental   Favors control

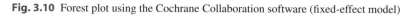

Fig. 3.10 Forest plot using the Cochrane Collaboration software (fixed-effect model)

Table 3.9 Meta-analysis results using the standardized mean difference instead of the weighted mean difference

| Year | Sample size | Standardized mean difference | 95% CI | | Weight (%) |
			Lower	Upper	
1997	42	−1.00	−1.64	−0.35	3.50
1998	31	−0.79	−1.52	−0.05	2.70
1999	44	−0.52	−1.12	0.08	4.00
1998	33	0.58	−0.12	1.28	2.95
2001	30	0.30	−0.43	1.02	2.78
2001	29	−0.36	−1.10	0.38	2.66
2002	27	0.15	−0.61	0.90	2.53
2002	31	−0.18	−0.89	0.52	2.90
2005	190	−0.09	−0.37	0.20	17.88
2008	80	0.17	−0.27	0.61	7.50
2006	145	0.14	−0.19	0.46	13.62
2007	394	−0.17	−0.37	0.03	36.97
Fixed-effect model		−0.11	−0.23	0.01	100.00
Random-effects model		−0.12	−0.32	0.08	100.00

ratios are frequently transformed using a natural log scale to facilitate analysis and presentation of the results (this transformation makes the scale symmetric). Thus, the horizontal axis of the Forest plot generally uses this scale, which may be misleading for the inexperienced reader. The same change in scale occurs for the Funnel plot. To test for Funnel plot symmetry in dichotomous data, Harbord et al., Peters et al., and Rücker et al. proposed alternative tests to the Egger test. Nevertheless, the same principles and interpretation of the results are still valid.

Needleman et al. [6] published a Cochrane review about guided tissue regeneration (GTR) for periodontal infra-bony defects compared to open flap debridement (control). The main outcome was clinical attachment gain that was dichotomized using a cut-off point of two sites gaining less than 2 mm of attachment. The Forest plot below was adapted from their study to illustrate an analysis of a dichotomous outcome with the Mantel–Haenszel method to pool the results across studies (Fig. 3.11). Results from 5 out of 6 studies favored GTR, but only one (the study by Tonnetti 1998) found a statistically significant difference compared to the control treatment. The meta-analysis demonstrated a final risk ratio of 0.54 indicating that the use of GTR

for periodontal infra-bony defects significantly reduces 46% the chance of having ≥2 sites gaining less than 2 mm. Additionally, it can be seen that they found some heterogeneity ($I^2=44\%$) and, consequently, a random-effects model was applied.

3.12 Concluding Remarks

Before concluding this chapter we would like to acknowledge that some of the concepts and statistics presented in this chapter have been simplified in order to improve understanding to a broader audience. Readers with greater statistical background or who are planning on conducting a meta-analysis are encouraged to look for more specialized information on this subject [1–5]. An updated list of books and websites is provided in the references. We also would like to acknowledge that the data sometimes violated some statistical assumptions. These minor violations were necessary in order to build an interesting dataset that could be used to show several important steps in meta-analysis.

Systematic reviews and meta-analyses are an integral part of evidence-based health care practice. In this

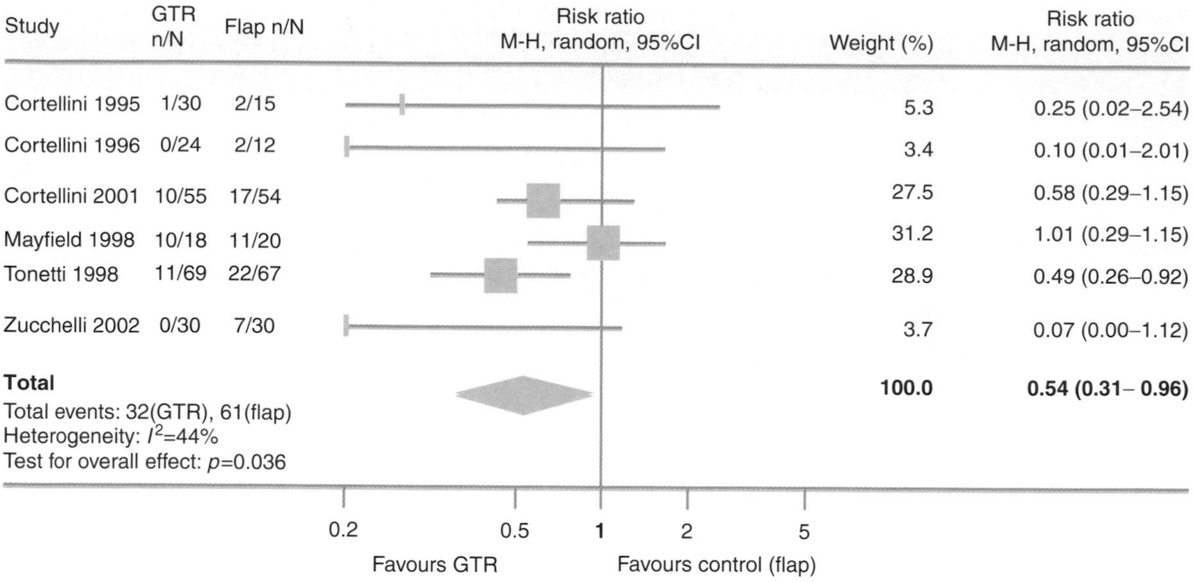

Study	GTR n/N	Flap n/N	Risk ratio M-H, random, 95%CI	Weight (%)	Risk ratio M-H, random, 95%CI
Cortellini 1995	1/30	2/15		5.3	0.25 (0.02–2.54)
Cortellini 1996	0/24	2/12		3.4	0.10 (0.01–2.01)
Cortellini 2001	10/55	17/54		27.5	0.58 (0.29–1.15)
Mayfield 1998	10/18	11/20		31.2	1.01 (0.29–1.15)
Tonetti 1998	11/69	22/67		28.9	0.49 (0.26–0.92)
Zucchelli 2002	0/30	7/30		3.7	0.07 (0.00–1.12)
Total				**100.0**	**0.54 (0.31– 0.96)**

Total events: 32(GTR), 61(flap)
Heterogeneity: I^2=44%
Test for overall effect: p=0.036

0.2   0.5   1   2   5

Favours GTR   Favours control (flap)

Fig. 3.11 Forest plot adapted from Needleman et al. [6]

context, we hope that this chapter will encourage more health care professionals to read and apply the evidence contained in systematic reviews and meta-analyses in their daily professional lives. Readers are also encouraged to remain updated since new developments over the years are likely to occur.

As a final message, we would like to call the reader's attention to the fact that we are approaching, at least in some areas of medicine and dentistry, a limit of how much information can be extracted from the current body of scientific evidence. Recent systematic reviews and meta-analyses have often been based in few studies of questionable quality yielding inconclusive results. Perhaps it is time to stop being creative with our systematic reviews and time to produce new and better evidence.

References

1. Borenstein M, Hedges LV, Higgins JPT, Rothstein HR (eds) (2009) Introduction to meta-analysis. Wiley, New York, 450pp
2. Centre for Reviews and Dissemination at University of York (2009) Systematic reviews – CRD's guidance for undertaking reviews in health care. Centre for reviews and dissemination: York Publishing Services Ltd, York, 3rd edn. 282pp
3. Egger M, Smith GD, Altman D (2001) Systematic reviews in health care: meta-analysis in context. BMJ Books, London, 512pp
4. Hartung J, Knapp G, Sinha BK (2008) Statistical meta-analysis with applications. Wiley, Hoboken, 248 pp
5. Higgins JPT, Green S (eds) (2008) Cochrane handbook for Systematic reviews of intervention. Wiley, Chichester, 672pp
6. Needleman I, Worthington Helen V, Giedrys-Leeper E, Tucker R (2009) Guided tissue regeneration for periodontal infra-bony defects (Cochrane Review). In: The Cochrane Library, Issue 1
7. Ng YL, Mann V, Gulabivala K (2008) Outcome of secondary root canal treatment: a systematic review of the literature. Int Endod J 41(12):1026–1046
8. Pavia M, Pileggi C, Nobile CG, Angelillo IF (2006) Association between fruit and vegetable consumption and oral cancer: a meta-analysis of observational studies. Am J Clin Nutr 83(5):1126–1134
9. Sterne J (ed) (2009) Meta-analysis: an updated collection from the Stata Journal. Stata Press, College Station, 259pp

Websites

The Cochrane Collaboration.http://www.cochrane.org/
The Cochrane Oral Health Group.http://www.ohg.cochrane.org/
The Centre for Reviews and Dissemination.http://www.york.ac.uk/inst/crd/index.htm
Comprehensive meta-analysis.http://www.meta-analysis.com/
The QUOROM statement (Quality of Reporting of Meta-analyses).http://www.consort-statement.org/
The GRADE working group (Grading of Recommendations Assessment, Development and Evaluation).http://www.gradeworkinggroup.org/

Making Evidence-Based Decisions in Nursing

4

Corazon B. Cajulis, Pauline S. Beam, and Susan M. Davis

Core Message

> Evidence-based practice in nursing, although supported in principle, its translation has been difficult and challenging. However, it has been improving in its popularity over time; indeed, a promising future for evidence-based nursing practice.

4.1 Introduction

Evidence-based practice has gained increased recognition within the past two decades as an important component of the current health care environment. Changes and competing demands from health care consumers, governmental, and private agencies are apparent in today's health care. These demands from the consumer of care and its agencies on safety and high quality care within a financial constraint are powerful reasons to link practice based on evidence. These demands are also taken largely into consideration during the process of clinical decision making.

Moving forward to making decisions based on the best available evidence takes considerable time. However, as nurses, we should realize that every clinical decision we make affects patient outcome as well as patient care resources; resources that may include personnel, time, and money. An expectation of positive patient outcome within the constraint of limited resources should engage us as health care providers to draw clinical decisions from best available evidence in providing an objective, effective, and efficient patient care.

The work of Florence Nightingale in the 1860s began the era of research in nursing. For years after it started, however, the pace of the nursing research movement was slow. It was only in the 1960s that nursing research was recognized as an important part in nursing practice. A change of focus in nursing research occurred in the 1970s; from topics regarding nurses, nursing education, and administration, to those improving patient care. This change signified a growing awareness by nurses of a need to base their practice from scientific evidence [55]. And so, in the 1980s and 1990s, nursing research became a major force in developing a scientific knowledge base for nursing practice [10]. By 2000, there was already a notable growing awareness and popularity of evidence-based practice in nursing [78].

Evidence-based practice is a problem-solving approach that utilizes best evidence together with clinical expertise to guide clinical decisions on options that are suited best for the patient. Sources of evidence may include evidence from research studies, expert opinions, and scientific principles [3, 15, 47, 56, 77, 79]. Moreover, accrued experiential knowledge, patient values/preferences, and expert opinions can all influence the nurse's clinical decision. It is crucial to acknowledge that integrating scientific evidence with experiential knowledge and patient values/preferences collectively represent a powerful base to achieving best care outcome for the patient.

C.B. Cajulis (✉)
P.S. Beam
S.M. Davis
Mount Sinai Medical Center, One Gustave Levy Place, New York, NY 10029, USA
e-mail: corazon.cajulis@msnyuhealth.org

F. Chiappelli et al. (eds.), *Evidence-Based Practice: Toward Optimizing Clinical Outcomes*,
DOI: 10.1007/978-3-642-05025-1_4, © Springer-Verlag Berlin Heidelberg 2010

4.1.1 How Do Nurses Make Clinical Decisions?

In nursing, there is no decision-making theory that can be singled out to describe how the nurses make clinical decisions. Although decision making in nursing is traditionally thought of as intuitive rather than rational, theories such as hypothetico-deductive clinical decision making and a model of pattern recognition and classification [5, 9, 21] are represented during the process of making decisions regarding patient care. Part of the reasons why this is so, is that when nurses make clinical decisions, they take into account the patient as a whole not as a fragmented entity.

Literature on nurse's clinical decision making suggested two primary approaches to clinical decision making [21]. One is a rationalist perspective. This perspective is described as using a framework of a logical process of using and analyzing information. Another approach is a phenomenological perspective. This perspective points the role of intuition in the process of decision making. Intuitive activities are based on previous knowledge in recognizing similarities and situations. These activities are at length outlined in Benner's theory of Novice to Expert [4]. Lauri and Salantera [38] pointed out that multiple research evidence indicated that nurses make clinical decisions based on the features of different decision-making theories; however, these are largely guided by the principles, rules, and plans of treatment. Research evidence further showed that nurses use information from different sources to draw clinical decisions about patient care [61, 76]. For example, in a study done by Pravikoff et al. [57], it was found that although nurses acknowledge their need for information, they preferred to ask their peers instead of accessing online databases for information regarding practice.

For the purpose of a better understanding of how nurses make clinical decisions, let us review the nursing process. Used by nurses as a basic problem-solving approach to patient care, the nursing process can be described from a perspective of an analytical decision making process [71]. It is a complex process that involves a series of decisions coordinated from each stage to achieve a desired goal of treatment [8, 22, 38]. This process has five components namely:

1. *Assessment*

The nurse collects the data from patient's own words (subjective) and from assessment and other sources (objective). Other sources of objective data may include the patient's medical records and information from other health care members and family members.

2. *Nursing diagnosis*

A nursing diagnosis is formulated from the data collected during the assessment stage. The nursing diagnosis is an identified problem, its cause, and its signs and symptoms.

3. *Planning*

Planning involves the development of a nursing care plan; a plan for intervention to address the identified nursing diagnosis. Goals to obtain the desired patient outcomes are also stated.

4. *Implementation*

This stage is the actual performance of the intervention. Coordination with other health care team members taking care of the patient occurs prior to the actual implementation of the intervention.

5. *Evaluation*

The outcomes of the plan of care are evaluated whether the goals are met or not met. If the goals are not met, a reevaluation of the plan of care is initiated and the process cycle starts again.

Integral to the process of decision making are clinical expertise, patient values and preferences, research-based evidence as well as health care resources, patient clinical state, setting, and circumstances [15, 49, 56]. The process of decision making in nursing involves multiple variables. Variables may include, but are not limited to, the nature of the nursing task at hand, the knowledge/skills, experience, and the ability of the nurse to cope with whatever clinical situation she is engaged in. Although, the nurse's experiential knowledge is not a sufficient basis for clinical decisions [76] and should not be used as a sole basis for decision making, this is considered important not as an evidence but rather as an influence in the process of decision making [64]. A research-based clinical decision is described as objective and rational decision; thus, reduces variations in care. Across clinicians (including nurses), when armed with evidence-based knowledge and experience in making decisions over the course of time, desirable outcomes tend to be maximized.

A network of activities occurs during the process of decision making. According to a study done by

Boblin-Cummings et al. [7], the nurse makes decisions on whom to involve, what resources to use, when and where to effectively implement the intervention. These decisions are being done simultaneously with multiple things to consider in mind prior to implementing an intervention. For example, in a clinical situation where a patient is having a sudden change in mental status, the nurse engages in a myriad of simultaneous activities from formulating a nursing diagnosis and planning of intervention to implementing the intervention. Formulating a nursing diagnosis requires synthesis of data collected from what the patient stated and from the nurse's assessment of the patient. Once the nurse identifies a working nursing diagnosis (what is going on with the patient), an action plan is made and an intervention is implemented to address the problem. Simultaneous decisions are made to address the sudden change in mental status. In addition to calling and involving other members of the health care team such as the physician/medical provider, the nursing assistant, or the nurse administrator, the nurse takes into consideration what resources she needs to provide that patient a safe, efficient, and effective care.

4.2 Why Is It Important to Nursing?

In today's ever changing health care, nurses must be actively involved in clinical decision making and problem-solving regarding patient care. With the explosion of information and technological advancement, it is no more acceptable not to consider incorporating evidence during the process of clinical decision making. The health care providers of today, including nurses, are expected to seek out, analyze, and utilize the best available evidence in making clinical decisions [78]. The American Nurses Association (ANA) [2] indicated a connection between evidence-based practice and the standards of care. For example, in order to meet the planning of care criteria as a standard for practice, current trends and research should be integrated in the care planning process. Furthermore, the ANA delineates that nurses are required to develop and maintain clinical and professional knowledge and skills in order to meet the standards of care and competence in practice. The incorporation of research is a requirement to meeting the standards of care and competence in nursing practice. This in itself is evidence-based practice.

Incorporating evidence in making clinical decisions is essential because they affect patient outcomes and resources as well as patient/family experience [7, 13, 76]. The use of evidence in nursing practice is also essential in achieving the Hospital Magnet status. Magnet designation or certification is the gold standard for nursing excellence. Achieving a Magnet status illustrates a strong and high quality nursing department; meaning that nurses exemplify the 14 forces of Magnetism. These forces include quality and evidence-based practice [25]. It has been demonstrated that when evidence-based practice approach to care is implemented, improved clinical outcomes are also at hand [30, 68]. The Institute of Medicine (IOM) reinforced the emphasis on making decisions based on research to improve patient care. The relevance of these decisions can be linked to the following reasons:

1. *Patient safety and quality improvement*

Patient safety has gained increased emphasis in our health care system. This emphasis is a key to the actions of government agencies, policy makers, and health care organizations. A 1999 report titled: To Err is Human: Building a Safer Health System, the Institute of Medicine (IOM) [35] identified that thousands of people die as a result of medical errors. Adverse drug events, injuries related to surgery, falls, pressure ulcers, and mistaken patient identity were all identified as common preventable medical errors. This report recommended a four-tiered approach to achieve and ensure basic patient safety. The recommendations included the creation of a governmental agency to improve and monitor safety in the health care delivery. It also included the development of a nationwide mandatory reporting system, raising of performance standards and expectations, and implementing safety system within the health care organization. In 2001, IOM published a report "Crossing the Quality Chasm: A New Health System for the twenty-first century." The report identified evidence-based decision making as one of the general principles of the redesigned health care system. The use of evidence in decision making aims to promote objectivity and to decrease variations in care. Care should not vary from clinician to clinician [36, 64].

The American Association of the Advancement of Science, the American Medical Association (AMA), and The Joint Commission (TJC) formed a partnership for patient safety initiatives on preventing injuries from medical errors [39]. TJC, an independent, not-for-profit organization that provides accreditation and certification to health care organizations is committed to improving patient safety and quality of care [73]. Most of the TJC standards are related to patient safety. These standards addressed patient safety issues such as medication use, infection control, prevention of injury from falls, surgery, medical equipment, etc.

Review of literature had shown that practice based on evidence not only saves money but also improves quality care. For example, a study done in 27 nursing units from 14 hospitals demonstrated that hourly rounding not only reduced patient falls and patient's use of call lights but also increased patient satisfaction [46]. The study further noted that an interdisciplinary rounding on some units like the intensive care unit (ICU) resulted in the reduction in incidence of pressure ulcers. Improving quality care makes patient safe. Prevention of errors or any events that jeopardize patient safety like falls, deep vein thrombosis (DVT), infection, PU are in themselves cost reduction and containment activities.

2. *Cost savings*

The US health care spends billions of dollars on extra-medical cost due to medical errors. About $17 billion are spent on injuries associated withpreventable medical errors. To name a few examples related to these medical errors:

* Medication errors affect 1.5 million people and cost approximately $3.5 billion/year [1, 63, 74]

The TJC identified medication reconciliation as one of the National Patient Safety Goals (NPSG) for 2008. Medication reconciliation is a process where medication orders for the patient are compared to the medications that the patient has been taking at home. This process prevents adverse medical events related to medication errors such as duplication, dosing, omission, and drug interaction.

* Pressure ulcers affect one million people with an annual cost of approximately $1.6 billion [58, 80].
* The direct cost of fall injuries for people who were 65 years and older exceeded $19 billion in 2000. It is estimated that in 2020, the cost will reach $ 54 billion [12].

Substantial changes in government and health insurance programs on reimbursement clearly provide a reason to also focus on cost saving and containment. In 2008, the Center for Medicare and Medicaid Services (CMS) [18] decided to deny reimbursements to hospitals for "reasonably preventable" (never events) treatment errors. With this decision, Medicare will no longer reimburse hospitals for treatment-related "never events" such as falls, hospital-acquired pressure ulcers, catheter-associated vascular and urinary tract infections, and surgical site infection.

Evidence from research findings on pressure ulcer (PU) prevention and treatment as well as fall prevention is searchable and available for nurses to use in practice. Results of studies regarding fall prevention like using evidence-based protocols or integrating an evidence-based fall prevention program to increase awareness had a positive result in decreasing falls [50]. Any falls and/or PU that are prevented is a cost saving.

3. *Patient and staff empowerment*

Research, support of information technology, and provision of safety information to both the providers and the consumers of care promote and support the empowerment of the consumer as well as the providers of care. The inclusion of patients in decision making regarding their care produces positive patient outcomes; outcomes that are necessary to improve compliance in care, quality, relationship with health care provider, and patient satisfaction. Patient empowerment enables patients or consumers to actively participate in making decisions regarding their health care needs. Likewise, providers are empowered to use available evidence to prevent patient care-related errors and to promote increased patient safety. It is the responsibility of the providers (i.e., nurses, doctors, and other health care members) to understand that clinical decisions and interventions that they make for their patients should not compromise patient safety. The use of evidence in clinical practice supports the empowerment of staff in making safe decisions for their patients. As nurses continue to base clinical decisions and actions on scientific evidence, they are better prepared to ask important questions in validating and addressing patient concerns. A well-informed practitioner uses the evidence to care for the patients. Knowledge of the evidence regarding specific intervention or patient care empowers the practitioner to make timely clinical decisions; decisions on interventions that are shown to be effective, safe, and efficient.

4. *Patient satisfaction*

Patient satisfaction is a very critical element of health care today; more so because of a national mandatory reporting of patient satisfaction. These scores can be viewed nationwide by any consumer of care. Patient satisfaction can potentially affect the financial aspect of the organization by the dollar reimbursement from both the government and private agencies. Better health outcomes and increased quality of care affect the overall patient satisfaction [53].

Building relationship with patients, engaging and empowering them to participate in decisions for their own health care is necessary in increasing patient perception of quality care and satisfaction. The use of a structured protocol or guidelines of nursing activities like the "hourly rounding" can improve quality of care and patient satisfaction as evidenced by a study done by Meade et al. [46]. Evidence-based protocols on pain management, immediate response to patient's call, compassionate care, listening to patient's concern, explaining care, treatment, and discharge plans are among the indicators of patient satisfaction. A satisfied customer perceives quality care and satisfaction with the care received.

4.3 Translating Knowledge Development into Knowledge Use

Translating knowledge in the form of evidence into nursing practice requires a health care environment that supports and facilitates transformative change. The resources required include an organizational culture that supports acceptance and change; leadership support; educational support; access to research databases; staff resources including, doctorally prepared nurse resources, clinical nurse leaders, advanced practice nurses, and engaged staff nurses; and the time, structure, and visibility to conduct evidence-based reviews and projects. Once support systems and resources are identified, selection of a nursing evidence-based practice model or models can support and guide the translation of knowledge developed into knowledge use in clinical decision making. Evidence-Based Practice models provide frameworks for systematically putting complex evidence-based knowledge into operation to achieve best practice. They provide a defined process for translating evidence into

practice. A number of evidence-based practice models (*addendum*) have been developed to define the steps necessary to achieve evidence-based nursing practice. While the models vary in context and in detail content, all of the models identify core steps necessary to the process:

1. Identify the issue (new knowledge, a practice question, practice assessment).
2. Find and critique the evidence.
3. Translate into practice by designing and implementing a practice change.
4. Evaluate, communicate, and maintain the change.

4.3.1 Identifying the Issue

Identification of the need to establish an evidence base in nursing practice may be triggered by the emergence of new knowledge related to patient care, a practice question being raised, or a purposeful review of current policies, procedures, and guidelines for an acceptable level of evidence (EBP models). Evidence-based models require the formulation of answerable questions to guide the search of databases and to design practice change. The PICO method provides a structure to develop and define many clinical questions in a way that supports an evidenced based approach to searching databases such as Medline [20].

P = Patient or problem is a description of the patient population or group of patients including important characteristics such as diagnosis, sex, or age.

I = Intervention is what you want to implement such as a medication, test, procedure, or exposure.

C = Comparison is the alternative intervention being compared to the new intervention.

O = Outcomes are what you hope to accomplish, measure, or improve.

PICO Example

Patient/problem	Diabetic ICU patients
Intervention	Nurse-driven continuous IV insulin protocol
Comparison	Intermittent subcutaneous insulin protocol
Outcome	Tightened glucose control

4.3.2 Finding and Evaluating the Evidence

Although much literature has been published on searching for and evaluating the available evidence to guide practice, a review is oftentimes needed for a better understanding of the search and evaluation of what constitutes "best evidence." As noted earlier, evidence can include research findings, expert opinion, and scientific principles (e.g., theories based on biological plausibility). A fundamental principal of the evidence-based practice paradigm is a hierarchy of evidence that places findings from rigorous scientific research at the top, and expert authority and unproven inference from scientific principles at the bottom. According to this paradigm, the best evidence on which to base clinical decisions arises from a methodologically strong and clinically relevant research [23, 33, 37]. A variety of evidence pyramids have been proposed to rank the relative strength of research methodologies in answering practice questions; the highest level of available evidence is usually preferred to inform decisions [17] (Fig. 4.1).

Although there is no absolute consensus within nursing or other disciplines about how best to define and rank evidence, it is generally accepted that the research methods that can provide the strongest evidence will vary depending on the question being asked [41, 44, 54]. The ability to identify the category of study that will best address a question is a core skill in evidence-based health care, and practitioners must be familiar with the study methodologies that offer the best evidence on the questions likely to arise in their practices and organizational settings.

Evaluating a study requires the identification of the appropriateness of a study's methodology to answer a question. The study's quality is then evaluated on the extent to which its design, conduct, and analysis minimized factors that might lead to bias or error [40]. If the study is of high quality and reported significant outcomes, practitioners must assess whether the findings can be used to improve outcomes for their individual patients in their unique practice environments. Textbooks and journal articles such as the User's Guides to the Medical Literature series published in the *Journal of the American Medical Association* (JAMA) offer guidance on in-depth critical assessment of research studies [23, 32, 33].

To make optimal evidence-based decisions, practitioners should consider the whole body of evidence on a topic and not just the results from a single study. Systematic reviews and clinical guidelines are the prime examples of evidence-based resources to support practice. Systematic reviews of the evidence are usually considered to offer the highest level of evidence to answer a question [33]. Systematic reviews use explicit and rigorous methods to summarize data from primary studies in order to answer a focused clinical question. They require a comprehensive literature search to locate as much research as possible, and use predefined quality criteria to select the studies to include in the review. The selected studies are then rigorously appraised and synthesized, sometimes using techniques of meta-analysis. Like any other evidence, users must critically appraise a systematic review's methodological rigor and the strength of its findings before applying those findings to patient care. Also, because systematic reviews often take months or years to conduct, users must make sure that their findings have not been superseded by newer evidence.

Clinical practice guidelines, like systematic reviews, are developed using systematic and explicit methods to locate, evaluate, and synthesize the evidence from as many studies as possible. Practice guidelines, however, usually go beyond systematic reviews in balancing a broader range of issues in a clinical context. The evidence basis of guidelines varies considerably; when research to support or refute a

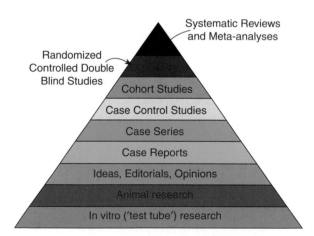

Fig. 4.1 The Evidence Pyramid. Available 25 February 2010 at http://library.downstate.edu/EBM2/2100.htm (with permission of the Medical Research Library of Brooklyn of the State University of New York (SUNY) Downstate Medical Center, New York, USA)

recommendation is lacking, authors must rely on expert consensus to make recommendations. The systematic evaluation of a body of evidence is usually done by small groups of experts, and guidelines are almost always developed under an organizational or society sponsorship [24].

It is clearly more difficult and time-consuming to evaluate a body of evidence than to evaluate the quality and strength of the evidence of an individual study. In most cases, an individual practitioner with clinical responsibilities will be unable to conduct a rigorous review of all of the research on a topic.

Finding the best evidence may seem challenging for health professionals. However, the rapid uptake of evidence-based health care has lead to the growth and development of specialized publications and databases that make it easier to find and apply the best evidence. Some of these resources have been specifically developed to support nursing decisions. To support optimal clinical decision and to standardize best practice, nurses frequently use protocols, clinical pathways, quality improvement (QI) programs, and similar guides. Other evidence-based resources available for nurses to support decision and practice include preprocessed resources (such as evidence-based topic overviews, structured abstracts, systematic reviews, and some textbooks), journal articles, and databases.

1. *Preprocessed resources*

It is generally most efficient to begin a search by examining "filtered" or "preprocessed" resources. Preprocessed resources are the ones where the authors have surveyed the literature, filtered out flawed studies, and selected those that are methodologically the strongest. Evidence-based topic overviews, structured abstracts, and systematic reviews are three examples of filtered resources [23, 27, 33]. In the United States, the National Guideline Clearinghouse (NGC) [34] an initiative of the Agency for Health care Research and Quality (AHRQ) and the Department of Health and Human Services (DHHS), provides a comprehensive database of clinical practice guidelines. NGC provides "structured abstracts" that facilitate the critical appraisal of a guideline's recommendations. The structured abstracts systematically summarize each guideline and describe the methodology that the guideline developers used to collect and select the evidence; to assess the quality and strength of the evidence; and to formulate the guideline's recommendations. A guideline comparison tool allows users

to generate side-by-side comparisons for any combination of two or more guidelines. Many guidelines can also be identified through databases such as Medline/PubMed [51] and the Cumulative Index to Nursing and Allied Health Literature (CINAHL) [16].

(a) Clinical topic review databases

This is a type of online "textbook" that has emerged over the last decade to support evidence-based practice. Clinical topic reviews filter and summarize the evidence to provide overviews to support decisions at the point of care. They are updated on an ongoing basis. UpToDate and BMJ Clinical Evidence are popular clinical topic review databases that have in-text citations to the evidence. BMJ Clinical Evidence provides systematic reviews on the prevention and treatment of clinical conditions, and ranks interventions on a scale ranging from "Beneficial" to "Likely to be ineffective or harmful" [6]. Although currently clinical topic review databases are oriented toward supporting medical practice, they provide in-depth information on a wide range of topics and may be especially useful to advanced practice nurses.

(b) Structured abstracts

Structured abstracts use systematic and explicit methods to summarize a study's objectives, methods, results, and conclusions. The abstract is enhanced by an expert commentary on the context, methods, and clinical applications of the study's findings. Journals of structured abstracts free practitioners from having to look through all the journals in their field to identify articles of possible importance, and they facilitate the appraisal of the evidence, thereby streamlining the translation of valuable new research to patient care. Journals of structured abstracts of particular interest to nurses are Evidence-Based Nursing and Database of Abstracts of Reviews of Effects (DARE) [28]. Many journals of structured abstracts, such as Evidence-based Nursing, are indexed in the Medline database. DARE, however, is not indexed in the Medline. DARE contains over 10,000 structured abstracts of systematic reviews, and as noted above, systematic reviews are considered to provide the best evidence to support clinical decisions.

(c) Systematic reviews

The single most important source of systematic reviews of health care treatments is the Cochrane Collaboration, an intentional consortium of review groups that develops and maintains systematic reviews and meta-analyzes. Cochrane Reviews are published in the Cochrane Database of Systematic Reviews (CDSR) [19]. Many consider the methodology used in Cochrane Reviews to be the gold standard for systematic reviews of treatments. Cochrane Review Groups of particular importance to nursing include the Cochrane Incontinence Review Group and the Cochrane Wounds Group. Completed Cochrane reviews can be found in the Cochrane Library, and they may also be identified through the Medline/PubMed and CINAHL databases, among others. Abstracts of Cochrane Reviews are freely available online, but a license is needed to obtain the full-text of the reviews. Systematic reviews that focus on nursing topics may be found in the JBI Library of Systematic Reviews [70] and the Worldviews on Evidence-Based Nursing Journal [67]. The Worldviews on Evidence-Based Nursing from The Honor Society of Nursing, Sigma Theta Tau International, is a source of knowledge synthesis articles as well as structured abstracts and original studies that aim to support decision making for clinical practice, nursing administration, nursing education, and public health care policies.

2. *Textbooks*

In keeping with the evidence-based practice movement, textbooks (many now available in digital format) increasingly integrate evidence from primary studies and systematic reviews into their recommendations [31]. Given the rapid pace of change in health care, a major weakness of textbooks has been their lack of currency. A few medical textbooks are now updated regularly, but at this time we are unaware of nursing textbooks that are updated on an ongoing basis.

3. *Primary studies*

If filtered resources do not answer a question, practitioners can obtain research evidence for decision making from primary research studies, which are usually published in the journal literature. The journal literature is usually accessed through electronic databases that contain citations and abstracts – and increasingly, links to the full-text – of the articles. The ability to search the journal literature for evidence is an important skill for evidence-based practice [11, 57].

4. *Database*

The most important databases for retrieving studies of interest to nursing are Medline and CINAHL, although depending on the topic, it may be necessary to examine psychology, education, population health, sociology, or social work databases. Since nursing topics are interdisciplinary, it may also be necessary to search more than one database. Interdisciplinary databases such as ProQuest and Web of Science may also be useful. Conducting a literature search may appear daunting to time-pressed clinicians overwhelmed by the vast quantity of electronic information. Only a small percentage of the published literature contains evidence that is ready for clinical application [43]. The goal of a database search is to identify that subset of evidence that addresses the clinician's question and that it is applicable in a local practice setting. At issue is the need to develop and maintain familiarity with the continuously evolving search interfaces of the databases most likely to provide evidence in a practice area.

Some nurses (generally, those prepared at the doctoral level) have the knowledge and skills of the statistical and analytical methods needed for in-depth appraisal of research evidence to determine best practices [62]. Nurses with other educational preparation can, however, learn to use the hierarchy of evidence to gauge the strength of a study. Nurses can assess whether the outcomes of the study would be significant to their patient population, and judge whether the findings could be applied in their clinical setting.

4.3.3 Making the Change

Knowledge for integration into practice can be generated through a new research and/or evidence-based project or through the synthesis of available research, or expertise of other sources of information [66]. Rogers's theory of diffusion of innovations [59] defines concepts and describes processes to promote knowledge diffusion and utilization. Diffusion or dissemination of knowledge is defined as the process by which an innovation or new idea is communicated over a time period among the members of the social system. The major components of diffusion include the following:

1. Innovation or idea perceived to be new by the individual or unit of adoption.

2. Communication is the process in which participants create and share information to reach a mutual understanding through one to one, one to group, or through journals, periodicals, books, the internet, or media channels.
3. Time spanning from introduction of an idea to rejection or adoption.
4. A social system or set of interrelated units connected to accomplish a goal.

Roger identifies five stages in the innovation to decision process:

1. Knowledge
2. Persuasion
3. Decision when the innovation or change is either rejected or accepted
4. Implementation
5. Confirmation (Fig. 4.2)

Opinion leaders present in health care can influence the rejection or adoption of an innovation during the knowledge phase. Rogers recognizes the importance of opinion leaders and the need to identify them in seeking adoption of evidence or research-based change. Advanced practice nurses among others are considered opinion leaders based on their clinical expertise and expanded education. Rogers describes the degree and agility with which adopters such as individual nurses will accept new ideas as (1) innovators or active seekers of new ideas, (2) early adopters who are often opinion leaders who learn about new ideas rapidly and then act as role models (3) the early majority or those who are active followers and will readily use a new innovation, (4) the late majority or those who are skeptical of new ideas and change but will change when the pressure is great and (5) laggards who are resistant to change and may or may not be persuaded to make the change and may leave the organization.

4.3.4 Evaluation and Maintenance

Knowledge generated, accepted, and successfully implemented requires ongoing evaluation to determine the quality, consistency, and applicability of the evidence over time and circumstance. The final stage in

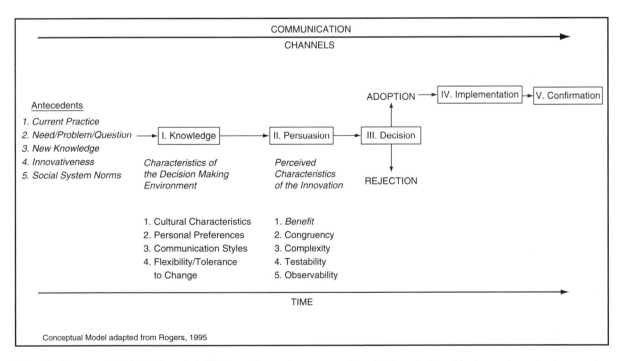

Fig. 4.2 Conceptual Model of Roger's Diffusion of Innovations process from first knowledge of the innovation to implementation and confirmation

the evidence-based practice model process is evaluation and maintenance. Outcomes of evidence-based practice may be evaluated on a broad range of endpoints including the impact on patients, practitioners, and the system [69]. Evaluation methods may include QI monitors, surveys, and endorsement by respected peers [60]. Maintaining change supported by an evidence base is achieved by providing resources to practitioners to sustain the change and integrating the evidence into protocols, texts, procedures, policies, and the educational process. Change is most likely adopted and sustained when people affected participate in the process to make the change [59].

4.4 Summary

Demands of the current health care system provide a powerful reason for evidence-based practice. For nurses, moving forward to evidence-based decision making can be challenging. However, it is undeniably a responsible approach to providing best possible care to patients. Nurses are required to make clinical decisions in the moment, to know what to do and how to do it instantly, without conscious deliberation [14]. The judgments that nurses make in the moment have a moral component that guides what must be done in a responsible way based on nursing knowledge [14]. Evidence-based guidelines appropriately applied to clinical decision making can reduce uncertainty and diminish variation in practice promoting quality and safety for patients [59].

Evidence-based nursing practice as a concept is widely embraced by nurses as a means to improve quality outcomes for patients receiving care. It is also considered to be important to the discipline of nursing for expressing nursing practice as scientific competence [14]. While integrating the best current evidence into the nursing practice of clinical decision making is supported in principle, the translation of evidence into nursing practice itself has been (viewed) as difficult and challenging. Barriers to change in health care practice can arise at any or multiple levels from the patient to individual professionals, the health care team, the organization, and the wider environment [29]. Barriers to the implementation of evidence in nursing practice include lack of authority to change practice, lack of organizational support, lack of professional mentoring, inadequate database researching skills, lack of access to applicable research evidence, and lack of defined processes for translating evidence into practice [52].

This inability to successfully integrate the best evidence into practice is the gap between nursing knowledge development and knowledge use [59].

Chinn and Kramer indentify four fundamental patterns of Nursing Knowledge development that nurses use in practice [14]. The most familiar pattern and the pattern of knowledge development most closely identified with evidence-based practice is empirics or the science of nursing. It is based on query on what is known, what it is, and how it works. This pattern of knowledge development is traditionally derived from testing hypotheses based on theory that offers an explanation. Empiric knowledge is articulated through competent action grounded in scientific knowledge. Additional patterns of knowledge development include ethics or the moral component of knowing, personal knowledge and aesthetics, or the art of nursing. The inquiry process in ethics is expressed in query as 'Is this action right? Is it responsible?' In personal knowledge, it is self reflection based on experience expressed as 'Do I know what I am doing? Am I doing what I know?' And in aesthetic knowledge, it is expressed as 'What does this mean? And how is it significant?' These four basic patterns of knowledge in nursing are interrelated and result in wholeness. The validation practices that confirm knowledge are ongoing to provide understanding as new circumstances emerge so that knowledge becomes a construct that varies across time, person, and place. Evidence-based nursing practice allows nurses to apply the best knowledge in time to the current situation, but continually question what is known to create new possibilities for moving patients toward health and wellbeing [14, 75].

The identification of "best" available evidence requires examination and evaluation of resources such as research findings, expert opinions, and scientific principles. These resources of evidence are integrated in clinical practice guidelines, practice protocols, and clinical pathways or flow charts. These resources are considered as decision support tools; decision support tools that nurses use to help or enhance clinical decisions for efficiency and better patient outcome [45, 65]. Evidence-based guidelines do not have to be solely from nursing literature but can be based on other disciplines as well [80]. The application of evidence from comprehensive systemic reviews can substantially produce a change in practice. The use of practice guidelines and protocols is believed to facilitate standardization of practice and effective care delivery [42, 48, 61, 68]. Clinical practice guidelines and systematic reviews are electronically searchable. The AHRQ [1] is an excellent site for clinical practice guidelines. The Cochrane library is a great source of systematic reviews on clinical practice and evidence. Quality improvement projects are another source of evidence that nurses use to guide and/or enhance their practice. Some examples of these projects are falls and pressure ulcers prevention, improving patient satisfaction, and infection control and prevention.

The nurse's clinical decision making process incorporates evidence, patient values, expert opinions, and own experiential knowledge. The process in itself is a combination of phenomenological and rational process taking into consideration the patient as a whole, to design an appropriate clinical decision regarding patient care. Evidence-based practice clearly has a great impact on practice, quality care, cost, as well as patient perception of satisfaction and patient's and health practitioner's empowerment.

The challenge remains, however, on how to overcome some barriers to the application of evidence in practice. In nursing, EBP application is at its early stages; however, it is becoming more promising and popular.

Acknowledgments Thanks to Dr. Carol Porter, DNP, RN Senior VP of Nursing, Chief Nursing Officer, Mount Sinai Medical Center, for her support to evidence-based practice in nursing.
Thanks to Dr. Francesco Chiappelli, PhD, for his guidance and patience during the completion of this section.

4.5 Addendum

Sample models:

(a) *ACE Star Model of Knowledge Transformation*
   ACE Star Model

Knowledge Transformation   ACE Star Model ©2004

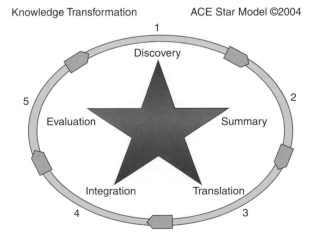

This model depicts forms of knowledge in a relational sequence. The model illustrates five major stages or star points of knowledge transformation [70].

1. Knowledge discovery – new knowledge becomes available (research).
2. Evidence summary – synthesis of all research knowledge into a single meaningful statement.
3. Translation – practice recommendations.
4. Integration – implementation of change into practice.
5. Evaluation – endpoints and outcomes.

(b) *John Hopkins Nursing Evidence-Based Practice Model (JHNEBP)*

This model incorporates the "best available evidence" as the core component necessary to make decisions that affect professional nursing in the domains of nursing practice, education, and research. Guidelines provide nurses with the tools necessary to acquire EBP knowledge and skills to implement change [26]. A three-step process is used:

1. Practice question – identifies EBP question, multi disciplinary team recruited.
2. Evidence – internal and external evidence collected, critiqued, summarized, recommendations developed.
3. Translation – action plan created, change implemented, evaluated, communicated.

(c) *The Iowa Model of Evidence-Based-Practice*

This model provides a guide for clinical decision making, details for implementation of evidence-based change, and enlists both the practitioner and the organizational perspectives [72]. In this model:

1. Problem-focused (PI data, risk issues) or knowledge-focused (new research, standards) triggers are identified
2. The question is this a priority for the organization is asked
3. A team is formed
4. Current knowledge and evidence is assembled, critiqued, and synthesized
5. A pilot to institute change is implemented
6. Change is instituted
7. Structure, process, and outcome data related to change is monitored and analyzed
8. Results are disseminated

(d) *Rosswurm and Larrabee Model*

The Rosswurm and Larrabee [60] model guides nurses through a systematic process for the change to evidence-based practice. This model recognized that translation of research into practice requires a solid grounding in change theory, principles of research utilization, and use of standardized nomenclature. The model has the following five phases:

1. Assess the need for change in practice.
2. Link the problem with interventions and outcomes.
3. Synthesize the best evidence.
4. Design a change in practice.
5. Implement and evaluate the practice.

References

1. Agency for Health Care Research and Quality (2000) Medical errors: the scope of the problem. Retrieved 12 June 2009 at http://www.ahrq.gov/qual/errback.htm
2. American Nurses Association (2004) Nursing: scope and standards of practice. Washington, DC
3. Balakas K, Potter P, Pratt E, Rea G, Williams J (2009) Evidence equals excellence: the adoption of an evidence-based practice model in an academic medical center. Nurs Clin Am 44(1):1–10
4. Benner P (1984) From novice to expert: excellence and power in clinical nursing practice. Addison Wesley, Menlo Park, CA
5. Benner P, Tanner C (1987) Clinical judgment: how expert nurses use intuition. Am J Nurs 87:23–31
6. BMJ clinical evidence (2006) [Earlier Title: Clinical evidence]. BMJ, London
7. Boblin-Cummings S, Baumann A, Deber R (1999) Critical elements in the process of decision making: a nursing perspective. Can J Nurs Leadersh 12(1):6–13
8. Bonnel C (1999) Evidence-based nursing: a stereotyped view of quantitative and experimental research could work against professional autonomy and authority. J Adv Nurs 30(1):18–23
9. Buckingham CD, Adams N (2000) Classifying clinical decision making: a unifying approach. J Adv Nurs 32(4):981–989
10. Burns N, Grove S (2005) The practice of nursing research, conduct, critique, and utilization. Elsevier, Saunders, St Louis
11. Cadmus E, Van Wynen EA, Chamberlain B, Steingall P, Kilgallen ME, Holly C et al (2008) Nurses' skill level and access to evidence-based practice. J Nurs Adm 38(11):494–503
12. Center for Disease Control and Prevention (2008) Cost of falls among older adults. Retrieved on 12 June 2009 at http://www.cdc.gov/nicpc
13. Chiappelli F (2008) Manual of evidence-based research for the health sciences. Nova, New York
14. Chinn P, Kramer M (2004) Integrated knowledge development in nursing. Mosby, St Louis
15. Ciliska DK, Pinelli J, DiCenso A, Cullum N (2001) Resources to enhance evidence-based nursing practice. AACN Clin Issues 12(4):520–528
16. CINAHL Information Systems. CINAHL. EBSCO Pub., Ipswich, MA
17. Cleary-Holdforth J, Leufer T (2008) Essential elements in developing evidence-based practice. Nurs Stand 23(2):42–46
18. CMS Office of Public Affairs (2008) CMS proposes to expand quality program to hospitals. Retrieved on 12 June 2009 at http://www.cms.hhs.gov
19. Cochrane Collaboration (1996) The Cochrane library. Wiley, Hoboken, NJ
20. Construct Well-Built Clinical Questions using PICO. Retrieved on 30 July 2009 at http://healthlinks.washington.edu/ebp/pico.html
21. Cranley L, Doran DM, Tourangeau AE, Kushniruk A, Nagle L (2009) Nurses's uncertainty in decision-making: a literature review. Worldviews Evid Based Nurs 6(1):3–15
22. De la Cuesta C (1983) The nursing process from development to implementation. J Adv Nurs 8(5):365–371
23. DiCenso A, Guyatt G, Ciliska D (2005) Evidence based nursing: a guide to clinical practice. Elsevier, Mosby, St Louis, Mo
24. Eddy DM (2005) Evidence-based medicine: a unified approach. Health Aff (Project Hope) 24(1):9–17
25. Garcis JL, Wells KK (2009) Knowledge-based information to improve the quality of patient care. J Health Care Qual 31(1):30–35
26. Gawlinski A, Rutledge D (2008) Selecting a model for evidence-based practice changes: a practical approach. AACN Adv Crit Care 19(3):291–300
27. GHaynes RB (2002) What kind of evidence is it that evidence-based medicine advocates want health care providers and consumers to pay attention to? BMC Health Serv Res 2(1):3
28. Great Britain, National Health Service, University of York (1994) DARE: University of York, NHS Centre for Reviews and Dissemination
29. Grol J, Grimshaw J (2003) From best evidence to best practice: Effective implementation of change in patient's care. Lancet 362:1225–1230
30. Grossman S, Bautista C (2002) Collaboration yields cost-effective, evidence-based nursing protocols. Orthop Nurs 21(3):30–36
31. Guyatt GH, Oxman AD, Vist GE, Kunz R, Falck-Ytter Y, Alonso-Coello P et al (2008) RADE: An emerging consensus on rating quality of evidence and strength of recommendations. BMJ (Clinical Research Ed) 336(7650):924–926
32. Guyatt GH, Rennie D (1993) Users' guides to the medical literature. J Am Med Assoc 270(17):2096–2097
33. Guyatt G, Rennie D, Evidence-Based Medicine Working Group, American Medical Association (2002) Users' guides to the medical literature: a manual for evidence-based clinical practice. AMA Press, Chicago, Ill
34. http://www.ngc.gov
35. Institute of Medicine (1999) To err is human: building a safer health system. National Academies Press, Washington DC
36. Institute of Medicine (2001) Crossing the quality chasm: a new health system for the 21st century. National Academies Press, Washington DC

37. Ismail AI, Bader JD (2004) Evidence-based dentistry in clinical practice. J Am Dent Assoc 135(1):78–83

38. Lauri S, Salantera S (1998) Decision-making models in different fields of nursing. Res Nurs Health 21:443–452

39. Leape LL, Woods DD, Hatlie MJ, Kizer KW, Schroeder SA, Lundberg GD (1998) Promoting patient safety by preventing medical error. J Am Med Assoc 280:1444–1447

40. Lohr KN (2004) Rating the strength of scientific evidence: relevance for quality improvement programs. Int J Qual Health Care 16(1):9–18

41. Mantzoukas S (2008) A review of evidence-based practice, nursing research and reflection: leveling the hierarchy. J Clin Nurs 17(2):214–223

42. Martin F (2008) Why we do what we do: implementation of practice guidelines by family nurse practitioners students. J Am Acad Nurse Pract 20:515–521

43. McKibbon A, Eady A, Marks S. (1999) PDQ: evidence-based principles and practice. Decker, Hamilton, ON

44. McQueen DV (2001) Strengthening the evidence base for health promotion. Health Promotion International 16(3): 261-268

45. McSweeney M, Spies M, Cann CJ (2001) Finding and evaluating clinical practice guidelines. Nurse Pract 26(9): 30–47

46. Meade C, Bursell A, Ketelsen L (2006) Effects of nursing rounds: on patient's call light use, satisfaction, and safety. Am J Nurs 106(9):58–70

47. Melnyk BM (2004) Integrating levels of evidence into clinical decision making. Pediatr Nurs 30(4):323–325

48. Meyers WC, Johnson JA, Klardie K, McNaughton MA (2004) Integrating the principles of evidence-based practice: prognosis and the metabolic syndrome. J Am Acad Nurse Pract 16(5):178–180, 182, 184

49. Michaels C, McEwen MM, McArthur DB (2008) Saying no to professional recommendations: client values, beliefs, and evidence-based practice. J Am Acad Nurse Pract 20:585–589

50. Murphy T, Labonte P, Klock M, Houser L (2008) Falls prevention for elders in acute care. Crit Care Nurs Q 31(1):33–39

51. National Center for Biotechnology Information (1996) PubMed. Bethesda, Md.: National Library of Medicine. Retrieved from http://www.ncbi.nlm.nih.gov/pubmed/

52. Oman K, Duran C (2008) Evidence-based policy and procedures: an algorithm for success. J Nurs Adm 38(1):47–51

53. Otani K (2004) The impact of nursing care and other healthcare attributes on hospitalized patient satisfaction and behavioral intentions. J Healthcare Manage 49(3):181–196

54. Pearson A, Wiechula R, Court A, Lockwood C (2007) A re-consideration of what constitutes "evidence" in the healthcare professions. Nursing Science Quarterly 20(1):85–88

55. Polit DF, Hungler BP (1999) Nursing research principles and methods, 6th edn. Lippincott, Philadelphia, PA

56. Portney LG (2004) Evidence-based practice and clinical decision making: it's not just the research course anymore. J Phys Ther Educ 18(3):46–51

57. Pravikoff DS, Tanner AB, Pierce ST (2005) Readiness of US nurses for evidence-based practice: many don't understand or value research and have had little or no training to help them find evidence on which to base their practice. Am J Nurs 105(9):40–51

58. Robinson C, Copas J, Kearns C, Kipp K, Labath B, Lonadier R, Lopez M, Nelson L, Newton S, Wentz D (2003) Determining the efficacy of a pressure ulcer prevention program by collecting prevalence and incidence data: a unit based effort. Ostomy Wound Manage 49(5):44–51

59. Rogers E (1995) Diffusion of Innovations. Retrieved on 30 July 2009 at http://www.stanford.edu/class/symbsys2005/diffusion%20

60. Rosswurm MA, Larrabee JH (1999) A model change to evidence-based practice. Image J Nurs Sch 31(4):317

61. Rycroft-Malone J, Fontela M, Seers K, Bick D (2009) Protocol-based care: standardization of decision-making. J Clin Nurs 18:1490–1500

62. Satterfield JM, Spring B, Brownson RC, Mullen EJ, Newhouse RP, Walker BB et al (2009) Toward a transdisciplinary model of evidence-based practice. Milbank Q 87(2): 368–390

63. Science Daily (2008) Medical errors cost $8.8 billion, result in 238,337 potentially preventable deaths, study shows. Retrieved 12 June 2009 at http://www.sciencedaily.com

64. Scott-Findlay S, Pollock C (2004) Evidence, research, knowledge: a call for conceptual clarity. Worldviews Evid Based Nurs 1(2):92–97

65. Shapiro SE, Driever MJ (2004) Clinical decision tools as evidence-based nursing. Western J Nurs Res 26(8):930–937

66. Sigma Theta Tau International (2008) Sigma Theta Tau International position statement on evidence-based practice February 2007 Summary. Worldviews Evid Based Nurs 5(2):57–59

67. Sigma Theta Tau International (2004) Worldviews on evidence-based nursing. Blackwell Publishing Inc. for Sigma Theta Tau International Malden, MA

68. Singleton J, Levin R (2008) Strategies for learning evidence-based practice: critically appraising clinical practice guidelines. J Nurs Educ 47(8):380–383

69. Stevens KR (2004) ACE star model of EBP: knowledge transformation. Academic Center for Evidence-based Practice. The University of Texas Health Science Center, San Antonio. Retrieved on July 30, 2009 at http://www.ace-star.uthscsa.edu

70. Systematic reviews – Joanna Briggs Institute. JBI library of systematic reviews. Adelaide South Australia, Australia

71. Taylor C (2000) Clinical problem solving in nursing: insights from the literature. J Adv Nurs 31(4):842–849

72. The Iowa model of evidence-based practice. Retrieved on 30 July 2009 at http://www.uihealthcar.com/depts/nursing/rqom/evdiencebasedpractice/iowamodel.html

73. The Joint Commission (2009) Medication reconciliation national patient safety goal to be reviewed, refined. Retrieved on 12 June 2009 at http://www.jointcommission.org/Patientsafety

74. The National Academies Press (2006) Preventing medication errors. Retrieved on 12 June 2009 at http://www8. nationalacademies.org

75. Thompson C (2001) JAN Forum: clinical decision making in nursing: theoretical perspectives and their relevance to practice- response to Jean Harbison. J Adv Nurs 35(1): 134–137

76. Thompson C (2003) Clinical experience as evidence in evidence-based practice. J Adv Nurs 43(3):230–237

77. Titler MG (2009) The evidence of evidence-based practice implemetation. In: Hughes R (ed) Patient safety and quality: an evidence-based handbook for nurses, Vol.1. AHRQ Publication Clearing House # 08-0043, Rockville

78. Trinder L (2000) Evidence-based practice: a critical appraisal. Blackwell, MA

79. Vratny A, Shriver D (2007) A conceptual model for growing evidence-base practice. Nurs Adm Q 31(2):162–170

80. Whittington K, Patrick M, Roberts JL (2000) A national study of pressure ulcer prevalence and incidence in acute care hospitals. J Wound Ostomy Continence 27(4): 209–215

A Model for Implementing Evidence-Based Decisions in Dental Practice

Clovis Mariano Faggion Jr., Stefan M. Listl, and Marc Schmitter

Core Message

> The purpose of this chapter is to present a useful evidence-based model, using treatment of peri-implantitis as an example, for searching, selecting, and appraising scientific literature and applying the information directly in the clinical setting.

5.1 Introduction

Dental undergraduate courses are intended to ensure that new dental practitioners are fully competent and confident in conducting clinical treatment. Dental courses, however, may not be long enough (most are 4–5 years in duration [1]) to enable students to learn all the theoretical and practical aspects of a great variety of dental procedures. Learning is a lifelong process in which the balance between clinical experience and a solid theoretical basis plays an important role in the development of skilled professionals. Besides clinical experience, dental surgeons facing complex clinical situations must develop evidence-based knowledge enabling resolution of problematic cases. When undergraduate training is complete, most dental practitioners seek knowledge, in training seminars and continuing dental educational courses, to enable them to plan and execute complex treatments [2]. In these courses, professional-centered education should be emphasized to stimulate clinicians to be active in the learning process [3]. Increasing evidence-based knowledge enables dentists in their careers to interact with colleagues, course instructors, and opinion leaders more as participants in a discussion than as mere listeners.

We propose in this chapter a model that may help dentists to improve their evidence-based knowledge [4], and thus, help them to make correct clinical decisions. Although we have used the treatment of peri-implantitis as an example to illustrate the usefulness of the model, the same rationale may be used in all facets of clinical dentistry.

C.M. Faggion Jr. (✉)
Department of Prosthodontics,
Dental School Ruprecht-Karls-University of Heidelberg,
Im Neuenheimer Feld 400,
69120 Heidelberg, Germany
e-mail: clovisfaggion@yahoo.com

S.M. Listl
Department of Conservative Dentistry,
Dental School Ruprecht-Karls-University of Heidelberg,
Im Neuenheimer Feld 400,
69120 Heidelberg, Germany

M. Schmitter
Department of Prosthodontics,
Dental School Ruprecht-Karls-University of Heidelberg,
Im Neuenheimer Feld 400,
69120 Heidelberg, Germany

5.2 Development of the Evidence-Based Model

Clinicians should have a basic understanding of statistical methods and study designs enabling critical assessment of the scientific literature. This knowledge should be good enough to enable the reader to understand whether or not a specific statistical approach was correctly used in the original study or systematic review. There are books [5, 6] that give a good introduction to important aspects of statistics in clinical research.

F. Chiappelli et al. (eds.), *Evidence-Based Practice: Toward Optimizing Clinical Outcomes*,
DOI: 10.1007/978-3-642-05025-1_5, © Springer-Verlag Berlin Heidelberg 2010

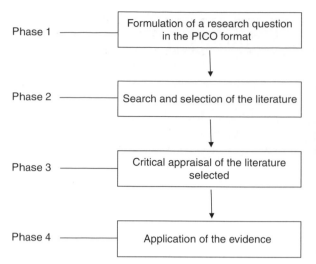

Phase 1 —————— Formulation of a research question
                in the PICO format

Phase 2 —————— Search and selection of the literature

Phase 3 —————— Critical appraisal of the literature
                selected

Phase 4 —————— Application of the evidence

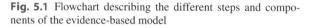

Fig. 5.1 Flowchart describing the different steps and components of the evidence-based model

The model is structured in four main parts: development of a PICO question, literature search and selection of studies, appraisal of the literature selected, and application of the evidence in a clinical setting by use of a decision tree (Fig. 5.1).

5.2.1 PICO Question

A well-developed question in the PICO format may facilitate optimization and application of the evidence-based approach to dental practice. This method also may provide a framework for more effective literature search [7].

The PICO question was formulated as follows:

P (patient): adults with peri-implantitis.
I (intervention): surgical intervention.
C (comparison): nonsurgical intervention.
O (outcomes): clinical attachment level gain, pocket probing depth (PPD) reduction, and implant survival.

"In patients with peri-implantitis which is the most effective treatment (surgical or nonsurgical approach) with regard to PPD reduction, probing attachment level (PAL) change, and dental implant survival?"

The question should be sufficiently focused to enable the clinician to search for evidence that answers the problem for a specific patient or population.

5.2.2 Search Process and Selection of the Studies

The literature search strategy should be sensitive enough to retrieve all relevant literature that can help answer our PICO question. It should also be specific enough to retrieve only literature relevant to the topic in question. The key to a good search strategy is the balance between these two concepts. A busy clinician does not have time to filter all irrelevant information from a very sensitive literature search.

For the topic presented, we used two pairs of key words, "peri-implantitis" and "review" and "peri-implantitis" and "review," in the PubMed and CENTRAL electronic databases on 1st January 2009. We limited our search to systematic reviews (SRs) in English. We also conducted a manual search to assess literature references in the SRs selected.

We searched for SRs of RCTs on treatment of peri-implantitis. Narrative reviews and consensus reports were excluded, as also were SRs that involved trials on animals.

5.2.3 Appraisal of the Studies Selected

After selection of the literature, we assessed its methodological quality using three standardized checklists:

1. The Critical Appraisal Skills Programme (CASP). This was developed by professionals with backgrounds in public health, epidemiology, or evidence-based practice. CASP tools specifically developed for assessing different research designs were divided into three sections related to internal validity, results, and relevance to practice (http://www.phru.nhs.uk/Pages/PHD/FAQs.htm). The authors of CASP claim the tools were developed to help with the process of critically appraising articles on seven types of research: systematic reviews, RCTs, qualitative research, economic evaluation studies, cohort studies, case-control studies, and diagnostic test studies. In our specific case, for obvious reasons, only the checklist related to assessment of systematic reviews was used (Table 5.1).
2. Quality of Reporting of Meta-analysis (QUOROM). This checklist was developed, by consensus, by a group of health professionals that included clinical epidemiologists, clinicians, statisticians, editors,

Table 5.1 CASP checklist

Did the review ask a clearly focused question?
Did the review include the right type of study?
Did the reviewers try to identify all relevant studies?
Did the reviewers assess the quality of the studies included?
If the results of the studies have been combined, was it reasonable to do so?
How are the results presented and what is the main result?
How precise are these results?
Can the results be applied to the local population?
Were all important outcomes considered?
Should policy or practice change as a result of the evidence contained in this review?

and researchers [8]. It consists of eighteen headings and subheadings (Table 5.2) and describes the ideal way of presenting the sections of a systematic review (abstract, introduction, methods, results, and discussion). Authors of QUOROM suggest the use of the checklist to provide sound and reproducible results in systematic reviews and meta-analysis of RCTs [8].

3. The Assessment of Multiple Systematic Reviews (AMSTAR). This checklist comprises 11 items derived from 37 items (Table 5.3). The tool is based on empirical evidence and expert consensus and has been externally validated [9].

Checklists were scored YES (assessed criterion was met in the systematic review), NO (assessed criterion

Table 5.2 QUOROM checklist

Title identifies the report as a meta-analysis (or systematic review) of RCTs
The abstract uses a structured format
The abstract describes the clinical question explicitly
The abstract describes the databases and other information sources
The abstract describes the review methods (the selection criteria (i.e., population, intervention, outcome, and study design), methods for validity assessment, data abstraction, study characteristics, and quantitative data synthesis in sufficient detail to enable replication)
The abstract describes the results (characteristics of the RCTs included and excluded, qualitative and quantitative findings (i.e., point estimates and confidence intervals), and subgroup analyses)
The conclusion of the abstract describes the main results
The introduction of the review describes the explicit clinical problem, the biological rationale for the intervention, and the rationale for the review
The methods section describes the search strategy (the information sources (in detail, e.g., databases, registers, personal files, expert informants, agencies, hand-searching), and any restrictions (years considered, publication status, language of publication)
The methods section describes the selection of studies (the inclusion and exclusion criteria (defining population, intervention, principal outcomes, and study design))
The methods section describes the validity assessment (the criteria and process used (e.g., masked conditions, quality assessment, and their findings))
The methods section describes data abstraction (the process or processes used (e.g., completed independently, in duplicate))
The methods section describes study characteristics (the type of study design, participants' characteristics, details of intervention, outcome definitions, and how clinical heterogeneity was assessed)
The methods section describes quantitative data synthesis (the principal measures of effect, method of combining results (statistical testing and confidence intervals), handling of missing data, how statistical heterogeneity was assessed, a rationale for any a-priori sensitivity and subgroup analyses, and any assessment of publication bias)
The results section shows a trial flow (flowchart figure)
The results section demonstrates study characteristics (descriptive data for each trial (e.g., age, sample size, intervention, dose, duration, follow-up period))
The results section describes quantitative data synthesis (report agreement on the selection and validity assessment; presents simple summary results (for each treatment group in each trial, for each primary outcome); presents data needed to calculate effect sizes and confidence intervals in intention-to-treat analyses (e.g., 2×2 tables of counts, means and SDs, proportions))
The discussion section summarizes key findings; discusses clinical inferences based on internal and external validity; interprets the results on the basis of all the available evidence; describes potential biases in the review process (e.g., publication bias); and suggests a future research agenda

Table 5.3 AMSTAR checklist

Was an "a-priori" design provided? The research question and inclusion criteria should be established before the review is conducted

Was there duplicate study selection and data extraction? There should be at least two independent data extractors and a consensus procedure for disagreements should be in place

Was a comprehensive literature search performed? At least two electronic sources should be searched. The report must include years and databases used (e.g., Central, EMBASE, and MEDLINE). Key words and/or MESH terms must be stated, and where feasible, the search strategy should be provided. All searches should be supplemented by consulting current contents, reviews, textbooks, specialized registers, or experts in the particular field of study, and by reviewing the references in the studies found

Was the status of publication (i.e., grey literature) used as an inclusion criterion? The authors should state that they searched for reports irrespective of publication type. The authors should state whether or not they excluded any reports (from the systematic review), on the basis of publication status, language, etc.

Was a list of studies (included and excluded) provided? A list of included and excluded studies should be provided

Were the characteristics of the included studies provided? In an aggregated form such as a table, data from the original studies should be provided on the participants, interventions, and outcomes. The ranges of characteristics in all the studies analyzed, e.g., age, race, sex, relevant socioeconomic data, disease status, duration, severity, or other diseases, should be reported

Was the scientific quality of the included studies assessed and documented? "A-priori" methods of assessment should be provided (e.g., for effectiveness studies if the author(s) chose to include only randomized, double-blind, placebo-controlled studies, or allocation concealment as inclusion criteria); for other types of studies, alternative items will be relevant

Was the scientific quality of the included studies used appropriately in formulating conclusions? The methodological rigor and scientific quality should be considered in the analysis and the conclusions of the review, and explicitly stated in formulating recommendations

Were the methods used to combine the findings of studies appropriate? For the pooled results, a test should be performed to ensure the studies were combinable and assess their homogeneity (i.e., chi-squared test for homogeneity, I2). If heterogeneity exists, a random effects model should be used and/or the clinical appropriateness of combining should be taken into consideration (i.e., is it sensible to combine?).

Was the likelihood of publication bias assessed? Assessment of publication bias should include a combination of graphical aids (e.g., funnel plot, other available tests) and/or statistical tests (e.g., Egger regression test)

Was the conflict of interest stated? Potential sources of support should be clearly acknowledged in both the systematic review and the studies included

was not met), cannot tell (when the information was unclear), or not applicable. The methodological quality was determined from the percentage of YES scores in each assessed study.

5.2.4 Statistical Analysis

We realize that interrater agreement is pivotal when a specific grade of reliability in the assessment of the quality of selected literature is expected. In other words, we become more confident when results may be reproduced by other colleagues using the same assessment strategy. Therefore, the quality of the methodology was assessed in duplicate by two referees and the interclass correlation-coefficient (ICC) was used to measure the level of agreement between the referees on all questions in the checklists. The level of agreement was considered good when the ICC was >0.8, substantial when it was 0.6–0.8, moderate when it was 0.4–0.6, fair when it was 0.2–0.4, and poor when it was <0.2 [10].

5.3 Results from Assessment of the Effectiveness and Methodological Quality of SRs

We included only SRs in our assessment because they are regarded the best available evidence for study therapies. After detailed assessment, two SRs [11,12] were retrieved from, initially, 90 potential studies.

5.3.1 Main Results of the Studies Selected

Kotsovilis et al. [11]: This SR demonstrated that the use of an ER:YAG laser might be superior to standard therapy (mechanical debridement/chlorhexidine) only with regard to bleeding on probing (BOP) reduction. These results are considered after six months of therapy. For the other therapy (minocycline+mechanical debridement), there was no clinically relevant difference from mechanical debridement only. Surgical therapy (e.g., open flap+guided tissue regeneration– GTR) resulted in greater PPD reduction and CAL gain than nonsurgical approaches, at least after 6 months.

Esposito et al. [12]: This SR demonstrated that PPD reduction and CAL gain occurred after regenerative procedures for a period of six months. Surgical therapy usually resulted in more PPD reduction and CAL gain than conservative approaches, for example, mechanical debridement with implant scalers.

There were also improvements in PPD reduction and PAL in more severe cases when antibiotics were combined with mechanical debridement.

The authors of both SRs agree that the RCTs included have several methodological limitations (for example, small sample size/lack of power calculation, lack of true randomization), which can interfere with the reliability of the evidence presented.

5.3.2 Agreement Between Referees

Inter-observer agreement on the individual items from the checklists ranged from substantial to good. ICC scores for CASP, QUOROM, and AMSTAR were 0.73 (CI = 0.22–0.91), 0.93 (CI = 0.87–0.97), and 0.60 (CI = 0.25–0.83), respectively.

5.3.3 Methodological Quality of SRs

When conducting clinical research, researchers should pay attention to several "rules" to avoid introducing bias into study results. For example, a clinical study can truly be nominated as an RCT only when all the procedures related to the randomization process (sequence generation, allocation concealment, and implementation) are well conducted. This information should also be reported by the researchers in the paper presenting the results of the research. Study results should usually be replicated by an independent group, using the same methodology as the group of researchers who conducted the original research. This characteristic of reproducibility makes the study results more reliable and convincing.

In good medical and dental journals, there is a trend toward requiring researchers to follow the CONSORT (Consolidated Standards of Reporting Trials) statement [13] when conducting RCTs. This statement comprises a checklist containing 22 items that can be compared directly for different sections of the study. The authors of CONSORT suggest the use of the checklist for two reasons:

1. Because empirical evidence indicates that not reporting the information is associated with biased estimates of the effect of treatment, or
2. Because the information is essential for judging the reliability or relevance of the findings.

Some evidence also suggests that the use of the CONSORT statement may be associated with improvements in the quality of reports of RCTs [13].

In the evidence-based model presented, only SRs were selected and, therefore, checklists developed for study reviews were used for the assessment of the methodological quality and the report. On average, more criteria were met in the Esposito study than in the Kotsovilis study and the assessment, therefore, suggests that the methodological quality of the former SR is better than that of the latter.

5.4 Applying Evidence in a Clinical Setting

Dental practitioners should use practical tools to apply evidence found in the scientific literature directly in the clinical setting. Guidelines or clinical recommendations have been suggested for assisting dentists in the decision-making process. These are usually supported by dental associations or organizations [14–17] and have been developed by a group of experts in the field.

Although guidelines can provide valuable information for dentists, they are very heterogeneous in quality and there is, currently, a lack of guidelines supporting most conventional dental procedures [18]. Furthermore, barriers may prevent the use of guidelines in private practice. For example, clinicians seem to be concerned that using guidelines may limit their autonomy in making clinical decisions [19]. Nevertheless, to increase the reliability of guidelines, they should be updated frequently—as soon as new information becomes available [20]. In dentistry, guidelines are not updated frequently [18] and clinicians are at risk of making decisions on the basis of out of date information. We will describe an approach that can have advantages in relation to guidelines.

5.4.1 Decision Tree Approach

Broadly defined, an algorithm is a step-by-step procedure for solving a specific problem. In medicine and dentistry, algorithms may play an important role in the decision-making process by providing a graphical description of several steps presented in tools created to link evidence to clinical practice, for example, guidelines [21].

Decision trees allow different "routes" of treatment depending on therapy response. For example, we can initially treat peri-implantitis with a more conservative approach, for example, mechanical debridement. This initial decision was based on information from a selected SR which concluded that mechanical debridement is effective in the treatment of peri-implantitis. If the first decision does not result in any improvement, or even results in worsening, of the clinical situation, the dentist may change the treatment by using more complex therapy (Fig. 5.2). In fact, the clinician can use a clinically relevant threshold (for example, a change of 1 mm PPD from baseline to after therapy) to define the success or lack of success of treatment.

5.4.2 Advantages of Decision Trees

- Decision trees can be developed as clinicians' "own" guidelines for every relevant dental procedure.
- Decision trees can be updated as soon as clinicians deem necessary.
- Clinicians can visualize the several treatment possibilities.

5.5 Discussion

To be useful, evidence should be systematically assessed and correctly applied to the clinical situation. It is intended that the model presented in this chapter should contribute to the evidence-based learning process for dental practitioners.

The huge number of dental studies reported every year makes understanding of all relevant literature by clinicians almost impossible. Systematic reviews and metaanalysis play a pivotal role in providing clinicians with the best available information for making decisions. Even systematic reviews are prone to bias [22] and dentists need to develop sufficient skill to enable critical assessment of the methodological quality of these studies. Many busy dental practitioners access only the abstract or authors' conclusions to obtain results and recommendations for clinical practice. This approach can be misleading, however, because information given in the abstract sometimes does not match the information in the full-text article. In addition, authors' conclusions can be biased and it is imperative that clinicians recognize the importance of scrutinizing all parts of the manuscript.

The proposed model adds important issues to assessment and application of evidence. For example, checklists such as CASP, QUOROM, and AMSTAR can provide information about the quality of the reporting and the methodology of the review. For both SRs, the methodological quality was regarded as good. In this specific instance, we had two systematic reviews with homogeneous results, and the checklists enabled us to decide whether or not the methodology of the studies was good. Checklists may, however, also be a valuable tool enabling decision between two SRs reporting heterogeneous results on the same topic. If we need to decide between two studies, the logical rationale would be to choose the study with the best methodology.

Inter-observer agreement is essential for reliable assessment of data, and clinicians should work in partnership with colleagues while selecting and assessing the scientific literature. In our assessment, ICC scores between two referees range from substantial to good. This indicates that reviewers were homogeneous in their assessment, suggesting that results from assessment using checklists may be reproducible.

Clinicians should, however, be aware that, although RCTs occupy a high position in the hierarchy of evidence [23], they do not always provide high-quality

Fig. 5.2 Example of evidence-based decision tree (algorithm) in the treatment of peri-implantitis. In this example, we assumed that treatment A is initially less expensive than B, and B less expensive than C. As we did not find any patient-oriented evidence for peri-implantitis treatment, this "route" was blocked. The first-line therapy is highlighted in *green*

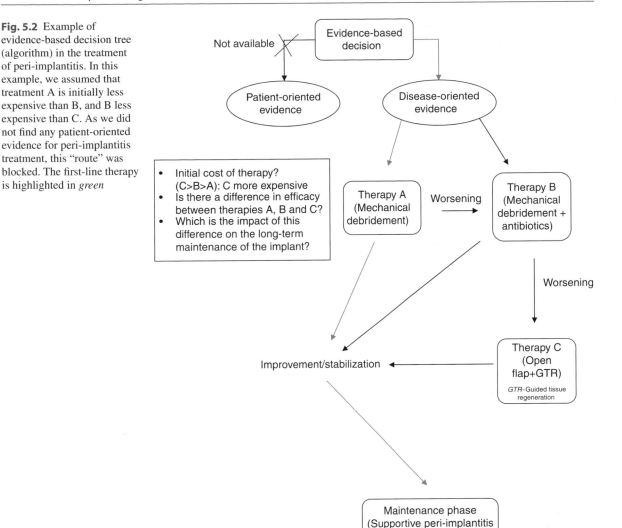

evidence. Sometimes the methodological development of a study is so poor that any definitive conclusion about its results may be misleading. This was true for studies included in both reviews which have several deficiencies in design (e.g., small sample size, short follow-up, lack of true randomization). It is crucial, therefore, to differentiate the methodological quality of SRs and the quality of evidence of studies included in the SRs. In contrast with results from poorly designed RCTs, robust treatment of effects derived from studies with lower hierarchy (for example, case-series) may generate more reliable evidence [24].

The decision to start with less complex therapy (mechanical debridement) for treatment of peri-implantitis seems reasonable, because more conser-vative therapy has been proved to be effective. Although outcomes from surgical procedures were better than those from nonsurgical procedures, we cannot deter-mine with precision whether surgical therapy will, in fact, be the best treatment in the long term. This can be proved only when true outcomes, for example implant failure, are assessed rather than surrogate outcomes, for example PPD and CAL changes [25]. Patient-oriented evidence (for example, evidence derived from true outcomes such as implant failure or quality of life) is, in fact, regarded as one of the key factors enabling determination of the strength of a recommendation based on a body of evidence [26]. Patient-oriented out-comes are a requirement for giving a recommendation an A grade (i.e., strong) [26].

The two SRs selected did not clearly report implant failure as primary outcomes, although some information on implant failure was presented. Hence, this disease-oriented evidence could only lead to a C grade recommendation (the weakest level in the SORT classification). Information on grading the quality of evidence and the strength of recommendations will be given later in the chapter.

This model is intended to fill the gap between what is frequently published and what is, in fact, relevant to clinical decisions. Applying the concepts of EBD to dental practice is a lifelong learning process in which dentists should also be skilled in subjects other than implant-placement technique. Knowledge of statistics and epidemiology is necessary to effectively understand the quality of published evidence.

5.6 Grading the Quality of Evidence and the Strength of Recommendations

Systems have been developed for making judgments about the quality of evidence and the strength of recommendations. The strength of a recommendation is the extent to which the clinician can be confident that following the recommendation will do more good than harm to the patient. In this context, it is important to make clear that high-quality evidence does not always lead to the strongest recommendation. For example, in the grading system called SORT, SRs graded as high-quality evidence of surrogate end points such as PPD or CAL changes result in grade C (the weakest recommendation), because these types of outcomes are related to efficacy instead of efficiency and in most cases they do not represent improvements in patient-oriented outcomes [26].

We will provide a brief discussion of two systems for grading evidence and recommending treatment strategies.

5.6.1 SORT

The strength of recommendation taxonomy, or SORT, approach is founded in three key elements: quality, quantity, and consistency of evidence [26]. The authors

of SORT, who represent the major family medicine journals in the United States and a large family medicine academic consortium, created a grading scale that could be used by readers with different expertise in evidence-based medicine and clinical epidemiology.

SORT classifies evidence into three levels:

- Level 1 – RCTs and SRs of RCTs with good quality, patient-oriented evidence
- Level 2 – SRs and RCTs of low quality, and cohort and case-control studies based on patient-oriented evidence
- Level 3 – Disease-oriented evidence (the lowest evidence, e.g., PPD and CAL changes)

The taxonomy includes ratings of A, B, or C for the strength of a recommendation of a body of evidence, with the A rating being the strongest recommendation. To distinguish between grades A and B, it is necessary to consider two other factors (quality of individual studies and consistency of evidence across all the studies being evaluated) to determine the final SORT grade.

5.6.2 GRADE

The grading of recommendations assessment, development, and evaluation (GRADE) developed from informal collaboration of people with an interest in addressing the shortcomings of current grading systems in health care. GRADE uses study design, study quality, consistency, and directness to judge the quality of evidence [24]. To grade the quality of evidence, the GRADE approach initially uses study design as reference. RCTs, therefore, start as high-level evidence, but other considerations such as limited study quality, inconsistency of results, imprecise or sparse data, and high risk of reporting bias can reduce the quality of the evidence.

The authors of GRADE suggest two degrees of recommendation—strong and weak. Four factors, however, may affect the strength of the recommendation [27]:

- The balance between desirable and undesirable effects—the larger the difference between the desirable and undesirable effects, the more likely a strong recommendation is warranted.

- The quality of the evidence—the higher the quality of the evidence, the more likely a strong recommendation is warranted.
- Values and preferences—the more variability in values and preferences, or the more uncertainty in values and preferences, the more a weak recommendation is warranted.
- Costs (resource allocation)—the higher the costs of an intervention, the less a strong recommendation is warranted.

5.6.3 The Usefulness of Both Systems in Dentistry

As already reported, assessment of the quality of reporting or the methodology of SRs (and other studies) by the use of checklists may be straightforward with good reliability between appraisers. In contrast, achieving good reliability in grading quality and providing levels of strength of recommendations from the evidence of the original studies or studies included in an SR are not easy tasks.

Determining the grade of evidence with the GRADE system depends on the assessment of at least nine variables [24] that can reduce or increase the initial assessment of the evidence on the basis of the type of study. Correct assessment of these variables seems to be more appropriate for researchers and guideline developers than for clinicians. The SORT approach dichotomizes levels of quality on the basis of study design and type of evidence (disease or patient-oriented) [26], consequently reducing the number of variables assessed. It may be easier to achieve reliability between appraisers by use of the SORT approach than by use of the GRADE system. Nevertheless, the inter-rater reliability of both approaches should be assessed by testing among dental practitioners.

Achieving good inter-rater reliability in the assessment of the strength of a recommendation seems to be even more difficult. We realize, however, that the strength of the recommendation is intended to help clinicians and patients to make the best clinical decision together. In this context, inter-rater agreement may not be pivotal, because the strength of recommendations is more based on individual patient needs. Nevertheless, we understand that the process of grading the quality of evidence should, at least, be reproducible, because

the level of evidence will affect the strength of the recommendation.

We suggest testing of both approaches by dental practitioners to assess the level of inter-rater reliability in determining quality of evidence. Strength of recommendations will be more based on the sensitivity of the clinician to the weight of all the variables in the process.

5.7 Economic Evaluation of Dental Health Services

5.7.1 The Rationale for Incorporating Costs in the Decision-Making Process

Imagine a patient who is missing a lower first molar. Intuitively, a clinician will first and foremost ask about the clinical prognosis for each of the treatment options available. At best, the corresponding information process will rely on an evidence-based approach and will tell us which of the interventions has the best clinical prospects. If we were to live in a world without budget restrictions, we would always go for this treatment, which is called the most *effective*. Most often, however, we face monetary limitations alongside a trade-off between health outcomes and costs. In the end, we need to decide whether the higher *effectiveness* of a treatment is worth the additional *costs* in comparison with the next best alternative. In other words, we must identify the most *cost-effective*, i.e., most *efficient*, treatment strategy. Generally speaking, health economic evaluation seeks to maximize the benefits which can be obtained from limited resources for health care or, vice versa, to minimize the costs in order to achieve a specific level of health outcome.

5.7.2 Cost-Effectiveness Analysis vs. Cost–Utility Analysis

A variety of approaches is available for economic evaluation of health care [28]. The two techniques most commonly applied are cost-effectiveness analysis

(CEA) and cost–utility analysis (CUA) [29]. Both methods are similar in requiring a definition of the costs to be included. The corresponding choice depends on the perspective of the decision maker. From the point of view of a health care provider, all costs of a particular intervention must be considered. A broad distinction can be made between *fixed costs*, for example rent of an operating theater, and *variable costs*, for example staff time, equipment used, or length of stay in a hospital or day unit (detailed discussion can be found elsewhere, e.g. [30]).

What makes CEA and CUA conceptually distinct is the definition of treatment consequences.

Whereas CEA builds upon natural units (e.g., implant surveillance or PPD), CUA relies on more general measures that enable comparison of different health conditions and their treatment. The most widely used concept within health care is quality-adjusted life years (QALYs). QALYs incorporate a morbidity weight, which adjusts the time lived with a qualitative measure [31]. Similarly, for dental health it was suggested to use quality-adjusted tooth years (QATYs) [32]. Their prospect is to reflect oral health outcomes as perceived by the patient and, thus, to make different dental conditions and treatments comparable against each other. For instance, a quality adjustment of tooth survival appears relevant when comparing conservative and surgical treatment of periodontal diseases. Specifically, patients may consider conservative intervention less detrimental for their quality of life than surgical intervention. Surgical treatment may, hence, be judged preferrable when relying on tooth survival

only, whereas adjusting tooth years for quality of life may result in the preferability of conservative treatment [33].

5.7.3 Decision Analytical Modeling

There are several ways of structuring the process through which different treatment alternatives lead to corresponding costs and health outcomes. Specifically, Markov models assume that a patient occupies one of a series of defined health states at a given point in time. Each health state specifies a certain cost and health outcome and, as time elapses, transitions from one health state to another occur with preset probabilities. Within this framework, the expected costs and health outcomes can be calculated when weighting the averaged time duration in each health state by the associated costs and health outcomes [33].

The most widely used modeling technique, however, relies on decision trees [34]. These represent individuals' possible prognoses, following some sort of intervention, by a series of pathways. By way of illustration (Fig. 5.3), consider a *stylized* example of CEA for restorative treatment of an upper premolar (assuming the baseline conditions are equal). Besides choosing no treatment, which also has no costs ("null strategy"), two treatment alternatives are considered:

- Strategy A costs $ 500 and will lead to tooth survival of 15 years.

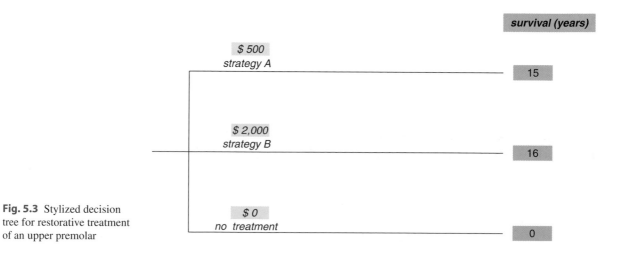

Fig. 5.3 Stylized decision tree for restorative treatment of an upper premolar

- Strategy B costs $ 2,000 and will lead to tooth survival of 16 years.

The given Information translates into a decision tree as illustrated in Fig. 5.1. The key question then is which of the given pathways is most *efficient*. This will be addressed in the next section.

5.7.4 Incremental Cost-Effectiveness Ratios (ICERs)

A frequently used decision rule for identification of the most *cost-effective* treatment strategy relies on the concept of ICERs [35]. Initially, all possible treatment pathways are ranked with regard to increasing costs of the intervention. Following this rank list, pairwise differences between costs ($\Delta C = C_{high-rank} - C_{low-rank}$) and treatment outcomes ($\Delta E = E_{high-rank} - E_{low-rank}$) are calculated. Finally, ICERs are defined by the ratio $\Delta C / \Delta E$. Within our stylized example, this leads to the values shown in Table 5.4.

Here, all ICERs increase with their rank. A strategy for which the ICER is higher than that of the succeeding strategy according to the rank list would be judged as *dominated* and no longer considered as an alternative treatment strategy. This is not the case here, however, and the interpretation is as follows—as long as a decision maker is willing to pay at least $1,500 for one more year of tooth survival, the most cost-effective strategy is treatment pathway (B). If, however, the decision maker is willing to pay more than $ 33.3 but less than $ 1,500 for one more year of tooth survival, treatment pathway (A) would be the most efficient strategy. Generally speaking, a treatment strategy can only be regarded as the most cost-effective when the corresponding ICER is exceeded by the decision maker's willingness to pay or, in other words, by the available resources.

Table 5.4 Costs, tooth survival, and ICERs of different restorative treatment strategies

	Costs ($)	Survival (years)	ΔC	ΔE	ICER
"Null strategy"	0	0	–		
(A)	500	15	500	15	33.3
(B)	2,000	16	1,500	1	1,500

5.8 Conclusions

This chapter presented a systematic approach to evaluating and applying research evidence directly in a clinical setting. Checklists for assessing the quality of the reporting and methodology of studies are important tools for helping clinicians in the decision-making process. Systems for assessing the quality of evidence and the strength of recommendations are also of value, but they should be further developed specifically for the dental field and tested in a clinical setting. Finally, economic aspects of dental treatment should also be taken into account at the moment of decision-making. There is a need for a model that incorporates information about evidence quality/strength of recommendation and the costs of dental procedures.

References

1. American Dental Association. Survey Publications (2009) Vol. 1 Academic Programs, Enrollment and Graduates. Available online at: http://www.ada.org/ada/prod/survey/publications_educational.asp#series
2. Vasak C, Fiederer R, Watzek G (2007) Current state of training for implant dentistry in Europe: a questionnaire-based survey. Clin Oral Implants Res 18(5):following 668
3. Spencer JA, Jordan RK (1999) Learner centred approaches in medical education. BMJ 318(7193):1280–1283
4. Faggion CM Jr. & Schmitter M (2010) Making appropriate evidence-based clinical decisions in implant dentistry, using treatment of peri-implantitis as an example. Int J Oral Maxillofac Implants forthcoming
5. Bland M (2000) An introduction to medical statistics. Oxford University Press, Oxford
6. Bulman JS, Osborn JF (2002) Statistics in dentistry. BDJ Books, London
7. Staunton M (2007) Evidence-based radiology: steps 1 and 2–asking answerable questions and searching for evidence. Radiology 242(1):23–31
8. Moher D, Cook DJ, Eastwood S et al (1999) Improving the quality of reports of meta-analyses of randomised controlled trials: the QUOROM statement. Quality of reporting of meta-analyses. Lancet 354(9193):1896–1900
9. Shea BJ, Bouter LM, Peterson J et al (2007) External validation of a measurement tool to assess systematic reviews (AMSTAR). PLoS ONE;2(12):e1350
10. Fleiss J (1986) The design and analysis of clinical experiments. Wiley, New York
11. Kotsovilis S, Karoussis IK, Trianti M, Fourmousis I (2008) Therapy of peri-implantitis: a systematic review. J Clin Periodontol 35(7):621–629
12. Esposito M, Grusovin MG, Kakisis I et al (2008) Interventions for replacing missing teeth: treatment of perimplantitis. Cochrane Database Syst Rev 16(2):CD004970

13. Moher D, Schulz KF, Altman D; CONSORT Group (Consolidated Standards of Reporting Trials) (2001) The CONSORT statement: revised recommendations for improving the quality of reports of parallel-group randomized trials. JAMA 285(15):1987–1991

14. ADA Council on Scientific Affairs. Dental mercury hygiene recommendations (2003). J Am Dent Assoc 134(11): 1498–1499

15. American Dental Association Council on Scientific Affairs (2006) Professionally applied topical fluoride: evidence-based clinical recommendations. J Am Dent Assoc 137(8):1151–1159

16. De Boever JA, Nilner M, Orthlieb JD, Steenks MH (2008). Educational Committee of the European Academy of Craniomandibular Disorders. Recommendations by the EACD for examination, diagnosis, and management of patients with temporomandibular disorders and orofacial pain by the general dental practitioner. J Orofac Pain 22(3):268–278

17. Academy of Osseointegration; Committee for the Development of Dental Implant Guidelines; American Academy of Periodontology, Iacono VJ, Cochran SE, Eckert MR, Wheeler SL (2008) Guidelines for the provision of dental implants. Int J Oral Maxillofac Implants 23(3):471–473

18. Faggion CM Jr (2008) Clinician assessment of guidelines that support common dental procedures. J Evid Based Dent Pract 8(1):1–7

19. van der Sanden WJ, Mettes DG, Plasschaert AJ et al (2003) Clinical practice guidelines in dentistry: opinions of dental practitioners on their contribution to the quality of dental care. Qual Saf Health Care 12(2):107–111

20. Shekelle PG, Ortiz E, Rhodes S et al (2001) Validity of the Agency for Healthcare Research and Quality clinical practice guidelines: how quickly do guidelines become outdated? JAMA 286(12):1461–1467

21. Oxman AD, Schünemann HJ, Fretheim A (2006) Improving the use of research evidence in guideline development: 8. Synthesis and presentation of evidence. Health Res Policy Syst 4:20

22. Sterne JA, Egger M, Smith GD (2001) Systematic reviews in health care: investigating and dealing with publication and other biases in meta-analysis. BMJ 323(7304):101–105

23. Concato J, Shah N, Horwitz RI (2000) Randomized, controlled trials, observational studies, and the hierarchy of research designs. N Engl J Med 342(25):1887–1892

24. Atkins D, Best D, Briss PA et al (2004) Grading quality of evidence and strength of recommendations. BMJ 328(7454): 1490

25. Hujoel PP, DeRouen TA (1995) A survey of endpoint characteristics in periodontal clinical trials published 1988-1992, and implications for future studies. J Clin Periodontol 22(5):397–407

26. Ebell MH, Siwek J, Weiss BD et al (2004) Strength of recommendation taxonomy (SORT): a patient-centered approach to grading evidence in the medical literature. J Am Board Fam Pract 17(1):59–67

27. Jaeschke R, Guyatt GH, Dellinger P et al (2008) Use of GRADE grid to reach decisions on clinical practice guidelines when consensus is elusive. BMJ 337:a744

28. Brazier J, Ratcliffe J, Salomon JA, Tsuchiya A (2007) Measuring and valuing health benefits for economic evaluation. Oxford University Press, Oxford

29. Drummond MF, Sculpher MJ, Torrance GW et al (2005) Methods for the economic evaluation of health care programmes. Oxford University Press, Oxford

30. Raikou M, McGuire A (2006) Estimating costs for economic evaluation. In: Jones AM (ed). The Elgar companion to health economics. Edward Elgar Publishing, Cheltenham (UK), Northampton (USA)

31. Pliskin J, Shepard D, Weinstein M (1980) Utility functions for life years and health status. Oper Res 28(1):206–224

32. Birch S (1986) Measuring dental health: Improvements on the DMF-index. Community Dent Health 3:303–311

33. Briggs A, Sculpher M (1998) An introduction to Markov modelling for economic evaluation. Pharmacoeconomics 13(4):397–409

34. Briggs A, Sculpher M, Claxton K (2006) Decision modelling for health economic evaluation. Oxford University Press, Oxford

35. Weinstein M (2006) Decision rules for incremental cost-effectiveness analysis. In: Jones AM (ed) The Elgar companion to health economics. Edward Elgar Publishing, Cheltenham (UK), Northampton (USA)

Evidence-Based Decisions in Human Immunodeficiency Virus Infection and Cardiac Disease

6

Raluca Arimie and Zohreh Movahedi

Core Message

> HIV infection and AIDS in the United States and worldwide still remains an important health issue. High number of infected persons, difficulty of treatment, and other co morbidity factors might increase the risk of cardiovascular diseases.

> Little is known about cardiovascular system involvement in HIV infected and AIDS patients. Patients with AIDS can have cardiac pathology related to opportunistic infections and tumors as well as that related to antiviral medication (highly active antiretroviral therapy, for short HAART).

6.1 Epidemiology

Globally, 33 million people were estimated to be living with HIV in 2007 and over one million HIV patients live in the United States. In 2008, Center for Disease Control (CDC) estimated that approximately 56,300 people were newly infected with HIV. Over half of these new infections (53%) occurred in gay and bisexual men. African American population was strongly affected and was estimated to have a high incidence rate which is more than 7 times higher than whites. There was estimation that 47% of the persons living with HIV were black, 34% were white, and 17% were Hispanic. Asians/Pacific Islanders and American Indians/Alaska Natives each represented roughly 1% of the HIV-infected population.

Most men (60%) acquired the infection by homosexual behavior, followed by 27% persons infected through high-risk heterosexual contact, 22% through injection drug use, 5% were exposed through both male-to-male sexual contact and injection drug use. Most women (75%) acquire the infection from heterosexual sex.

Young people aged 15–35 account for an estimated 25% of new HIV infections.

Approximately, one-fourth (25%) of HIV-infected persons are believed to be unaware of their infection [15].

It is very interesting that in Africa, the incidence of AIDS-related cardiac disease is very high compared to that seen in western developed countries. For instance, in the period from 1993 to 1999 in Burkina Faso (West Africa), 79% of the AIDS patients exhibited heart involvement, including myocarditis and cardiomyopathy, whereas in an Italian study in the period from 1992 to 1995, the incidence of AIDS-related cardiac disease was 6.5%.

The frequency of cardiac manifestations is influenced by different variables including: survival prolongation in HIV-infected patients, because of advances in antiretroviral treatment and reduction in the occurrence of opportunistic infections [89].

With the introduction of highly active antiretroviral therapy (HAART), patients are living longer and other comorbidities such as hypertension, metabolic abnormalities including hyperglycemia, hyperlipidemia, and

R. Arimie (✉)
Z. Movahedi
Department of Cardiology,
Internal Medicine, University of California Los Angeles,
1245 16th Street, # 307, Santa Monica, CA 90404, USA
e-mail: rarimie@mednet.ucla.edu

F. Chiappelli et al. (eds.), *Evidence-Based Practice: Toward Optimizing Clinical Outcomes*,
DOI: 10.1007/978-3-642-05025-1_6, © Springer-Verlag Berlin Heidelberg 2010

Fig. 6.1 As the frequency of the use of antiretroviral therapy, including PIs, increased in HIV–infected patients, their mortality during this same time period decreased [107]

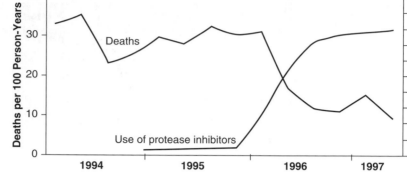

lipodystrophy increase the risk of cardiovascular diseases [30, 107].

Since the introduction of the HAART, the mortality rate has decreased and is shown in Fig. 6.1 [78].

6.2 Pericarditis

The most frequent clinical manifestation of cardiovascular disease in patients with AIDS is pericardial disease. Pericardial effusion is the most frequent type of effusion associated with HIV in about one third of cases [16]. Echocardiographic studies have identified a pericardial effusion in approximately 20% of these patients [53, 97].

Incidence of pericardial effusion in HIV patients before the introduction of treatment with HAART was found to be 11% per year in one study [47]. The incidence after introducing HAART is unknown [88].

The picture of clinical pericarditis is similar to that of pericarditis from etiologies other than HIV. Some patients are symptomatic with fever, pleuritic chest pain. However, most patients present with an asymptomatic increase in the cardiac silhouette on chest X-ray.

Patients with pericardial effusion have shorter 6 month survival rate than AIDS patients without pericardial effusion (36% vs. 93%) [88]. Overall, the development of pericardial effusion in a patient with AIDS is a bad prognostic sign, even if asymptomatic [14, 46].

6.3 Coronary Artery Disease

6.3.1 Clinical Features of CAD in HIV Patients

Typical HIV patient with coronary artery disease is a male, smoker, with very low HDL cholesterol, and significantly younger than non-HIV patients with coronary artery disease. The main studies addressing these features are summarized in Table 6.1 [88].

HIV-infected patients with acute coronary syndromes differ in several ways from other ACS patients. Apart from being more than a decade younger than controls, the HIV patients were more likely to be male and current smokers and have low HDL cholesterol. Although they have less extensive coronary disease, they have a significantly higher rate of restenosis after PCI than other ACS patients.

The most common presentation of CAD among patients with HIV disease is myocardial infarction (MI), and 67% of HIV patients presented with acute MI. It is interesting that majority of cases are males; only 9% were females.

In a small French study, patients treated with PIs had almost a threefold increase in the risk of MI compared with untreated HIV-infected patients, suggesting that rapidly forming drug-induced plaques are unstable and prone to rupture [75].

A retrospective analysis of two large cohorts of patients with HIV infection over the course of an

Table 6.1 Clinical features of coronary disease in HIV patients [35]

Study	Patients (n)	Age (years)	Current smoking (%)	CD4 count (cells/mm^3)	PI use (%)	MI on presentation (n) (%)	Single-vessel disease (n) (%)
David et al. [53]	16	43*	81	234 (74–731)*	69	8/16 (50)	NA
Matetzky et al. [88]	24	47±9	58	318±210	71	24 (100)	5/21 (24)
Escaut et al. [46]	17	46±6	71	272±185	65	11/17 (65)	9/17 (53)
Mehta et al. [82]	129[a]	42±10	NA	313±209	NA	82/106 (77)	26/76 (35)
Ambrose et al. [14]	51	48±9	55	426±290	59	34/51 (67)	21/45 (47)
Varriale et al. [54]	29	46±10	55	>500 in 18/29	66	29 (100)	NA
Hsue et al. [108]	68	50±8	68	341 (3–4360)*	49	37/68 (54)	20/56 (36)

NA not reported

*Median value; all other values are means

[a]Patients drawn from 25 previous reports

8-year period showed that MI rates in patients receiving PI therapy were 5 times greater than MI rates in those not on such therapy [59]. This relative increase risk was explained partly by dyslipidemia [110].

Regarding cholesterol profile in HIV patients with acute coronary syndrome, mean HDL cholesterol level was very low, reported between 28 and 35 mg/dL, which is significantly lower than those of HIV patients without coronary artery disease and lower than non-HIV control patients with coronary artery disease. In one study, mean LDL was much higher in these HIV patients in comparison with those without coronary artery disease.

In one report, HIV patients diagnosed with acute coronary syndrome, on an average are 11 years younger than control non-HIV patients with acute coronary syndrome.

The HIV patients have frequent single coronary artery disease, low TIMI score (blood flow in the coronary artery which is determined by angiogram). Coronary angiogram and revascularization has the same indications as in non-HIV patient with coronary artery disease. Coronary angioplasty and stent placement have very good immediate results. Interestingly, HIV-infected patients who had undergone coronary percutaneous intervention had a significantly higher rate of restenosis compared with their HIV-negative counterparts, after both balloon angioplasty and bare metal stent placement; data are not available for the drug eluting stent [88]. For example, in one study, restenosis has developed in 15 of 29 HIV patients compared with 3 of 21 non-HIV patients. It means that the rate of restenosis in HIV patients is 52% vs. 14% in non-HIV patients ($p=0.006$) [54].

Regarding coronary artery revascularization by coronary bypass surgery, no long-term follow-up data are available [88]. Median age for bypass surgery HIV patients was 44 years [54].

6.3.2 Cardiovascular Risk Factors in HIV Patients

Many studies have demonstrated high rates of cardiovascular risk factors in patients with HIV infection. Some of these, such as dyslipidemia, diabetes mellitus, hypertension, chronic inflammation, altered immune system function, and metabolic syndrome, may be related to HIV infection or to HIV therapies. Others, such as high smoking rates, are independent of HIV infection. More than half of HIV patients are smokers at the time of the coronary event. Dyslipidemia and alterations in serum lipid values have been reported in HIV-infected patients.

Lower CD4 count in untreated HIV patients are associated with lower total cholesterol, lower HDL, and higher TG [43].

The proportion of patients receiving Protease Inhibitors (PIs) ranged from 49 to 71%.

In one study, a 10-year coronary heart disease risk of >20% was twice as common among patients receiving combination antiviral therapy (ART) as in a matched control group without HIV infection, 11.9% vs. 5.3%, respectively [54].

In one report of HIV-infected patients, total choles-terol exceeded 240 mg/dL in 27% of those receiving a PI, 23% of those receiving an NNRTI, 44% of those receiv-ing a PI and an NNRTI, and 10% of those receiving only an NRTI, compared with 8% of patients not receiving ART [70]. Triglyceride levels above 200 mg/dL were present in 40% of PI-treated patients, 32% of those treated with NNRTIs, 54% of those receiving both PIs and NNRTIs, 23% of NRTI-treated patients, and 15% of the untreated.

Insulin resistance and hyperglycemia appear to be more common in persons with HIV infection than in uninfected individuals. Patients receiving ART may have even higher rates of insulin resistance and diabe-tes, and certain ARV medications, such as Indinavir, may confer greater risk than others [81, 111].

Hypertension occurs in up to one third of patients with HIV infection [37, 57]. NNRTIs or PIs have been linked to hypertension in some studies but not in others [13, 17, 57]. The hypertension associated with HIV appears to be linked to insulin resistance and the meta-bolic syndrome [37].

6.3.3 Pathogenesis of Atherosclerosis in HIV Patients

HIV disease is in itself atherogenic which is associated with accelerated T-cell proliferation, heightened T-cell activation, and high levels of inflammatory markers [45, 48]. T lymphocytes play a key role in partheno-genesis [44, 56, 112]. CD4 cell activation promotes atherosclerosis through proinflammatory cytokines such as tumor necrosis factor and interleukins [36]. Chronic low-grade inflammation accelerates athero-sclerosis [71]. C-reactive protein levels are higher in HIV patients than in control subjects [55]. Some data indicate that C-reactive protein is an active participant in the process of atherosclerosis [84, 113].

Monocyte chemoattractant protein-1 is a potent activator of macrophages and monocytes, stimulating them to migrate to the subendothelial space where they begin phagocytosis of modified lipoproteins to become lipid-laden foam cells, an early step in atherogenesis. Among HIV patients with subclinical atherosclerosis by carotid and femoral ultrasound, monocyte chemoat-tractant protein-1 plasma levels were higher compared with HIV patients without atherosclerosis [1].

Coagulation abnormalities are another factor that would predispose HIV patients to thrombotic events [99]. Protein S deficiency is the most common, reported in 73% of HIV-infected men in 1 study [103]. Serum levels of Von Willebrand factor are higher in untreated HIV patients than in control sub-jects, reflecting endothelial activation, but tend to decrease toward normal with HAART. Platelet acti-vation also increases in HIV patients [5]. Smoking cigarettes activates platelets and increases coagula-bility, and smoking rates are very high in HIV patients [88].

So, endothelial dysfunction, inflammation associ-ated with platelets activation and hypercoagulation can explain the increased atherogenesis and thrombosis of the arterial wall in HIV positive patients.

On the other hand, PIs induce deleterious metabolic effects such as dyslipidemia and insulin resistance which has been shown to induce atherosclerosis in HIV patients [12].

6.3.4 Endothelial Dysfunction and HIV Infection

HIV can damage endothelium through several mecha-nisms. Tat protein is a small cationic polypeptide released from infected cells, interacts with different types of receptors present on the surface of endothelial cells, activating signal transduction pathways and triggers the expression of adhesion molecules, vascu-lar endothelial growth factor, and platelet activation factor [94].

Moreover, the death of CD4 T lymphocytes caused by HIV increased the amount of shed membrane parti-cles which induce endothelial dysfunction by reduction in nitric oxide and prostacyclin-induced vasodilatation [6, 74].

6.3.5 Endothelial Dysfunction and HIV Medications

The use of PIs in HIV patients is associated with endothelial dysfunction as assessed by brachial artery flow-mediated vasodilatation. This is mediated, probably, by the atherogenic dyslipidemia induced by PIs [104].

6.3.6 Surrogate Measurement of Atherosclerosis in HIV Patients

6.3.6.1 Carotid Intima-Media Thickness (IMT)

In one study, mean carotid IMT was thicker in HIV patients than in control subjects ($p < 0.001$) [17]. Predictors of thicker IMT in HIV patients included: older age, higher LDL cholesterol, cigarette pack-years, and hypertension. Also, there was a rapid progression of carotid IMT in HIV patients after 1 year, but not in control subjects ($p = 0.002$). The rapid progression of carotid IMT in HIV patients and their thicker baseline values strongly suggests very high rates of coronary and cerebrovascular events.

In this study, carotid IMT correlated with classic risk factors and with low nadir CD4 count [55].

6.4 Metabolic Abnormalities Associated with Antiretroviral Therapy

There are many studies suggesting that chronic HIV therapy is associated with the development of metabolic disturbances, which may have a negative effect on cardiovascular risk.

Hypertension associated with HIV appears to be linked to insulin resistance and metabolic syndrome [37].

Higher rate of MI in young HIV-infected patients receiving PIs have focused interest on the association between HIV infection coronary artery disease and antiretroviral medications. The main studies addressing this issue are summarized in Table 6.2 [88]. Taken

Table 6.2 Studies comparing coronary event rates in HIV patients with vs. without PIs [35]

Study	Patients (n)	Age (years)	Follow-up	Events	Results
Bozette et al. [30]	36,766	NA	40 months	1,207 admissions for CVD	No increase in CVD admissions with PIs or with increase in duration of PI treatment
Coplan et al. [78]	10,986	37 (mean)	1 year	29 MIs	Risk of MI not increased in PI- vs. non-PI-treated patients; OR, 1.69; 95% CI, 0.54–7.48
Holmberg et al. [16]	5,672	42.6 (mean)	3.1 years	21 MIs	Risk of MI increased in PI- vs. non-PI-treated patients; OR, 7.1; 95% CI, 1.6–44.3
DAD Study Group [47]	23,468	39 (median)	1.6 years on PIs	126 MIs	Risk of MI increased with increased exposure to PI combination therapy ($p < 0.001$)
Mary-Krause et al. [97]	34,976	37.7 (mean)	33 months	60 MIs	Risk of MI increased in PI- vs. non-PI-treated patients; OR, 2.56; 95% CI, 1.03–6.34
Klein et al. [33]	4,159	42.6 (mean)	3.6 years	72 CHD events, including 47 MIs	Event rates in PI- vs. non-PI-treated patients similar but increased in HIV patients vs. controls
Barbaro et al. [32]	1551	35.5 (median)	36 months	25 coronary events, including 13 MIs	Risk of MI increased in PI- vs. non-PI-treated patients; RR, 11.5; 95% CI, 2.7–48.5

CVD cardiovascular disease; *OR* odds ratio; *CHD* coronary heart disease together, these studies suggest that the rate of MI is higher in HIV patients taking PIs and this risk increases by lengthening the duration of treatment.

In HIV-infected patients, clinical studies of the effects of PIs on lipid levels have shown that PIs increased total cholesterol by 66%, LDL cholesterol by 37%, and triglycerides by 80% at 48 weeks [61]. PIs appear to have drug-specific effects on lipid and glucose metabolism. Some PIs, such as Atazanavir, do not appear to perturb lipid or glucose levels. However, in studies of HIV-uninfected subjects, Ritonavir increased triglycerides and lowered HDL cholesterol slightly, with no increase in LDL cholesterol, whereas Indinavir did not affect lipoproteins but caused insulin resistance [81, 91, 95]. Lopinavir/Ritonavir increased triglycerides without affecting LDL or HDL cholesterol or insulin resistance [67]. Amprenavir had no effect on lipoproteins [95].

Long-term consequences of these metabolic abnormalities result in an increase in coronary events and stroke [88].

In HIV-infected patients, Lipodystrophy can be a possible side effect of Antiretroviral Therapy which is characterized by peripheral fat wasting with fat accumulation in the neck, dorsocervical region, abdomen, and trunk. Its development and severity is strongly associated with the type and duration of therapy.

Lipodystrophy was seen in 20–35% patients after 1–2 years of HAART. Lipodystrophy in HIV patients is associated with metabolic abnormalities such as insulin resistance, impaired glucose tolerance, elevated triglyceride, low HDL, and hypertention.

The most likely regimen to induce severe lipodystrophy is the combination of PI + 2 NRTIs (particularly stavudine+didanosine) [88].

6.5 Treatment of Coronary Risk Factors in HIV Patients

There are no definitive studies at present showing that treatment of traditional coronary risk factors improves outcomes in patients with HIV infection.

The Adult AIDS Clinical Trials group recommends that dyslipidemia be managed according to the guidelines of the National Cholesterol Education Program Adult Treatment Panel III [26]. Certain considerations should guide the selection of lipid-lowering agents in

HIV-infected individuals who are taking PIs. Both PIs and Statins (with the exception of Pravastatin) are metabolized by the cytochrome P450 system. In non-HIV-infected individuals, the combination of Ritonavir/Saquinavir has been shown to increase the area under the curve (AUC) by 30-fold for Simvastatin and by 79% for Atorvastatin, whereas the AUC decreased by 50% for Pravastatin [29]. Simvastatin and lovastatin are contraindicated in patients taking PIs, whereas atorvastatin should be used cautiously, and, if used, should be initiated at low dosage [26]. Pravastatin is safe, but has lower potency with respect to LDL cholesterol lowering. The cholesterol absorption inhibitor Ezetimibe has not been studied in HIV-infected patients, but represents an attractive approach to LDL cholesterol lowering because of its lack of drug–drug interactions. A newer PI, Atazanavir, does not appear to be associated with lipid abnormalities [96]. Thus, switching patients with hyperlipidemia who are on other PIs to Atazanavir represents an alternate approach to lipid management.

Many HIV-infected patients also have elevated triglyceride levels. Fibrates (bezafibrate, fenofibrate, and gemfibrozil) appear to reduce triglycerides effectively in HIV-infected patients receiving ART [7, 40]. Fibrates should be used cautiously in combination with statins because of the increased risk of myopathy. Fibrates are conjugated by glucuronidation with renal elimination. Ritonavir and Nelfinavir are inducers of glucuronidation and could decrease the effect of the Fibrates [27].

Niacin is an alternate option for triglyceride reduction, but may be a poor choice for many HIV patients because of its propensity to worsen blood glucose levels [88].

Hypertriglyceridemia is often accompanied by the other components of the metabolic syndrome: low HDL cholesterol, increased remnant lipoproteins, small LDL particle size, abdominal obesity, hypertension, insulin resistance and glucose intolerance, a proinflammatory state, and a prothrombotic state [41].

There have been a limited number of studies investigating cigarette smoking in HIV-infected patients. The prevalence of cigarette smoking in HIV patients has been reported to be as high as 70–80% in some areas, and HIV-infected persons appear less likely to have contemplated tobacco cessation compared with other smokers [80].

The primary treatment target for the metabolic syndrome is obesity, and the recommended measures include diet and exercise [42]. Even modest reductions in body weight may improve dyslipidemia, hypertension, and glucose intolerance, as well as levels of inflammatory and thrombotic markers [42]. Also smoking cessation should be a major focus of attention in the clinical care of HIV-infected smokers.

6.6 Myocardial Disease

There are three major forms of myocardial disease in patients with AIDS:

- Focal myocarditis
- Echocardiographic evidence of left ventricular dysfunction
- Clinical cardiomyopathy

Clinical dilated cardiomyopathy is seen in approximately 1–3% of patients with AIDS for an annual rate of 1–2% [2, 68, 69, 93, 98].

By multivariate analysis, low socio-economic status, long duration of HIV infection, low CD4 count, HIV viral load, and low plasma level of selenium were factors significantly associated with dilated cardiomyopathy.

It is not clear if HIV-associated disease is due to direct myocardial infection, an autoimmune process induced by HIV or other cardiotropic viruses or coexisting opportunistic infection [51].

In autopsy studies, in the pre-HAART era, myocarditis was identified in more than half of 71 patients evaluated and biventricular dilatation was present in 10% of cases [3].

Histological studies showed evidence of myocyte hypertrophy and myocarditis [24].

Before the use of HAART, congestive heart failure due to HIV-induced left ventricular dysfunction was diagnosed in 2% of all HIV patients, most commonly with lowest CD4 count. Global left ventricular dysfunction was detected by echocardiogram in 15% of randomly selected HIV patients, in one study [50].

Since the introduction of HAART regimens, there has been a marked reduction in the incidence of myocarditis and opportunistic infections, which has led to a nearly 30% reduction in HIV-associated cardiomyopathy [90].

Zidovudine (ZDV) has been demonstrated to cause mitochondrial myopathy in skeletal muscles, and may cause similar dysfunction in myocardial muscle

[25]. Studies performed on transgenic mice suggest that ZDV is associated with diffuse destruction of cardiac mitochondrial ultrastructures and inhibition of cardiac mitochondrial DNA replication [70]. A study of six patients with cardiac dysfunction reported clinical association between cardiac disease and therapy with ZDV and dideoxyinosine (didanosine) [49]. Three patients improved after ZDV was discontinued. However, another study evaluated left ventricular dysfunction by echocardiography in 60 HIV-infected patients with left ventricular dysfunction who were receiving ZDV and in 38 HIV-infected patients not on ZDV. It found that patients receiving ZDV did not have worse left ventricular function or more frequent evidence of diastolic dysfunction than did patients who were not on ZDV [10]. These findings are consistent with those of a previous study by the same investigators showing that ZDV does not affect left ventricular function during short-term use [11].

6.7 Pulmonary Hypertension

Pulmonary hypertension, with and without cor pulmonale and right heart failure, have been described in patients with AIDS. The incidence of HIV-related pulmonary hypertension before the use of HAART has been 0.5% [52, 76, 83, 85, 100, 102].

The etiology of this problem is not well understood. The pathogenesis is unknown, but could relate to infection with human herpesvirus 8 (HHV-8) [22].

Many of these patients have had multiple pulmonary infections, often with Pneumocystis carinii and many of those were intravenous drug users (IDUs) [87]. As a result, interstitial disease and vascular bed destruction by multiple pulmonary infections were thought to be important. However, hyperplasia of vascular smooth muscle cells in the small pulmonary arteries occurs in HIV infection even without multiple pulmonary infections. Those changes may cause release of cytokines. There is a homology between a receptor-active region of the envelope protein gp120 of HIV virus and neuropeptide Y (NPY). NPY is mitogenic for vascular smooth muscle cells. In an in- vitro preparation; the gp 120 protein was a more potent mitogen than NPY [64]. Gp120 is a viral protein necessary for the binding and entrance of HIV into macrophages and has been shown to target human lung endothelial cells, increase markers of apoptosis, and stimulate the secretion of endothelin-1 [60].

The oral endothelin receptor antagonist, Bosentan has improved exercise tolerance and hemodynamic measurements in a small study of HIV patients [101].

6.8 Valvular Disease

Three main types of valvular disease have been associated with HIV infection:

- Nonbacterial thrombotic endocarditis (NBTE)
- Infective endocarditis (IE)
- Mitral valve prolapse

Nonbacterial thrombotic (marantic) endocarditis consists of sterile vegetations, which can occur on any of the valves. It may present as systemic embolization, but is otherwise clinically silent; no valvular disturbance occurs. Before 1989, NBET was found in 10% of autopsies in the United States in AIDS patients. The incidence has markedly decreased since then, possibly due to the virtual disappearance of cachexia in these patients. There have been no cases reported in AIDS patients since 1989 [31].

IE in HIV patients occurs almost exclusively in IDUs [19, 23, 31, 38, 77].

One retrospective study demonstrated that the incidence of IE in HIV-infected patients has declined with the introduction of HAART. Presenting symptoms were similar to those seen in HIV-uninfected patients and included fever, chills, and shortness of breath. In one multivariate analysis, an increased risk of IE was associated with a low CD4 count (<50 cells/μL), high HIV RNA levels (>100,000 copies/mL), and a history of IDU.

The treatment approach to IE in HIV-infected patients is similar to the approach to those who are HIV-seronegative; clinicians must consider the possibility of methicillin resistant *S. aureus* endocarditis [19].

6.9 Cardiac Tumors

Kaposi's sarcoma is the most frequent neoplasm in HIV patients, [62] and cardiac involvement has been reported in autopsy studies [9].

Among the patients with AIDS, Kaposi's sarcoma can involve the myocardium or the pericardium, and can cause pericardial effusion and in some cases, tamponade were reported [18, 105].

Non-Hodgkin lymphoma is a malignancy often seen in the patient with AIDS. The tumor is usually widespread, but can present as a primary cardiac lymphoma. When lymphoma involves the heart, it is usually diffusely infiltrative, but can form nodules and even intracavitary masses. Cardiac lymphoma can cause heart failure, superior vena caval syndrome, atrial and ventricular arrhythmias, and heart block. With intracavitary growth, the masses cause mechanical obstruction to the blood flow across the valves. In such cases, surgical resection is indicated. Chemotherapy and radiation therapy have produced variable results [21, 39, 63, 72, 79, 92, 106].

6.10 Long QT Syndrome

QT prolongation and *torsade de pointes* (TdP) have been described in patients with HIV infection, even in the absence of drug therapy. In one study, 29% of hospitalized patients with HIV infection had QT prolongation [65]. Postulated mechanisms include myocarditis, a subclinical cardiomyopathy, and autonomic neuropathy [109].

In addition, Pentamidine may promote TdP both directly and by causing hypomagnesemia, and HIV PIs can directly cause the long QT syndrome by blocking the HERG channel [4, 28, 58]. A patient with prolonged QT interval and torsades de pointes associated with Atazanavir was reported, emphasizing the importance of monitoring such patients who have risk factors for QT interval prolongation [73].

6.11 Autonomic Dysfunction

In the pre-HAART era, studies demonstrated autonomic nervous system (ANS) involvement affecting both parasympathetic and sympathetic divisions in a significant proportion of patients [20, 34]. One study found that compared to controls, HIV-infected patients taking potent ART regimens for at least three years had an increased resting heart rate and decreased short-term heart rate variability indicating parasympathetic dysfunction [66].

Autonomic dysfunction can lead to QTc prolongation and malignant ventricular arrhythmias.

6.12 Peripheral Arterial Disease

Little is known about PAD in HIV-infected patients. The prevalence of this disorder was investigated in 92 consecutively enrolled HIV-infected adults (mean age 50 years) by using a claudication questionnaire and by measuring the systolic ankle-brachial blood pressure index (ABI) at rest and after exercise [86]. Patients with PAD by ABI were further evaluated with duplex scanning of the lower limb arteries. Twenty-one percent of HIV-infected patients had peripheral vascular disease compared to the expected prevalence in the general population of 3% at age 60 [8].

References

1. Alonso-Villaverde C, Coll B, Parra S, Montero M, Calvo N, Tous N, Joven J, Masana L (2004) Atherosclerosis in patients infected with HIV is influenced by a mutant monocyte chemoattractant protein 1 allele. Circulation 110:2204–2209
2. Anderson DW, Virmani R, Reilly JM et al (1988) Prevalent myocarditis at necropsy in the acquired immunodeficiency syndrome. J Am Coll Cardiol 11:792
3. Anderson DW et al (1988) Prevalent myocarditis at necropsy in the acquired immunodeficiency syndrome. J Am Coll Cardiol 11:792–799
4. Anson BD, Weaver JG, Ackerman MJ et al (2005) Blockade of HERG channels by HIV protease inhibitors. Lancet 365:682
5. Aukrust P, Bjornsen S, Lunden B, Otterdal K, Ng EC, Ameln W, Ueland T, Muller F, Solum NO, Brosstad F, Froland SS (2000) Persistently elevated levels of von Willebrand factor antigen in HIV infection: downregulation during highly active antiretroviral therapy. Thromb Haemost 84:183–187
6. Aupeix K et al (1997) The significance of shed membrane particles during programmed cell death in vitro, in HIV-1 infection. L Clin Invest 99:1546–1554
7. Badiou S, Merle De Boever C, Dupuy AM, Baillat V, Cristol JP, Reynes J (2004) Fenofibrate improves the atherogenic lipid profile and enhances LDL resistance to oxidation in HIV-positive adults. Atherosclerosis 172:273–279
8. Bernal E, Masia M, Padilla S et al (2008) Low prevalence of peripheral arterial disease in HIV-infected patients with multiple cardiovascular risk factors. J Acquir Immune Defic Syndr 47:126
9. Cammarosano C et al (1985) Cardiac lesion in acquired immune deficiency syndrome (AIDS). J Am Coll Cardiol 5:703–706
10. Cardoso JS, Moura B, Martins L, Mota-Miranda A, Rocha Goncalves F, Lecour H (1998) Left ventricular dysfunction in human immunodeficiency virus (HIV)-infected patients. Int J Cardiol 63:37–45
11. Cardoso JS, Moura B, Mota-Miranda A, Goncalves FR, Lecour H (1997) Zidovudine therapy and left ventricular function and mass in human immunodeficiency virus-infected patients. Cardiology 88:26–28
12. Carr A et al (1999) Diagnosis, prediction and natural course of HIV-1 protease-inhibitor-associated lipodystrophy, hyperlipidaemia, and diabetes mellitus: a cohort study. Lancet 353:2093–2099
13. Cattelan AM, Trevenzoli M, Sasset L, Rinaldi L, Balasso V, Cadrobbi P (2001) Indinavir and systemic hypertension. AIDS 15:805–807
14. Cegielski JP, Lwakatare J, Dukes CS et al (1994) Tuberculous pericarditis in Tanzanian patients with and without HIV infection. Tuber Lung Dis 75:429
15. Centers for Disease Control (2005) Basic statistics from the Divisions of HIV/AIDS Prevention. Available at: http://www.cdc.gov/hiv/stats/htm
16. Chen Y et al (1999) Human immunodeficiency virus-associated pericardial effusion: report of 40 cases and review of the literature. Am Heart J 137: 516–521
17. Chow DC, Souza SA, Chen R, Richmond-Crum SM, Grandinetti A, Shikuma C (2003) Elevated blood pressure in HIV-infected individuals receiving highly active antiretroviral therapy. HIV Clin Trials 4:411–416
18. Chyu KY, Birnbaum Y, Naqvi T et al (1998) Echocardiographic detection of Kaposi's sarcoma causing cardiac tamponade in a patient with acquired immunodeficiency syndrome. Clin Cardiol 21:131
19. Cicalini S, Forcina G, De Rosa FG (2001) Infective endocarditis in patients with human immunodeficiency virus infection. J Infect 42:267
20. Cohen JA, Laudenslager M (1989) Autonomic nervous system involvement in patients with human immunodeficiency virus infection. Neurology 39:1111
21. Constantino A, West TE, Gupta M, Loghmanee F (1987) Primary cardiac lymphoma in a patient with acquired immune deficiency syndrome. Cancer 60:2801
22. Cool CD et al (2003) Expression of human herpesvirus 8 in primary pulmonary hypertension. N Engl J Med 349:1113–1122
23. Currie PF, Sutherland GR, Jacob AJ et al (1995) A review of endocarditis in acquired immunodeficiency syndrome and human immunodeficiency virus infection. Eur Heart J 16 Suppl B:15
24. D'Amati G et al (2001) Pathological findings of HIV-associated cardiovascular disease. Ann N Y Acad Sci 946:23–45
25. Dalakas MC, Illa I, Pezeshkpour GH, Laukaitis JP, Cohen B, Griffin JL (1990) Mitochondrial myopathy caused by long-term zidovudine therapy. N Engl J Med 322:1098–1105
26. Dube MP, Stein JH, Aberg JA, Fichtenbaum CJ, Gerber JG, Tashima KT, Henry WK, Currier JS, Sprecher D, Glesby MJ (2003) Guidelines for the evaluation and management of dyslipidemia in human immunodeficiency virus (HIV)-infected adults receiving antiretroviral therapy: recommendations of the HIV Medical Association of the Infectious Disease Society of America and the Adult AIDS Clinical Trials Group. Clin Infect Dis 37:613–627

27. Dube MP et al (2003) For the Adult AIDS Clinical Trials Group Cardiovascular Subcommittee. Guidelines for the evaluation and management of dyslipidimia in human immunodeficiency virus (HIV)-infected adults receiving antiretroviral therapy: recommendations of the HIV Medical Association of the Infectious Disease Society of America and the Adult AIDS Clinical Trials Group. Clin Infect Dis 37: 613–627

28. Eisenhauer MD, Eliasson AH, Taylor AJ et al (1994) Incidence of cardiac arrhythmias during intravenous pentamidine therapy in HIV-infected patients. Chest 105:389

29. Fichtenbaum CJ, Gerber JG, Rosenkranz SL, Segal Y, Aberg JA, Blaschke T, Alston B, Fang F, Kosel B, Aweeka F (2002) Pharmacokinetic interactions between protease inhibitors and statins in HIV seronegative volunteers: ACTG Study A5047. AIDS 16:569–577

30. Fisher SD, Lipshultz SE (2001) Epidemiology of cardiovascular involvement in HIV disease and AIDS. Ann N Y Acad Sci 946:13–22

31. Fisher SD, Lipshutz SE (2001) Epidemiology of cardiovascular involvement in HIV disease and AIDS. Ann N Y Acad Sci 946:13

32. Flum DR, McGinn JT, Tyras DH (1995) The role of the 'pericardial window' in AIDS. Chest 107:1522–1525

33. Freedberg RS, Gindea AJ, Dieterich DT, Greene JB (1987) Herpes simplex pericarditis in AIDS. N Y State J Med; 87:304–306

34. Freeman R, Roberts MS, Friedman LS et al (1990) Autonomic function and human immunodeficiency virus infection. Neurology 40:575

35. Friis-Moller N, Reiss P, Sabin CA, Weber R et al (2007) Class of antiretroviral drugs and the risk of myocardial infarction. N Engl J Med 356(17):1723–1735

36. Frostegard J et al (1999) Cytokine expression in advances human atherosclerotic plaque: dominance of proinflammatory (TH1) and macrophage-stimulating cytokines. Atherosclerosis 145:33–43

37. Gazzaruso C, Bruno R, Garzaniti A, Giordanetti S, Fratino P, Sacchi P, Filice G (2003) Hypertension among HIV patients: prevalence and relationships to insulin resistance and metabolic syndrome. J Hypertens 21:1377–1382

38. Gebo KA, Burkey MD, Lucas GM et al (2006) Incidence of, risk factors for, clinical presentation, and 1-Year outcomes of infective endocarditis in an urban HIV cohort. J Acquir Immune Defic Syndr 43:426

39. Goldfarb A, King CL, Rosenzweig BP et al (1989) Cardiac lymphoma in the acquired immunodeficiency syndrome. Am Heart J 118:1340

40. Grinspoon S, Carr A (2005) Cardiovascular risk and body-fat abnormalities in HIV-infected adults. N Engl J Med 352:48–62

41. Grundy SM, Brewer HB, Cleeman JI, Smith SC, Lenfant C (2004) Definition of metabolic syndrome: Report of the National Heart, Lung, and Blood Institute/American Heart Association conference on scientific issues related to definition. Circulation 109:433–438

42. Grundy SM, Hansen B, Smith SC Jr, Cleeman JI, Kahn RA (2004) Clinical management of metabolic syndrome: report of the American Heart Association/National Heart, Lung, and Blood Institute/American Diabetes Association conference on scientific issues related to management. Circulation 109:551–556

43. Grunfeld C et al (1992) Lipids, lipoproteins, triglycerides clearance, and cytokines in HIV infection and the acquired immunodeficiency syndrome. J Clin Endocrinol Metab 74:1045–1052

44. Hansson GK, Jonasson L, Lojsthed B, Stemme S, Kocher O, Gabbiani G (1988) Localization of T lymphocytes and macrophages in fibrous and complicated human atherosclerotic plaques. Atherosclerosis 72:135–141

45. Hazenberg MD et al (2000) T-cell division in human immunodeficiency virus HIV-1 infection is mainly due to immune activation: a longitudinal analysis in patients before and during highly active antiretroviral therapy (HAART). Blood 95:249–255

46. Heidenreich PA, Eisenberg MJ, Kee LL et al (1995) Pericardial effusion in AIDS. Incidence and survival. Circulation 92:3229

47. Heidenreich PA et al (1995) Pericardial effusion in AIDS. Circulation 92:3229–3234

48. Hellerstein M et al (1999) Directly measures kinetics of circulating T lymphocytes in normal and HIV -1-infected humans. Nat Med 5:83–89

49. Herskowitz A, Willoughby SB, Baughman KL, Schulman SP, Bartlett JD (1992) Cardiomyopathy associated with antiretroviral therapy in patients with HIV infection: a report of six cases. Ann Intern Med 116:311–313

50. Herskowitz A et al (1993) Prevalence and incidence of left ventricular dysfunction in patients with human immnunodeficiency virus infection. Am J Cardiol 71:955–958

51. Herskowitz A et al (1994) Myocarditis and cardiotropic viral infection associated with severe left ventricular dysfunction in late-stage infection with human immuno-deficiency virus. J Am Coll Cardiol 24:1025–1032

52. Himelman RB, Dohrmann M, Goodman P et al (1989) Severe pulmonary hypertension and cor pulmonale in the acquired immunodeficiency syndrome. Am J Cardiol 64:1396

53. Hsia J, Ross AM (1994) Pericardial effusion and pericardiocentesis in human immunodeficiency virus infection. Am J Cardiol 74:94–96

54. Hsue PY et al (2004) Clinical features of acute coronary syndrome in patients with human immunodeficiency virus infection. Circulation 109:316–319

55. Hsue PY et al (2004) Progression of atherosclerosis as assessed by carotid intima-media thickness in patients with HIV infection. Circulation 109:1603–1608

56. Hunt PW, Martin JN, Sinclair E, Bredt B, Hagos E, Lampiris H, Deeks S (2003) T cell activation is associated with lower CD4+ T cell gains in human immunodeficiency virus-infected patients with sustained viral suppression during antiretroviral therapy. J Infect Dis 187:1534–1543

57. Jung O, Bickel M, Ditting T, Rickerts V, Welk T, Helm EB, Staszewski S, Geiger H (2004) Hypertension in HIV-1-infected patients and its impact on renal and cardiovascular integrity. Nephrol Dial Transplant 19:2250–2258

58. Justo D (2006) Methadone-induced long QT syndrome vs methadone-induced torsades de pointes. Arch Intern Med 166:2288

59. Jutte A, Schwenk A, Franzen C, Romer K, Diet F, Diehl V, Fatkenheuer G, Salzberger B (1999) Increasing morbidity from myocardial infarction during HIV protease inhibitor treatment? AIDS 13:1796–1797

60. Kanmogne GD, Primeaux C, Grammas P (2005) Induction of apoptosis and endothelin-1 secretion in primary human lung endothelial cells by HIV-1 gp120 proteins.Biochem Biophys Res Commun 333:1107

61. Kannel WB, Giordano M (2004) Long-term cardiovascular risk with protease inhibitors and management of the dyslipidemia. Am J Cardiol 94:901–906

62. Kaplan LD et al (2003) Case 31-2003: a 44-year old man with HIV infection and a right atrial mass. N Engl J Med 349:1369–1377

63. Kelsey RC, Saker A, Morgan M (1991) Cardiac lymphoma in a patient with AIDS. Ann Intern Med 115:370

64. Kim J, Ruff M, Karwatowska-Prokopczuk E et al (1998) HIV envelope protein gp120 induces neuropeptide Y receptor-mediated proliferation of vascular smooth muscle cells: relevance to AIDS cardiovascular pathogenesis. Regul Pept 75–76:201

65. Kocheril A, Bokhari SAJ, Batsford WP (1997) Long QTc and torsades de pointes in human immunodeficiency virus disease. Pacing Clin Electrophysiol 20:2810

66. Lebech AM, Kristoffersen US, Mehlsen J et al (2007) Autonomic dysfunction in HIV patients on antiretroviral therapy: studies of heart rate variability. Clin Physiol Funct Imaging 27:363

67. Lee GA, Seneviratne T, Noor MA, Lo JC, Schwarz JM, Aweeka FT, Mulligan K, Schambelan M, Grunfeld C (2004) The metabolic effects of lopinavir/ritonavir in HIV-negative men. AIDS 18:641–649

68. Leidig GA Jr (1991) Clinical, echocardiographic, and electrocardiographic resolution of HIV related cardiomyopathy. Mil Med 156:260

69. Levy WS, Simon GL, Rios JC, Ross AM (1989) Prevalence of cardiac abnormalities in human immunodeficiency virus infection. Am J Cardiol 63:86

70. Lewis W, Grupp IL, Grupp G, Hoit B, Morris R, Samarel AM, Bruggeman L, Klotman P (2000) Cardiac dysfunction occurs in the HIV-1 transgenic mouse treated with zidovudine. Lab Invest 80:187–197

71. Libby P (2000) Imflammation in atherosclerosis. Nature 420:868–874

72. Little RF, Gutierrez M, Jaffe ES et al (2001) HIV-associated non-Hodgkin lymphoma: incidence, presentation, and prognosis. JAMA 285:1880

73. Ly T, Ruiz ME (2007) Prolonged QT interval and torsades de pointes associated with atazanavir therapy. Clin Infect Dis 44:e67

74. Martin S et al (2004) Shed membrane particles from T lymphocytes impair endothelial function and regulate endothelial protein expression. Circulation 109:1653–1659

75. Mary-Krause M, Cotte L, Simon A, Partisani M, Costagliola D (2003) Increased risk of myocardial infarction with duration of protease inhibitor therapy in HIV-infected men. AIDS 17:2479–2486

76. Mesa RA, Edell ES, Dunn WF, Edwards WD (1998) Human immunodeficiency virus infection and pulmonary hypertension: two new cases and a review of 86 reported cases. Mayo Clin Proc 73:37

77. Miró JM, del Río A, Mestres CA (2002) Infective endocarditis in intravenous drug abusers and HIV-1 infected patients. Infect Dis Clin North Am 16:273

78. Mocroft A, Vella S, Benfield TL, Chiesa A, Miller V et al (1998) Cahging patterns of mortality across Europe in patients infected with HIV-1. Lancet 352:1725–1730

79. Montalbetti L, Della Volpe A, Airaghi ML et al (1999) Primary cardiac lymphoma. A case report and review. Minerva Cardioangiol 47:175

80. Niaura R, Shadel WG, Morrow K, Tashima K, Flanigan T, Abrams DB (2000) Human immunodeficiency virus infection, AIDS, and smoking cessation: the time is now. Clin Infect Dis 31:808–812

81. Noor MA, Lo JC, Mulligan K, Schwarz JM, Halvorsen RA, Schambelan M, Grunfeld C (2001) Metabolic effects of indinavir in healthy HIV-seronegative men. AIDS 15:F11–F18

82. Ntsekhe M, Mayosi BM (2009) Cardiac manifestations of HIV infection: an African perspective. Nat Clin Pract Cardiovasc Med 6:120

83. Opravil M, Pechere M, Speich R et al (1997) HIV-associated primary pulmonary hypertension. A case control study. Am J Respir Crit Care Med 155:990

84. Pasceri V et al (2000) Direct proinflammatory effect of C-reactive protein on human endothelial cells. Circulation 102:2165–2168

85. Pellicelli AM, Barbaro G, Palmieri F et al (2001) Primary pulmonary hypertension in HIV patients: a systematic review. Angiology 52:31

86. Periard D, Cavassini M, Taffe P et al (2008) High prevalence of peripheral arterial disease in HIV-infected persons. Clin Infect Dis 46:761

87. Petitpretz P, Brenot F, Azartam R et al (1994) Pulmonary hypertension in patients with human immunodeficiency virus infection: comparison with primary pulmonary hypertension. Circulation 89:2722

88. Hsue PY, Waters DD (2005) What a cardiologist needs to know about patients with human immunodeficiency virus infection. Circulation 112: 3947–3957

89. Pugliese A, Gennero L, Vidotto V et al (2004) A review of cardiovascular complications accompanying AIDS. Cell Biochem Funct 22(3):137–141

90. Pugliese A et al (2000) Impact of highly active antiretroviral therapy in HIV-positive patients with cardiac involvement. J Infect 40:282–284

91. Purnell JQ, Zambon A, Knopp RH, Pizzuti DJ, Achari R, Leonard JM, Locke C, Brunzell JD (2000) Effect of ritonavir on lipids and post-heparin lipase activities in normal subjects. AIDS 14:51–57

92. Roldan EO, Moskowitz L, Hensley GT (1987) Pathology of the heart in acquired immunodeficiency syndrome. Arch Pathol Lab Med 111:943

93. Roy VP, Prabhakar S, Pulvirenti J, Mathew J (1999) Frequency and factors associated with cardiomyopathy in patients with human immunodeficiency virus infection in an inner-city hospital. J Natl Med Assoc 91:502

94. Rusnati M et al (2002) HIV-1 Tat protein and endothelium: from protein/cell interaction to AIDS-associated pathologies. Angiogenesis 5:141–151

95. Sadler BM, Piliero PJ, Preston SL, Lloyd PP, Lou Y, Stein DS (2001) Pharmacokinetics and safety of amprenavir and ritonavir following multiple-dose, co-administration to healthy volunteers. AIDS 15:1009–1018

96. Sanne I, Piliero P, Squires K, Thiry A, Schnittman S (2003) Results of a phase 2 clinical trial at 48 weeks (AI424-007): a dose-ranging, safety, and efficacy comparative trial of atazanavir at three doses in combination with didanosine and stavudine in antiretroviral-naive subjects. J Acquir Immune Defic Syndr 32:18–29

97. Schuster M, Valentine F, Holzman R (1985) Cryptococcal pericarditis in an intravenous drug abuser. J Infect Dis 152:842

98. Shannon RP, Mathier MA, Manleod S et al (1999) Macrophages not cardiomyocytes are the reservoir for lentivirus in SIV cardiomyopathy. Circulation 100:1

99. Shen YM, Frenkel EP (2004) Thrombosis and a hypercoagulable state in HIV-infected patients. Clin Appl Thromb Hemost 10:277–280

100. Silva-Cardoso J, Moura B, Ferreira A et al (1998) Predictors of myocardial dysfunction in human immunodeficiency virus-infected patients. J Card Fail 4:19

101. Sitbon O et al (2004) Bosentan for the treatment of human immunodeficiency virus-associated pulmonary arterial hypertension. Am J Respir Crit Care Med 170:1212–1217

102. Speich R, Jenni R, Opravil M et al (1991) Primary pulmonary hypertension and HIV infection. Chest 100:1268

103. Stahl CP, Wideman CS, Spira TJ, Haff EC, Hixon GJ, Evatt BL (1993) Protein S deficiency in men with long-term human immunodeficiency virus infection. Blood 81:1801–1807

104. Stein JH et al (2001) Use of Human immunodeficiency virus-1 protease inhibitors is associated with atherogenic lipoprotein changes and endothelial dysfunction. Circulation 104:257–262

105. Stotka JL, Good CB, Downer WR, Kapoor WN (1989) Pericardial effusion and Pericardial effusion and tamponade due to Kaposi's sarcoma in acquired immunodeficiency syndrome. Chest 95:1359

106. Sturm A, Noppeney R, Reimer J et al (2001) AIDS and non-Hodgkin's lymphoma: initial cardiac manifestations of highly malignant B-cell lymphoma 18 years after HIV infection. Dtsch Med Wochenschr 126:364

107. Tershakovec AM, Frank I, Rader D (2004) HIV-related lipodystrophy and related factors. Atherosclerosis 174(1):1–10

108. Trachiotis GD et al (2003) Cardiac surgery in patients infected with the human immunodeficiency virus. Ann Thorac Surg 76:1114–1118

109. Villa Foresti V, Confaloneri F (1995) Autonomic neuropathy and prolongation of the QT interval in human immunodeficiency virus infection. Clin Auton Res 5:48

110. Wafaa E-S, Reiss P, De Wit S, Monforte AD, Thiebaut R, Morfeld L, Weber R, Pradier C, Calvo G, Law M, Kirk O, Sabin C, Friis-Moller N, Lundgren J (2005) Relationship between prolonged exposure to combination art and myocardial infarction: effect of sex, age, and lipid changes. In: Program and abstracts of the 12th conference on retroviruses and opportunistic infections; 22-25 February 2005, Boston. Abstract 42

111. Wlodarczyk D (2004) Managing medical conditions associated with cardiac risk in patients with HIV. In: Peiperl L, Volberding PA (eds) HIV insite knowledge base [textbook online]. UCSF Center for HIV Information, San Francisco. Available at: http://hivinsite.ucsf.edu/InSite?page=kb-03-01-20#S2.3X.

112. Zhou X, Nicoletti A, Elhage R, Hansson GK (2000) Transfer of CD4+ T cells aggravates atherosclerosis in immunodeficient apolipoprotein E knockout mice. Circulation 102:2919–2922

113. Zwaka TP et al (2001) C-reactive protein-mediated low density lipoprotein uptake by macrophages: implications for atherosclerosis. Circulation 103:1194–1197

Bringing Evidence Basis to Decision Making in Complementary and Alternative Medicine (CAM): Prakriti (Constitution) Analysis in Ayurveda

7

Sanjeev Rastogi and Francesco Chiappelli

Core Message

> › Ayurveda, the traditional health care system rooted in India, is one among the oldest yet living traditional healthcare system. Ayurvedic clinical practice utilizes a comprehensive clinical examination of the patient to reach at a judgment about the pathogenesis and its possible mode of management. The chapter discusses the extent to which this can practically be utilized in routine clinical settings of Ayurveda to reach at evidence-based decision.

7.1 Introduction

Decision-making in health care practice is a complex process. This essentially involves collection of information regarding the disease through a comprehensive enquiry of symptoms, signs, and physical telltale of disease and also a direct or indirect visualization of pathological process through several investigations. These pieces of information are then analyzed in a way to reach at a point, which may indicate the possible

S. Rastogi (✉)
Department of Kaya Chikitsa, State Ayurvedic College and Hospital, University of Lucknow, Tulsi Das Marg, Lucknow 226004, India
e-mail: rastogisanjeev@rediffmail.com

F. Chiappelli
Divisions of Oral Biology and Medicine, and Associated Clinical Specialties (Joint), University of California at Los Angeles, School of Dentistry, CHS 63-090, Los Angeles, CA 90095-1668, USA
e-mail: fchiappelli@dentistry.ucla.edu

cause of pathology and therefore can help in decision making to its management.

An increasing insurgence of fast emerging biotechnological application to medical diagnostics, however, substantially influenced the conventional decision making in medical practice. Overuse and overdependence on the technology to reach at a decision have unfortunately increased the health care cost exponentially with an unequal distribution of their utilization among the people from different socio-economic groups.

Contrary to the concurrent decision making of conventional medicine, a decision making in complementary and alternative medicine (CAM) largely depends upon enquiring the disease through subjective and objective clinical examination followed by its interpretation through intrinsic understanding about the pathogenesis and management. CAM encompasses a vast array of traditional health care practices prevalent in many countries. Ayurveda from India and traditional Chinese medicine (TCM) (including acupuncture) from China are between two most widely acknowledged forms of traditional health care practice for their completeness of theory and practice style [37]. Besides making a substantial contribution to the health care needs in the country of their origin, they are contributing to global healthcare needs.

Conventional diagnostic decision making in TCM and acupuncture largely depends upon a comprehensive physical examination of a patient with an intention to enquire about variables pathognomonic to different pathological states. This examination includes enquiry about physical and physiological features compounded with a comprehensive tongue and pulse examination. A cross analysis of the information obtained through physical examination and symptom enquiry helps one to reach at a decision determining the final course of therapy [38].

Ayurvedic clinical practice, similarly, utilizes a comprehensive clinical examination of the patient to reach at a judgment about the pathogenesis and its possible mode of management. Interestingly, Ayurveda principally distinguishes between the examination of the disease (Roga *pariksha*) and the examination of the person who is afflicted with the disease (Rogi *pariksha*). Eventually, the examination of the former is primarily meant to examine the disease process whereas the latter is to examine the vitality of the patient. This bimodal clinical examination in Ayurveda is proposed to bring out the information crucial for the tailoring of the management as per the individual conditions [34]. A *Rogi pariksha* consequently is a comprehensive examination of various host-related factors having important roles to play in the determination of the choice of therapy, dosage, minimization of adversities, and prognosis of a disease in relation to its affliction to an individual. A *rogi pariksha,* therefore eventually includes examination about constitution of the patient (*prakriti*), age (*vaya*), disease (*vikriti*), tolerance (*satmya*), psychological status (satva), digestive capacity (*aharashakti*), capacity for exercise (*vyayama shakti*), quality of tissue (*sara*), physical proportion of body (*sanhanana*), and strength (*bala*). Together, they all compose a tenfold (*dashavidha*) examination, which remains the mainstay of decision making in Ayurvedic clinical practice [27].

Irrespective of the classical textual descriptions available in ancient Ayurvedic scriptures such as Charaka Samhita (200 BC), Sushruta Samhita (600 BC), and Astanga Samgraha (fourth century AD) supporting this form of evidence analysis [25], the same has become increasingly difficult to be translated into practice. Among the several reasons which are limiting the clinical application of these seemingly important methods of evidence search in Ayurveda, the foremost ones are unavailability of tools to transform these measured variables into accurate, consistent, and reproducible piece of information. In the absence of such dependable tools, any information observed in relation to disease and its management remains an individual observation and not an evidence. A decision-making based upon such information is liable to have inaccuracies leading to uncertainties of results.

Prakriti or the constitutional specificity of a person is a perpetual concept of Ayurveda. Conceptually, it brings about a phenotypical classification of human population based on the predominance of certain biohumors *(dosha)* in every individual leading to a constitutional specificity and on which the physical, physiological, and mental traits of a person depends. A *prakriti* examination forms an essential component of the tenfold examination plan of Ayurvedic decision making. Recent years have shown a renewed scientific interest to the idea of Ayurvedic phenotyping of human population and to see if it has a genomic and biochemical basis [15].

As a *prakriti* examination is primarily the identification of the predominance of certain biohumors of the body, which in turn are responsible for the state of health, or disease in a person, its accuracy in observation may have important bearings on the part of decision making in Ayurvedic therapeutics.

It is this concept of *prakriti* in Ayurveda that we would be focusing upon in this chapter. Besides identifying its fundamental importance in Ayurvedic diagnostics and therapeutics, we would also be examining as to how this can practically be utilized in routine clinical settings of Ayurveda to reach at evidence-based decision. A deliberation about *prakriti,* however, cannot be fully accomplished unless we reach at a basic understanding of the constructs of Ayurvedic fundamentals. It is in this purview that we would briefly introduce Ayurvedic principles of health and disease that examine as to how the concept of *prakriti* derived, before we actually enter into the main focus of this chapter.

7.2 Ayurveda: The Science of Life: Background

Oriental world is known for its ethno-cultural traditions rooted in identical philosophical and social ideologies. These traditions are deeply intertwined to their social fabric for their direct influence upon life and related issues and hence are carried forward through the successive generations since antiquity. Healthcare, being an important and integral component of human life, essentially forms the core of this ethno-cultural ethos of traditional societies. Having originated, transformed, and nurtured in relation to the actual need of the society, these health care systems are grown as the systems taking care of the health and diseases but essentially with a care for socio-economic and geographic factors affecting the life of the people in a particular area of its practice. This is how, the traditional health care systems, at places, are found interfered with seemingly unrelated topics from ethics, agriculture, and sociology. That was primarily to provide a broader base to medical science and to link it with every issue having a potential to affect human health directly or indirectly.

Ayurveda, the traditional health care system rooted in India, is one among the oldest yet living traditional healthcare system. This is practiced predominantly in Indian subcontinent but sporadically throughout the globe. Ayurveda, in connotation to the TCM, has a strong theoretical and practical basis; hence it is recognized as a whole system of medicine [37]. Primarily looking into the integration of body, mind, and spirit as a means to prevent and treat a disease, Ayurveda has gone through phased development of its fundamental constructs historically. Beginning with *Athrvaveda*, which is found to have the basic seeds of health care philosophy, it was further adopted and enriched by various schools of thoughts through many centuries to be evolved into the shape it is observed today [14].

Ayurveda, being the science primarily concerned with human being as the subject of its study, begins exhortatively to understand a human being in terms of its compositional details and then proceeds further into identifying a compositional harmony and anomaly as the cause of health and disease in human being. Interventions to bring about health in a sick are essentially the measures intended to restore the lost harmony among the primary components of the body. Approaching from simple to complex, Ayurveda further specifies the disharmony with reference to etiopathogenesis of a disease by the identification of the presenting symptoms of the person. An intervention essentially looks for the restoration of lost harmony which is achieved by addition, supplementation, or removal of the components leading to imbalance [3].

For a better understanding of Ayurveda, however, we still need to know the following:

1. What are these components which form a human body?
2. How their imbalance and rebalance leads to sickness and health?
3. How can diseases be diagnosed in terms of a compositional imbalance?
4. How a specific intervention may be determined to act upon a specific type of imbalance?

Ayurveda tries to answer these many queries through an innovative proposition of certain postulates. Theory of five elements (*pancha mahabhut*), uniqueness of body constitution (prakriti), three physiological principles

(tridosha), and property of a drug (*rasa*) are some of these dictums which are extensively used in Ayurveda to understand the causes of disease and health. Besides these theories, Ayurveda also propagates the concept of similarity of macrocosm and microcosm (loka purusha samya) for their mutual dependence.

These thoughts and constructs of Ayurveda, though unfamiliar to conventional medical science, are gradually being recognized for having seeds of more explicit human biology yet to be understood by the scientific world [4].

Utilization of these postulates to bring evidences for their possible utilization in patient care is a cumbersome thought requiring more rigorous fundamental and scientific research than it may seem. Among all the postulates of Ayurveda, Prakriti, a fundamental conceptualization of Ayurveda about constitutional identity of each individual seems to be more near to scientific understanding for its tangibility and application. Prakriti identification is proposed to be of explicit value in individualized health care. This is also proposed to be of value in predictive medicine by presenting a clue to disease susceptibility and incidence pattern in a given constitution type [8]. Considering the pragmatic importance of prakriti in patient care, it would be important to understand the concept of prakriti as is perceived in Ayurveda and to see as to how this is being proposed for its utilization in patient care. It would be of further importance to see if a Prakriti analysis could be used as a dependable tool for evidence-based decision making in Ayurvedic clinical practice.

7.2.1 Concept of Prakriti in Ayurveda: The Empirical Basis

Among us, we find people with variable physical, mental, and spiritual capabilities and also with variable disease susceptibility and tolerance. Why are we all not alike? Ayurveda is the first science which has identified these subtle intraspecific differences among the human beings and also brought about a far-sighted application of this difference into medicine. An individual constitutional specificity is called prakriti in Ayurveda. A germplasm derivation (beej) of the parent is hypothesized as the primary determinant of qualitative and physical specification in an individual. An environmental and dietary influence upon growing fetus through maternal life style is also proposed to affect net *prakriti* determination [23, 28] By a germplasm specification, ayurveda actually proposes to identify the predominance of biohumors (*dosha*) in developing fetus, which are held responsible for specific physiological and metabolic functions of the body. Therefore, *prakriti* of a child is conceived to be determined by the actual *dosha*, which is predominant in germplasm at the time of conception [23]. With this elaboration, *prakriti* appears to be the sum of inheritance in an individual primarily through parental genes and partially through the interplay of environment and maternal diet during the antenatal period. Conceptually, *prakriti* remains unchanged throughout the life once it is finally determined. Interestingly, the idea of differential gene expression as a potential reason for the phenotypical differences among the people from the same pedigree has much resemblance to the idea of *Dosha* predominance of Ayurveda as a key factor in *prakriti* determination. It is known that despite the similarity of the human genome, it is the differential gene expression, which makes a phenotypical differentiation among individuals [26].

A *prakriti* identification is given paramount importance in Ayurvedic clinical practice primarily for its application to Ayurvedic diagnostics, disease management, and prognostication of a disease with reference to an individual. Additionally, this is also proposed to be of help in susceptibility identification of diseases in an individual.

As *prakriti* is primarily conceived as a state of three doshas in their differential proportion identical to every individual [29], it would be imperative to know as to what Ayurveda understands through the concept of *tridosha* and how they can truly be associated to the concept of *prakriti*.

7.2.1.1 Conceptual Evolution of Fundamentals in Ayurveda

To get a real understanding of the Ayurvedic theory of disease and subsequent management, it is important to observe them in the spirit of how they have evolved. Being a natural science, dictums of Ayurveda have a direct observational relationship to nature, how life would have evolved on earth, and hence what are the components of life? This is the point where Ayurveda begins its stipulations. By enriching this thought through a physical (five element), biophysical, and

physiological (tridosha) construction in human beings, it tries to understand the cause of health and disease. Moreover, by extrapolation of the similar physical and biophysical thoughts to naturally available substance, Ayurveda tries to find the remedies for any imbalance of the body created thereupon leading to disease.

To begin with, Ayurveda by default relies upon certain postulates, which are primarily rooted in sankhya school of eastern philosophy. These are

1. Nonexistence cannot give rise to existence (*Na sato vidyate bhavo nabhavo vidyate satah*) [13].
2. Life is a process of becoming visible (*vyakta*) from invisible *(avyakta)* interspersed with many intermediary stages.

Ayurveda identifies the eternal availability of basic life building blocks in the universe with a condition that beginning of life process is subject to the availability of optimal conditions (that is how, despite the eternal availability of the basic material, the life process on earth could begin only a few billion years ago). Primitive earth was proposed to be composed of three primary properties (triguna) namely *sata, raja,* and *tama. Sata* here symbolizes the energy needed for creation, *raja* symbolizes the movements responsible for aggregation or segregation reactions leading to the creation of complex molecules, and tama finally symbolized physical material. A reorganization of *tama* under the influence of *raja* and *sata* is proposed to be a process, which finally led to origin of life in due course of time.

After passing through many invisible stages characterized by the formation of five elements from primitive inert material through a differential combination and condensation first into *tanmatra* (smallest possible component of *pancha bhuta* which has its property but is not physically visible) and then into *panchabhuta*, the visible stage of life began through the formation of *pancha maha bhuta* (Pancha = five, Maha = big, *Bhuta* = primitive form or elements namely *akasha* (void), *vayu* (air), *agni* (fire), *jala* (water) and *prithvi* (earth)) as the condensation and combination products of five elements. Ayurvedic version of the formation of life states for many intermediary stages before the physically visible substance is available in the form of *Mahabhuta*. Modern science supports these postulates by observing that a differential combination of formative particles (electron, proton, and neutron) can evolve different atoms, elements, and compounds under suitable conditions. If we reduce a matter into its formative components, we would essentially be getting the elements which are essentially similar in every substance and only differing in their quantitative ratio. Ayurveda paraphrases this truth by postulating that every matter available on the earth is composed of five elements (*sarvam dravyam hi panch-bhautikam*) and it is their differential ratio, which brings about the differences among individuals.

It is equally important to reemphasize here that *pancha-mahabhuta* as proposed in Ayurveda are not the primary constructs and instead are the condensation product of *pancha-bhuta* which in turn are the combination of *pancha-tanmatras* with a differential representation of each of the five *tanmatra* to a single *bhuta*. As a consequence, every living structure comes to be an amalgamation of five *mahabhuta* which themselves are a combination *pancha tanmatras*. This is how we get a complex mixture of feature in every living being which ipso facto represents the predominance of their formative substances [30].

It is the harmonic balance of these *panchamahabhuta* in a living body which is held responsible for the state of health, and hence every health care intervention as is perceived in Ayurveda is focused toward the ultimate goal of restoring the lost balance of *panchamahabhuta* in an individual.

As a disease per se is proposed to be the manifestation of the lost balance of *panchamahabhuta* in a living body, for a health care intervention, it is imperative to know precisely about the qualitative and quantitative imbalances occurring among various *mahabhuta* within the body.

Theory of *tridosha* intercepts here as the biological application to the theory of *mahabhuta*. *Tridosha* (Vata, Pitta, and Kapha) for instance, symbolize the physico-biological properties among living beings made of various combinations of pancha *mahabhuta*. *Tridosha*, hereby, represents the physiological functions in a living body, which ipso facto are the function of the component material of the same. Individual grouping of *vata, pitta,* and *kapha* among *tridosha* is primarily the categorization of physiological functions with reference to their elemental predominance. A functional enquiry, thereby is adopted as a tool in Ayurveda to acquire knowledge about deficits or excess of some of the component material of a living body which in turn is leading to a disease and whose restoration is required to bring back the healthy state.

Through preceding parts of our discussion in this chapter we come to know about the generalization of the Ayurvedic theory of *panchamahabhuta* which is said to be applicable to every living and nonliving being of the universe alike [31]. Interestingly, this generalization has given way to the foundation of another important theorem of Ayurveda saying that every substance available in this world is having a potential to be used as a medicine (*nanaushadhibhutam jagat kinchit*) [32]. It is again the panchabhautic composition of various natural substances, which proffer them to be used as medicine in order of their predominance and applicability to various disease conditions.

7.2.1.2 *Prakriti*: The Proto Typical Composition

Literally, *prakriti* symbolizes more than a single meaning. Conventionally, this is used synonymously to nature. From preliminary understanding of Ayurveda, this is supposed to be a representation of individual physical and mental characteristics, which are grouped in order of the predominance of *dosha* in an individual. Either of these inferences, however, does not represent the concept of prakriti in toto. *Prakriti (pra* = primary or first, *kriti* = creation) ideally stands for a primary creation or prototype. This prototype here refers to the primary compositional subtyping of a living being at the time it was born. This subtyping of composition is different in different people as per the actual ratio of the formative components in their body. Remaining in this naïve state of originality is being healthy as Ayurveda identifies. Essentially, in a bid to maintain its original existence, a living being continuously interacts between oneself (microcosm) and environment (macrocosm). This interaction is essentially driven toward the ultimate goal of maintaining the prototypical composition. Hence, in a broader sense, a disease is the state where the inherent mechanism of *prakriti* maintainance fails. This failure, in turn gives way to interactions unfavoring the prakriti sustenance and finally giving rise to the features which are not consistent to the ingenious *prakriti* of a given individual. These features are nothing but the morbid feature explaining the underlying malfunctioning of the system maintenance.

Incidently, *vikriti (vi= special, kriti = creation)*, the antonym to *prakriti* is conventionally used in ayurveda to symbolize the pathological conditions. In a broader sense, however, it simply represents the state where a *prakriti* maintenance failed and led to the state which is not indigenous. The duo of *prakriti* and *vikriti* in

Ayurveda are used with a wider reference and has practical applications in the identification of the ideal health conditions and their deviations leading to diseases.

Prakriti, for practical purposes, can be quantified through the measurement of *dosa* activity in body, which in turn is the functional representation of the differential combination of five elements. *Prakriti* is also considered as an inheritable feature but is simultaneously said to be influenced by the intimate environment and the diet of the mother during the intrauterine phase. Being an inherent feature, it is proposed that we get borne with a predetermined *prakriti*. This is why we are able to find some obvious differences in the appearance and behavior of newborn babies who have not yet interacted with the environment. Tracing the origin of *prakriti* to its *panchbhautic* ancestry defines certain patterns of their combinations. For practical purposes of Ayurvedic diagnostics, these patterns of *prakriti* are identified as seven subtypes representing specific *dosha* predominance in each type. A subtyping with reference to three *dosha* namely *vata, pitta,* and *kapha* can be identified as under.

- One *dosha* predominance –identified as *vata, pitta,* and *kapha* predominant *prakriti*.
- Two *dosha* predominance – identified as a dual combination of *dosha* in order of their predominance such as *vata-pitta, vata-kapha,* and *pitta-kapha*.
- Three *dosha* predominance – refers to an equi-state representation of each *dosha*.

For all practical purposes of acquiring health and to remain healthy, the golden rule of Ayurveda is to stick to the original prototypical features and to avoid the activities coming against this basic composition. This is how Ayurvedic health care philosophy seems revolving around disease prevention through the avoidance of aggravating factors and health maintenance through the observation of health promotive practices aiming to maintain one's *doshik* equilibrium intact.

7.2.1.3 Linking *Prakriti* with *Tridosha*: Understanding Ayurvedic Physiology

In preceding parts of our discussion (Sect. 7.2.1.1) we realized that Ayurveda developed most of its principles in accordance with the practical needs of understanding human physiology and function. *Tridosha* theory

similarly is developed as a tool first to identify and then to quantify the grade of pathology and the consequent need of health care interventions. We have perceived through Ayurvedic fundamentals that consequent to the process of evolution of nonliving or living beings in the universe, we all get organized as a composite of *panchamahabhuta*, though in variable order and amount, leading to differences among apparently similar or dissimilar things.

In a living being, a compositional enquiry can be made through the observation of functions. Considering the function as a direct representative to its compositional integrity, a functional enquiry is hence observed as a more practical approach in Ayurvedic diagnostics.

For any living system, ability to interact constantly with the environment with an intention to keep its integrity maintained is of prime concern. Three basic functions are presumed to be fundamental for a living system [5]. These are input–output, throughput (turn over), and storage. These functions of an open system have a striking resemblance to the function of *vata, pitta,* and *kapha* respectively. Interestingly, the functions of *vata, pitta,* and *kapha* can be dissected as the embodiment of *panchamahabhuta* grouped as per their functional attributes. *Vata* principally represents movements, which in turn is the function of *akasha* and *vayu*. *Pitta* principally represents the turnover, dissociation or disintegration, which in turn is the function of Agni, and finally *kapha* principally represents synthesis and storage, which in turn is the function of *jala* and *prithvi* (Table 7.1).

A theory of *tridosha*, thereby, seems to be the physiological application of the theory of *panchamahabhuta* where a compositional enquiry can be made by the observation of functions, and a judgment about compositional imbalance can be made through the malfunction of the system. Because of their potential to represent compositional specificity, a *dosha* activity observation in healthy state in a person can give us an idea about its normal *panchabhautic* status i.e., *prakriti*. This is how a judgment about *prakriti* can be made through the observation of biological functions in a healthy person.

Table 7.1 *Panchamahabhuta* roots to *Tridosha*

Predominant *Mahabhuta*	Representative *Dosha*
Akash + Vayu	*Vata*
Agni	*Pitta*
Jala + Prithvi	*Kapha*

Incidentally, it should also be known that every single voluntary act of human being, every single interaction with environment, and every edible has also been defined for their possible effects upon the *panchbhautic* composition of an individual. It is in this purview, the dietary or voluntary recommendations are made in Ayurveda for their possible role in health maintenance or in disease management.

7.3 Evidence Basis to *Prakriti:* The Scientific Correlates

Prakriti in Ayurveda is essentially explained in terms of relative *dosha* activity. *Dosha*, in light of the preceding discussions, can well be considered as the physiological extension to *panchmahabhuta* theory. This ingenious hypothesis of Ayurveda helps to understand the process of disease and health within the limited knowledge resources available in nature.

Being an identical reflection to functioning *dosha*, *prakriti* is supposed to represent physical, mental, and physiological specifications in any individual. On the other hand, *dosha* and hence the function of the body is proposed to be the reflection of *prakriti*.

An individual *prakriti* finally manifests through a mechanism involving an interplay of inherited principles, environment, maternal dietary factors, and age of the mother at the time of conception and the same in turn is reflected through physical and physiological features of the newborn.

It can be hypothesized that possibly the *panchbhautic* composition and hence the corresponding *dosha* activities are resumed at the earliest stages of fetal growth (from the status of zygote formation itself). This in turn can affect the fetal growth through the process of cell differentiation determining the physical and functional fate of a cell, tissue, or organ in individual body. Surprisingly, this hypothesis seems similar to the idea of differential gene expression in living cells, which possibly explains to the different fate of cells under the influence of signals leading to the differential expression of genes finally leading to the corresponding activation of mRNA and the production of resultant proteins [2].

Every living cell of an organism is known to be composed of a complete set of substances required to form an entire new organism. This phenomenon is called totipotencey. What a cell will become in the course of normal development depends upon the determination of different cell types (cell fates), which operates through a progressive restriction to their developmental potentials. When a cell chooses a particular fate, it is said to be determined, although it still looks similar to its undetermined neighbors. Determination implies a stable change, as the fate of determined cells does not change. It is possibly at this stage that the *prakriti* of an individual is finally determined. Differentiation follows determination, as the cell now undergoes a cell-specific developmental program.

7.3.1 Mechanism of Prakriti Determination Through Cellular Differentiation

How does a cell become different from its parent cell? How do two identical daughter cells become different from one another? How might one daughter cell become a neuron, while the other daughter cell becomes a skin cell? A *prakriti* differentiation among individuals and siblings can aptly be defined through this primary cellular mechanism of cell differentiation. In some cases, determination results from the asymmetric segregation of cellular determinants. However, in most cases, determination is the result of inductive signaling between cells.

Asymmetric segregation of cellular determinants is based on the asymmetric localization of cytoplasmic molecules (usually proteins or mRNAs) within a cell before it divides. During cell division, one daughter cell receives most or all of the localized molecules, while the other daughter cell receives less (or none) of these molecules. This result in two different daughter cells, which then take on different cell fates based on differences in gene expression. The localized cytoplasmic determinants are often mRNAs encoding transcription factors, or the transcription factors themselves. Unequal segregation of cellular determinants is observed during early development of the *C. elegans* and *Drosophila* embryos. From Ayurvedic perspective proposing for a five elemental composition to every living cell, this could be the differential distribution of these formative elements among daughter cells leading to their differential fate through variable *dosha* activity resulting through the differential gene expression.

Table 7.2 Phenotypical representation of *panchbhautic* predominance

Elements	Physical feature	Physiological feature	Mental feature
Akasha	Ear, small ness, fine ness	Acoustic capacity	Capacity to distinguish between right and wrong (*vivek*)
Vayu	Skin, gross and subtle movements, dryness	Touch perception, circulation, internal movements	Impulse generation, motivation
Agni	Appearance, eyes	Warmth, digestion, metabolism, vision	Objective perception
Jala	Tongue, softness and suppleness, oilyness	Taste perception	Flexibility
Prithvi	Nose, physical strength, heaviness, toughness	Olfactory perception	Rigidity

The *prakriti* is conceived to be decided at cell determination stage when this is no more changeable. Further to the determination, at the stage of differentiation, it is possibly the elemental predominance, which acts as the signal to differential expression of genes and hence making a path to the morphological and function differentiation of the cells. Without any convincing data to support with, *panchamahabhuta* theory of Ayurveda seems to operate at a level deeper than differential gene expressions. It tries to underline the various reasons, which may possibly act as the signals to make a cell differentiated. These signals can aptly be called as *panchbhut* in Ayurveda, and a *prakriti* may be proposed as a net characterization of determined cells, which are differentiated gradually to express them morphologically and functionally in course of their development.

7.3.2 Mechanism of Cell Differentiation: Ayurvedic View

Ayurveda prima-facie considers the maternal (*matraja bhava*), paternal (*pitraja bhava*) inheritance and maternal dietary influence (*rasaj bhava*) as responsible for distinctive features in every fetus [12]. These influencing factors with reference to the *prakriti* determination may act via signals which either operate through a differential elemental distribution or support to a particular element group. Ayurveda proposes an elemental predominance representation through the physical, physiological, and mental features attributed to the corresponding element [33]. Following is a summary of

Ayurvedic perception of how *panchabhuta* are represented phenotypically in growing fetus and how they are responsible for bringing specific features to growing fetus (Table 7.2).

It is proposed that *panchamahabhuta* are responsible for the arousal of specific perceptions and corresponding sense organs in the body. Apart from physical specifications as softness, roughness, physical dimensions, toughness, and gross appearance, they are also responsible for some specific physiological and mental functions.

7.3.3 Evidences from the Genomic Studies

Because of its invasion into almost every theoretical and practical aspect of Ayurveda, *prakriti* fundamentally and *dosha* as its applied extension, presented themselves as the central dogma of Ayurveda. Fascinated by its possible application to Ayurvedic diagnostics and for its being as an evidence to help decision making for personalized treatment, it has recently evoked the scientific community to look at the issue in their own perspectives [9]. It was vividly approached to see if the *prakriti* has a genomic basis [12, 35]. In a meticulous approach to quantify *tridosha* through biostatistical methods, Joshi [7] succeeded to conclude that *tridosha* has a concrete empirical basis which can be utilized for its scientific establishment. Inspired by the initial findings of Patwardhan [12] showing a positive correlation between different *prakriti* and HLA alleles, an intense brainstorming among biologists ensued and resulted in coinage of a term Ayurvedic biology [36] as a bid to differentiate Ayurvedic understanding of health and disease from that of conventional biology. Clearly underpinning the importance of *prakriti* to Ayurvedic understanding, Valiathan, the proponent of Ayurvedic biology, stated, "Since innate disposition determines the manifestation of disease and individual response to treatment, one of the first things a physician does is to determine the *prakriti* of his patient. This is necessary to personalize the treatment in accordance to the basic principles of Ayurveda. It is clearly suggested that *dosa prakriti* represents phenotypes" [36]. These initial visions and subsequent efforts by Indian academy of science (IAS) and Indian National Science Academy (INSA) provoked the Government of India to launch an innovative project intended to make genomic variation analysis and gene expression profiling of human *dosha prakriti* based on the principles of Ayurveda. Consequential to the approaches made to define Ayurvedic genomics [11, 12], a further advancement is made by the identification of biochemical correlates and whole genome expression to the extreme constitutional types as described in Ayurveda [15]. This landmark study interestingly was able to reveal differences at gene expression level, biochemical level, and also genomic level in different phenotypic groups as per the Ayurvedic classification. Differential gene expression is possibly the concept, which looks more appealing with reference to *prakriti* as it permits various internal and external factors to operate at different levels to make a final cumulative conglomeration of features in the form of phenotype. Some approaches have recently been made to identify the role of various signals in differential gene expression during the developmental phases. It was noted in these studies that specific signals were able to produce specific gene expressions determining the physiological fate of the cell line [24]. This is again in accordance with the fundamentals of *prakriti*, which repeatedly says that various factors operating at the time of conception and also during the developmental phase of the fetus finally determine the *prakriti* of an individual.

It would be of interest to note that the concept of *prakriti* is luring scientists for its novelty since long. Almost a decade back, it was seriously thought as an important factor determining the final outcome of any therapeutic intervention in a given population. Dahanukar and Thatte [1] in a revealing study were able to correlate the therapeutic outcomes with phenotypical specifications as described in Ayurveda [1]. Incidentally,

it can also be noted that similar phenotype-response correlation studies are usually done in almost every postgraduate research work conducted so far at various Ayurvedic institutes in India [19].

7.4 Clinical Application of *Prakriti* Identification: Translating Theory into Practice

Prakriti typology is finally determined as per the differential distribution of three *dosha* in an individual. A unilevel increase of *dosha* is called mono-doshic *prakriti*, which in turn can be *vata, pitta,* or *kapha* predominant respectively. An exigency of any two *dosha* among the three is called bidoshik (*dvandaja*) *prakriti*. There can be three such combinations including *vata-pitta, vata–kapha,* and *pitta-kapha* among this category of *prakriti*. Finally, a homogenous distribution of three *dosha* in an individual forms another category called as homogenous constitution (*sam prakriti*) (Fig. 7.1). *Sam prakriti* representing a homogenous distribution of *dosha* is considered as an ideal *prakriti* because of its proximity to health owing to the balance of physiological activities consequential to a *dosha* balance there in .In real clinical situation, however, this is a rarity and a heterogeneous distribution of *dosha* is commonly observed. Interestingly, a heterogeneous

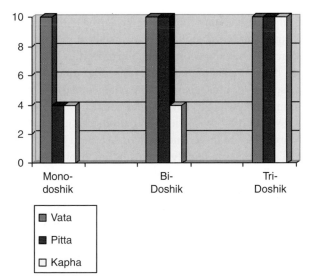

Fig. 7.1 *Prakriti* typology: a proposal to differential distribution of *dosha*

distribution of *dosha* is marked in ayurveda for its disease proneness consequential to its association with particular *dosha* and simultaneous dissociation with others. Among many possible variables of heterogeneous *prakriti*, a single dosha predominance prakriti is further identified as *sadatura* (ever sick people) for its exceeding proneness and quick adherence toward diseases. It is conventionally belived that the people with a specific *dosha* predominance have an increased preponderance of suffering the disease due to the same *dosha* if there are discrepancies in diet and routine favoring the exigency of the same. Similarly, as an important health promotive measure,they are advised to go for a balanced diet with special care to not exceed the factors which may lead to an excess of the predominant *dosha* in their *prakriti*.

Prakriti identification, besides its role in the identification of the disease susceptibility, has also been identified as a key factor in the prognostication of a disease. Coneventionally, a disease where the causative *dosha* is found similar to that of primary constitution of the patient is presumed to be difficult to treat. Conversely, an antagonizing combination of the two is proposed as an indicator to a fair to good prognosis.

It is a known fact that a drug does not lead to similar effects upon its every recipient. These variations of drug effect among individuals are primarily due to the pharmacodynamic differences among individuals getting reflected through variable handling of the drug by their own biological system. *Prakriti* of an individual again intercepts at this point by determining as to what would be the possible impact of a drug in a given individual. It is interesting to note that the adversities of a drug are more common in people where the properties of a drug are similar to that of the patient *prakriti*. A *pitta prakriti* person, for example may be more prone for the adversity from a drug which is having *pitta* augmentive property. Individual drug sensitivities and adversities are tried to be explained in this connotation of Ayurveda [16, 21].

Despite its seemingly promising implications upon clinical practice, a serious attempt to bring *prakriti* examination in routine medical practice has sparingly been attempted. A definitive role of *prakriti* to the prevalence and prognosis of rheumatoid arthritis(RA) was identified in 2001 by Rastogi et al. [19].This report identified a *vata-pitta* constitutional subtype as more prone yet fairly treatable fraction among the RA population. RA was found to be less severely manifested in this population subgroup. Conversely, a *vata–kapha* subgroup of RA population is found to be worst hit owing to its severe presentation leading to a bad prognosis. A similar approach was applied recently in a clinical trial upon lymphatic filariasis treated with an ayurvedic traditional herbal formulation (ATF) [10]. A *prakriti* examination was done here to exclude the patients in whom the components of the treatment were presumed to be contraindicated on classical grounds. A *dosha* explanation about the disease and its linkage to the patient's *prakriti* is approached in many isolated cases where successful management of a difficult disease is attributed to the customized ayurvedic therapy in accordance with this identification [17, 20, 22].

7.4.1 Approaching Prakriti Identification in Clinic: Where is the Tool of Practice?

Preliminary clinical studies directed toward the identification of the role of *prakriti* in customized disease prevention and management and its corresponding genomic exploration is tempting enough to bring *prakriti* analysis as a requisite tool of evidence generation in Ayurvedic clinic. To reach at this ultimate goal, initially we require more data toward its conventional applicability. Following a substantial data generation of this account, we need to develop and standardize a tool which can universally be applied for *prakriti* analysis in Ayurvedic clinics. Once this tool is developed and tested statistically for it applicability, validity and significance, this can be universally applied as a tool of evidence generation for the decision making. As *prakriti* is a culmination of *dosha* preponderance, it is reflected through the physical, physiological, and psychological features specific to the respective *dosha*. Classical texts of Ayurveda have gone in length to bring out a handy description of readily identifiable *prakriti* features for their presence or absence and a consequent *prakriti* analysis in an individual (Table 7.3). In routine Ayurvedic clinics, conventionally, it is the subjective approach of Ayurvedic physician which makes a judgment about patient's *prakriti* during his routine clinical examination with reference to the classical descriptions of *prakriti* features. For ease of the application and documentation, this approach was gradually shifted into a semi-objective, questionnaire-based model where individual features pertaining to a specific *dosha* were identified in a print format for their presence or absence in any individual. For *prakriti* diagnosis, a mix of these two approaches can be seen in concurrent Ayurvedic practice.

A questionnaire based model seems to be a more objective, handy, and reproducible tool for making a *prakriti* diagnosis in routine Ayurvedic clinic. Making of a standardized format of the questionnaire for an unambiguous diagnosis of *prakriti,* however, is another lacuna which needs to be addressed before the practical application of this tool can be expedited. Various ambiguities can be identified among *prakriti* analysis questionnaire models used so far in practice or research.

Identififying the patient's categorical (physical, physiological, and mental) features first and then to transpolate them upon the individual *dosha* preponderance is the prospective approach of diagnosing *prakriti.* In routine clinical practice, some easily identifiable presenting features from different categories are identified as principle variables. These features are then graded for their affinity toward any of the three *dosha.* Finally, a screening of total responses is made which gives a cumulative idea of the possible predominant *dosha* representing *prakriti.* In this prospective exercise, however, a questionnaire is expected to give false positive results for some *dosha* group, where the responses are applied upon variables because of a compulsive grading.

A thorough search through classical ayurvedic literature identifies that the categorical features which are defined in relation to their affinity for one specific *dosha* may not necessarily be applicable to other group of *dosha.* These variables may either be common and varying only in their grade to define a *dosha* affinity or can be an altogether different variable specific to one *dosha* and nonavailable to the other *dosha.* It is for this reason that a compulsive search for one among the three *dosha* through a process of grade variation with reference to every variable identified essentially has a possibility to lead to incorrect results. *Pitta* for instance being moderate in its physical presentation and also for few of its unique features not available to *vata* and *kapha,* has the highest possibility for being presented as false positive. On the other hand, *vata* and *kapha* share many variables which differ only in grade to define a *dosha* affinity. This possibility of false positive inferences favoring *pitta* in *prakriti* diagnosis using the conventional tools is also supported through the *prakriti* distribution pattern among the studied population in few of the recent studies [12].

7.4.2 Diagnosing Prakriti: The Retrospective Approach

Against the currently utilized prospective model for *prakriti* diagnosis, a retrospective approach promises for more. The latter model primarily proposes for the recognition of *dosha* through their distinguishing features followed by a search for their presence in a patient through a closed ended binomial (yes/no) questionnaire. Eventually, this model offers an equal opportunity for a symptom to be completely refused or accepted if it does not or does have a resemblance to the individual presentation. The retrospective approach is advantageous to prospective approach on two important grounds. First, it offers a clear choice for the specific features and so selection is relatively straight forward. Second, it also offers a liberty to refuse a feature if the same is not applicable in individual conditions. Both of these factors can significantly lower the possibility of symptom overlap and compulsive reporting which is an inherent feature of the prospective approach. Moreover, the retrospective approach also offers a direct linking of *dosha guna* (characteristics) to that of their physical manifestation. In this way, in case of any predominance for some specific *dosha,* it is also possible to visualize what basic components of *dosha* are responsible for its predominance, and consequently a preventive strategy can be planned in accordance. While describing the identifying features for different *prakriti,* Charaka has clearly identified different components of *dosha* which are actually leading to their manifestations (Table 7.3). It is important to mark that making a *prakriti* diagnosis through retrospective way not only gives us an idea of what is the predominant *dosha,* but also essentially enumerates the actual factors leading to this manifestation.

Considering the limitation of previous approaches, a novel prototype tool for *prakriti* diagnosis has been proposed with an address to the standardization issue [18]. By considering the classical description of *prakriti* based upon each component of individual type, a model was prepared primarily to look into the presence or absence of some feature in some individual. To find a numerical value to the responses and so to get a cumulative idea of the ratio of *dosha* features present, each set and subset of a feature was provided with a numerical value to make a cumulative sum equal in every individual *dosha* (Table 7.4). A liberty to accept or reject any feature here eliminated the

Table 7.3 *Dosha guna* (genotype) and their manifestation (phenotype)

Genotype	Phenotype
Kapha	
Snigdha	Oily body
Shlakshna	Smooth body
Mridu	Soft texture Fair complexion Good looking face features
Madhur	Good sexual induration More offspring Increased amount of semen
Sara	Compact body
Sandra	Well-formed body parts (proportionate) Well-nourished body parts
Manda	Slow physical movements Slow conversation Slow eating
Staimitya	Delayed (well thought) beginning of actions Cool temperament
Guru	Slow walking speed
Sheeta	Less appetite Less thirst Less sweating Less prone to heat-induced discomforts
Picchila	Compact joints (not prominent)
Accha	Pleasing face Pleasing complexion Pleasing voice
Pitta	
Ushna	Intolerant to heat Soft textured Fair complexion Increased presence of moles Good appetite Good thirst Premature graying and fall of hair
Tikshna	Voracious eater and drinker (eat good quantity in a time) Good digestive capability Sharp reacting, argumentative Intolerant to discomforts
Drava	Lax and soft flesh and joints Profuse sweat, urine, and stool formation
Visra	Increased and bad odor from armpit, head, and body
Katu	Less sexual induration Less no. of children Less amount of semen
Amla	Less sexual induration Less no. of children Less amount of semen

Table 7.3 (continued)

Genotype	Phenotype
Vata	
Ruksha	Dry body Poorly formed and poorly nourished body Dry, poor, interrupted, and unpleasant voice Reduced sleep
Laghu	Quick but incoherent movements Quick but incoherent appetite Quick but incoherent speech
Chala	Unstable joints and body parts (moves them while sitting)
Bahu	Increased number of visible tendons and veins on extremities Over talkative
Shighra	Quick indulgence in some activity Increased amount of anxiety Quick reactions in the form of attachment, detachment, or fearfulness Quick understanding and grasping Less memory
Sheet	Intolerant to cold (does not like) Prone to cold-induced ailments (common cold, URTI)
Parush	Rough hair, nail, body, foot, and hand
Vishad	Prominent body parts (as joints) Crepitus in joints while moving

Table 7.4 Prototype *prakriti* analysis questionnaires (PAQ)

Genotype	Phenotype	Yes/No(scores)
Kapha trait		
Snigdha	Oily skin (scratch the mid flexor aspect of right forearm with some blunt object. If mark is visible, it is dry, if not it is oily)	60
Slakshna	Smooth skin	60
Mridu	Less tolerant to difficulties Fair complexion Good looking face features	20 20 20
Madhur[a]	Good sexual induration[b] More offspring (0–1=no, 2 or more=yes, including abortions or still birth)	30 30
Sara	Compact muscular body[c] Stable body(almost consistent body weight)	30 30
Sandra	Well formed, proportionate body parts Well-nourished body parts	30 30
Manda	Slow physical movements Slow conversation Slow eating	20 20 20
Staimitya	Delayed (well thought) beginning of actions Cool temperament (less anxiety)	30 30
Guru	Slow walking speed	60

(continued)

Table 7.4 (continued)

Genotype	Phenotype	Yes/No(scores)
Sheeta	Less appetite	15
	Less thirst	15
	Less sweating	15
	Tolerant to heat	15
Picchila	Compact joints (not prominent)	60
Accha	Pleasing face	20
	Pleasing complexion	20
	Pleasing voice	20
Total score[d]		
Pitta trait		
Ushna	Intolerant to heat	15
	Soft textured	15
	Fair complexion	15
	Increased presence of moles	15
	Good appetite and thirst	15
	Premature graying and fall of hair	15
Tikshna	Voracious eater (eat good quantity in a time)	18
	Voracious drinker (drink good quantity in a time)	18
	Good digestive capability	18
	Sharp reacting, argumentative	18
	Intolerant to discomforts	18
Drava	Lax and soft flesh and joints	45
	Profuse sweat, urine, and stool formation	45
Visra	Increased and bad odor from armpit, head, and body	90
Katu[a]	Less sexual induration[b]	45
	Less no. of children (0–1 = Yes, 2 or more = No, including abortions or still birth)	45
Amla[a]	Less sexual induration[b]	45
	Less no. of children (0–1 = Yes, 2 or more = No, including abortions or still birth)	45
Total score[d]		
Vata trait		
Ruksha	Dry skin	30
	Poorly formed and poorly nourished body	30
	Dry, poor, interrupted, and unpleasant voice	30
	Reduced sleep	30
Laghu	Quick but incoherent movements	40
	Quick but incoherent appetite	40
	Quick but incoherent speech	40
Chala	Unstable joints and body parts (moves them while sitting)	120
Bahu	Increased number of visible tendons and veins on extremities	60
	Over talkative	60
Shighra	Quick indulgence in some activity	20
	Increased amount of anxiety	20
	Quick reactions in the form of attachment, detachment	20
	Fearfulness or timidness	20
	Quick understanding and grasping	20
	Less memory	20

Table 7.4 (continued)

Genotype	Phenotype	Yes/No(scores)
Sheet	Intolerant to cold (does not like)	60
	Prone to cold-induced ailments (Common cold, URTI)	60
Parush	Rough hair, nail, body, foot, and hand	120
Vishad	Prominent body parts (as joints)	60
	Crepitus in joints while moving	60
Total score[d]		

[a]Quantity of semen is deleted as a feature of *Madhur (Kapha), Katu, and Amla (Pitta)* properties because of its inability to be identified precisely in males and inapplicability to females

[b]These features are specific to married people. For unmarried people alternative questions are to be framed

[c]Physical features like compact body and musculature are to be judged in accordance with the gender and geographical standards

[d]Total score is 960 for each *Dosha*. Individual scores are calculated as per the responses, and then predominance may be determined

problem of compulsive responding and consequent false positive or negative inference in favor of or against some particular *dosha*. This tool is further proposed to be verified through testing of its verifiable features and also through reliability testing as are applicable in the statistical testing of questionnaire-based tools.

7.5 Conclusion: Steps Ahead Toward an Evidence-Based Ayurveda

After getting a preliminary acquaintance with Ayurvedic fundamentals and also their possible scientific correlates, more comprehensive and conclusive studies require to be planned for underpinning any possible application of *prakriti* to routine clinical practice. The empirical conceptualization of *prakriti,* supported through biochemical and genomic studies, can prove to be of value in customization of therapy as per the actual need of the individual. Much of the drug associated adversities can be prevented through the application of *prakriti* in the identification of possible drug sensitivity in an individual. A biochemical understanding of *prakriti* can be of value for dose determinations as per the individual *prakriti*. Therefore, a more effective management plan simultaneous to minimization of dosage in susceptible people can be made by effective utilization of *prakriti* analysis in ayurvedic clinical practice. This can also be of value in choosing the right medicine for the right person to work in best harmony.

A disease susceptibility prediction among individuals could be among few of the most fascinating applications of *prakriti* identification for allowing a targeted prevention before a disease actually surfaces.

Cells of a multicellular organism are genetically homogeneous but structurally and functionally heterogeneous owing to the differential expression of genes. Many of these differences in gene expression arise during development and are subsequently retained through mitosis. Stable alterations of this kind are said to be epigenetic, because they are heritable in the short term, but do not involve mutations of the DNA itself. Research over the past few years has focused on two molecular mechanisms that mediate epigenetic phenomena: DNA methylation and histone modifications. Epigenetic effects by means of DNA methylation have an important role in development, but can also arise stochastically as animal age. Identification of proteins that mediate these effects has provided insight into this complex process and diseases that occur when it is perturbed. External influences on epigenetic processes are seen in the effects of diet on long-term diseases such as cancer. Thus, epigenetic mechanisms seem to allow an organism to respond to the environment through changes in gene expression. The extent to which environmental effects can provoke epigenetic responses represents an exciting area of future research [6]. Epigenetic studies can find a place in identifying the possible correlation of *prakriti* subtypes and dietary or environmental factors which are making them susceptible to some specific diseases. All this, however, requires a great deal of effort from both extremes of health science, the modern and the occidental, that too in a concerted way to reach a point where this can become implicated and beneficial to everyone, irrespective of their belief, origin, or medical system which they trust upon.

References

1. Dahanukar SA, Thatte UM (1997) Current status of ayurveda in phytomedicine. Phytomedicine 4:359–368
2. Differential gene expression (2009) Downloaded from http://koogle.kenyon.edu/courses/biol114/Chap11/Chapter_11.html. Accessed 30 March 2009
3. Gupta AD (2007) (ed) Ashtanga Hridayam, Chaukhambha prakashana, Varanasi pp 8–10
4. Hankey A (2005) CAM modalities can stimulate advances in theoretical biology. Evid Based Complement Alternat Med 2:5–12
5. Hankey A (2005) A test of system analysis underlying the scientific theory of Ayurveda's Tridosha. J Altern Complement Med 11:385–390
6. Jaenisch R, Bird A (2003) Epigenetic regulation of gene expression: how the genome integrates intrinsic and environmental signals. Nat Genet 33:245–254
7. Joshi RR (2004) A biostatistical approach to Ayurveda: quantifying the Tridosha. J Altern Complement Med 10:879–889
8. Lavekar GS (2006) Holistic concepts of research and development of Ayurvedic herbal drugs. In: Sharma R, Arora R (eds) Herbal drugs: a twenty first century perspective. Jaypee brothers, New Delhi, pp 522–534
9. Mashelkar RA (2008) Second World Ayurveda Congress (Theme: Ayurveda for the Future) – Inaugural Address: Part II. Evid Based Complement Alternat Med 5:243–245
10. Narahari SR, Ryan TJ, Aggithaya MG, Bose KS, Prasanna KS (2008) Evidenced based approaches for the Ayurvedic traditional herbal formulations: towards an Ayurvedic CONSORT model. J Altern Complement Med 14:769–776
11. Patwardhan B, Bodekar G (2008) Ayurvedic genomics: establishing a genetic basis for Mind Body Typologies. J Altern Complement Med 14:571–576
12. Patwardhan B, Joshi K, Chopra A (2005) Classification of human population based on HLA gene polymorphism and the concept of Prakriti in Ayurveda. J Altern Complement Med 11:349–353
13. Prabhupada ACBS (1972) Bhagavad Gita as it is, 2/16, Macmillan, Accessed at http://www.asitis.com/2/16.html. Accessed on 29 March 2009
14. Prasad PV (2000) Atharvaveda and its materia medica. Bull Indian Inst Hist Med Hyderabad 30(2):83–92
15. Prasher B, Negi S, Aggarwal S, Mandal AK, Sethi TP, Deshmukh SR et al (2008) Whole genome expression and biochemical correlates of extreme constitutional types defined in Ayurveda. J Transl Med 6:48

16. Rastogi S (2008) Ayurvedic approach to multiple chemical sensitivity In Clinical Roundup: how do you treat chemical sensitivity in your practice? Alter Complement Therap 14(6):310–314. doi:10.1089/act.2008.14605
17. Rastogi S (2008) CAM management of peripheral arterial occlusive disease (PAOD): A Case Report. Complement Health Pract Rev 13(3): 198-203. doi: 10.1177/1533210108325383
18. Rastogi S (2010) Building bridges between Ayurveda and Modern Science, Int J Ayurveda Res 1:39–44
19. Rastogi S, Singh RH (2002) A clinical study of the factors influencing therapeutic out come in Rheumatoid arthritis. J Res Ayurveda Siddha. 23:10–19
20. Rastogi S, Rastogi R, Singh RH (2006) What are we losing by ignoring Ayurveda? New Approaches Med Health 14(1):26–29
21. Rastogi S, Ranjana, Singh RH (2007) Adverse effects of Ayurvedic drugs: an overview of causes and possibilities in reference to a case of Vatsanabha (Aconite) overdosing. Int J Risk Safety Med (3):117–125
22. Rastogi S, Chawla S, Singh RK (2009) Ayurvedic management of unilateral loss of vision following a blunt injury to eye: a case report. Complementary Health Pract Rev (14): 84–92
23. Shastri AD (ed) (2006) Sushruta Samhita, Sharira sthana 4/63, Chaukhaba Sanskrit sansthan, Varanasi
24. Siddiqui MA, Singh G, Kashyap MP, KhannaVK, Yadav S, Chandra D, Pant AB (2008) Infuence of cytotoxic doses of 4-hydroxynonenal on selected neurotransmitter receptors in PC-12 cells. Toxicol In vitro (22):1681–1688
25. Singh RH (1994) Kaya chikitsa,Varanaseya Sanskrit sansthan, Varanasi 213–326
26. Storey JD, Madeoy J, Strout JL, Wurfel M, Ronald J, Akey JM (2007) Gene-expression variation within and among human populations. Am J Human Genet (80):502–509
27. Thatte U, Bhalerao S (2008) Pharmacovigilance in Ayurvedic medicine in India. Indian J Pharmacol 40:S10–S12
28. Tripathi BN (ed) (1983) Charaka Samhita,Vimana stahna 8/95, Chaukhambha surbharti publication, Varanasi 758–765
29. Tripathi BN (ed) (1983) Charaka Samhita,Vimana sthahna 6/14, Chaukhambha surbharti publication, Varanasi 706
30. Tripathi BN (ed) (1983) Charaka Samhita, Sutra sthana 8/30, Chaukhambha surbharti publication, Varanasi 206
31. Tripathi BN (ed) (1983) Charaka Samhita, Sutra sthana 26/10, Chaukhambha surbharti publication, Varanasi 470
32. Tripathi BN (ed) (1983) Charaka Samhita, Sutra sthana 26/12, Chaukhambha surbharti publication, Varanasi 471
33. Tripathi BN (ed) (1983) Charaka Samhita, Sharira sthana 4/12, Chaukhambha surbharti publication, Varanasi 879
34. Tripathi RD (ed) (2006) Ashtanga sangraha, (Sutrastahana), Chaukahambha Sanskrit pratishathana,Varanasi, P19
35. Valiathan MS (2006) Ayurveda: setting the house in order. Guest Editorial. Curr Sci 90:5–6
36. Valiathan MS (2006) Towards ayurvedic biology: a decadal vision document. Indian academy of sciences, Bangalore
37. What is cam? downloaded from http://nccam.nih.gov/health/whatiscam/ Accessed on 09 May 2009
38. Zicheng Y, Dayong C, Wenlong W (eds) (1997) Diagnostics of traditional Chinese medicine. Wuhan university press, Wuhan

Evidence-Based Clinical Decisions in Oral Surgery

Oladimeji Adeniyi Akadiri and Wasiu Lanre Adeyemo

Core Message

> Advocacy for evidence-based clinical decisions in oral surgery is gaining momentum, but as yet, there are not enough randomized clinical trials to support evidences at the highest level in many aspects of the field. In this chapter, an appraisal of evidences in two aspects of oral surgery namely; third molar surgery and jaw augmentation is presented.

8.1 Introduction

Conventional model for clinical decision making in medical practice is based on knowledge acquired from traditional medical training, individual's clinical observations and experiences, knowledge of pathological mechanisms of diseases, and published but not necessarily validated literature [63, 76]. On the other hand, evidence-based medicine is the integration of best research evidence with clinical expertise and patient values in making decisions about the care of individual patients [25,191]. Over the last 15 years, the advocacy for evidence-based practice has gained significant

momentum, and there is growing compliance in every medical and surgical specialty [134].

In tracking down the best evidence, systematic reviews and meta-analysis of critically appraised randomized controlled trials (RCT) offer the highest quality, and these study designs are being increasingly adopted in various fields of medicine. Despite the increasing adoption of RCT in other areas of medicine, it was stated that RCTs form only 3–9% of clinical study design among all specialties of surgery [71, 210, 212, 213]. The evidence available in oral and maxillofacial surgery was particularly found to be relatively weak in comparison with other specialties due to the limited number of RCTs and meta-analysis of RCTs (MA-RCT) [123, 130, 134]. Hence, well-conducted RCTs need to be generated on many subjects in oral and maxillofacial surgery to further promote evidence-based research and practice in the field.

The subsequent sections of this chapter contain discussions on evidence in relation to two subject areas of oral and maxillofacial surgery, third molar surgery and jaw augmentation procedures.

8.2 Evidence-Based Decisions in Third Molar Surgery

The impacted mandibular third molar is arguably the most widely researched subject in oral surgery. In spite of this enormous interest, there is yet to be a conclusive consensus on several aspects of the subject. Most previously published guidelines were based on consensus reached among experts at meetings convened by some professional associations such as American Association of Oral and Maxillofacial surgeons (AAOMS) and Scottish Intercollegiate Network (SIGN), or health

O.A. Akadiri (✉)
Department of Oral and Maxillofacial Surgery, College of Health Sciences, University of Port Hacourt, Post Box 212, Choba, Port Harcourt, Rivers State, Nigeria
e-mail: oaakadiri@yahoo.com

W.L. Adeyemo
Department of Oral and Maxillofacial Surgery, College of Medicine, University of Lagos, PMB 12003, Lagos, Nigeria
e-mail: lanreadeyemo@yahoo.com

care regulatory bodies such as National Institute of Health (NIH) and National Institute for Clinical Excellence (NICE), etc. Some of the decisions were not evidence-based and have generated controversies that have lingered over several decades.

In the light of modern practice that emphasizes evidence-based decisions in clinical practice, evidences in regard to decisions for or against removal of a mandibular third molar, radiographic assessment of the third molar, assessment of surgical difficulty, prophylactic use of antibiotic, control of short-term postoperative morbidity, and prevention of lingual nerve injury are discussed.

8.2.1 Removal of Impacted Mandibular Third Molar

It is generally agreed that impacted third molars associated with obvious pathology require removal [11, 46, 137, 168]. The controversy has been about the removal of asymptomatic third molars. With the advent of sophisticated technology in anesthesia, antibiotics, and surgical equipment, there was a corresponding surge in the rate of third molar removal [113, 170]. At that time, a huge amount of asymptomatic third molars, including fully formed teeth, partially formed teeth, and tooth germs, were frequently removed [113]. This generated concerns among some opinion groups who argued against prophylactic removal. Some of the strongest arguments proffered are:

1. That an impacted third molar in a young person may still change position and some will eventually erupt into normal positions [93, 226].
2. The inherent risk of complications in third molar surgery is considerable; therefore, it should not be embarked upon without a strict indication [88, 106].
3. A huge cost is incurred by patients, government, and third party payers due to the removal of impacted third molars [30, 31].

On the contrary, proponents of prophylactic removal argued that (1) there is a risk of cyst and tumor arising from the follicle of an impacted tooth if left in situ [51], (2) the risk of surgical complications is higher in the older age group [33, 34, 215], (3) there is a risk of late anterior crowding [132, 194], and (4) retained impacted third molar predisposes to mandibular angle fractures [128]. The questions are how many of these arguments

have been substantiated by research evidence?, and what does the currently available evidence favor?

By critical literature reviews and critical appraisal of evidence using EVB techniques, it has been shown that the risk of pathology (cyst and tumor) in impacted mandibular third molar exists, but it is too low to justify prophylactic removal [216, 224]. Since there is no reliable way to predict pathologic changes, continued monitoring with periodic clinical and radiographic examination was recommended [116]. The likelihood of anterior crowding secondary to an impacted third molar has been debunked [139, 185, 193]. However, there are evidence in support of greater incidence of complications in older patients (≥25 years) and proneness to mandibular fracture in the presence of an impacted third molar which is also age-related [33, 34, 123, 215]. On the contrary, some authors have reported that the retention of an impacted third molar protects against mandibular condylar neck fracture [136], which is a more difficult fracture to manage compared to the angle fracture [1]. The argument that impacted third molars do change positions has been verified, but this hardly happens beyond age 25 years [93, 226]. A small proportion does erupt into proper position in the arch, but eruption to the occlusal plane does not guarantee proper periodontal support for the maintenance of a tooth in good health [226].

It is also true that a huge amount of money is expended on third molar surgery, but it is still not clarified how much of this was particularly expended on the removal of asymptomatic teeth. Some authors have observed that the annual expenditure on third molar surgery is still low compared to expenditures on some other diseases in same countries [82] and that the economic cost of progressive monitoring of an impacted third molar is equally enormous [16]. Therefore, it may be irrational to deny a patient the opportunity of early removal of an impacted tooth because of cost if the ultimate health benefit of the procedure can be justified. What then could be a strong justification for the removal of asymptomatic impacted mandibular third molar?

By reviewing a wide range of articles including RCT, cohort studies, and large scale case-controlled studies from various respectable and trustworthy databases such as Ovid Medline, PubMed, Google Scholar, and the Cochrane Database, a special task force constituted by the AAOMS in 2007 highlighted important periodontal considerations in third molar surgery [10]. This include the effect of surgery on the distal periodontium of the second molar and the impact of retained third molar on the periodontal health and general health status of a patient.

The loss of periodontal attachment on the distal aspect of the second molar associated with third molar surgery was proven and no single surgical approach was able to minimize the loss, but potentially successful treatment techniques such as root planning and plague control, guided tissue regeneration (GTR), and/or use of demineralized bone powder (DBP) were identified.

On the other hand, retained impacted third molar was associated with greater periodontal disease severity in the second molar and other posterior teeth with progressive loss of attachment and pocket formation. The supportive influence of third molars on periodontal microflora, especially putative pathogens, and on molecular markers of inflammation was substantially established and the positive effect of removal of third molar on reduction of periodontal disease severity, pathogenic microbial count, and inflammatory mediators was as well established.

An important research conducted by Dr. Ray White and his team corroborated the implication of retained impacted third molar in the etiology and severity of periodontal diseases with proven evidence of association with systemic consequences such as premature delivery, low birth weight, and cardiovascular effects [69, 70, 107, 230–232].

In view of the foregoing, the current argument is that the concept of prophylactic removal is a misnomer [16, 82]. Since, there is established evidence of ongoing periodontal pathology associated with an impacted third molar. The absence of clinical symptoms does not necessarily rule out pathology, since symptoms often arise after the disease has advanced significantly. A new concept, *"therapeutic removal of asymptomatic third molar,"* has been suggested [16, 82].

Based on the recent evidence-based research, the journal of Oral and maxillofacial surgery proposed the following guidelines for the management of asymptomatic third molar [16]:

1. All third molars should be considered for removal in young adults in order to mitigate the risks of systemic inflammation and local progression of emergent periodontal disease.
2. Patients who elect to retain their third molars need to be monitored for the progression of periodontal disease.
3. Patients with retained third molars should be informed of research regarding increased risks for systemic disease.

It would appear in the light of current evidence that most of the traditional arguments in support of prophylactic removal of impacted lower third molars can no longer be substantial reasons for removal of asymptomatic impacted lower third molars. However, a new perspective is emerging to justify the routine extraction of this tooth; this is based on the consideration for periodontal health and its consequent potential for systemic complications.

A possible guide to treatment decisions is to inform every patient with impacted third molars about the newly established potential consequences of retained impacted third molar and allow patient to participate in decision making. Based on this thinking, the conclusions highlighted by JOMS [16] are reasonable. However, considering that the well-established systemic complications of periodontitis were related to obstetrics patients, further evidence is required to convince that these considerations should not be limited to impacted teeth in females.

8.2.2 Imaging Techniques in Third Molar Management

Before removing an impacted lower third molar, it is always advisable to conduct a thorough radiographic evaluation of the tooth. By doing so, a surgeon is able to assess the risk of inferior alveolar nerve (IAN) injury, determine the potential surgical difficulty, and plan appropriate technique for removal.

Dental panoramic tomography (DPT) is the recommended standard [190, 233], where this is not available, periapical radiograph (PAR) is used to assess individual third molar [6]. The relative merit of the DPT rests in its ability to present the radiographic picture of the entire jaws in one film, thereby reducing overall radiation dose while making comprehensive assessment for risk of nerve injury, associated pathology, and difficulty possible [1, 22]. The demerit has to do with the variable distortion of images associated with the technique [21].

Some advanced imaging techniques have also been used in third molar management. Most important is computerized tomography (CT). Others such as digital panoramic radiography [23] and Magnetic resonance imaging [156] are less frequently used. The former requires more sophisticated technology and is not universally available, while the latter is applicable only for the evaluation of the lingual nerve position and risk to injury, but as yet the clinical efficacy is not proven.

CT axial and coronal slices are frequently adequate, but 3-D reconstruction offers additional benefits in some situations [143]. Special techniques such as volumetric CT [175] and tuned aperture computerized tomography (TACT) [146] are also employed for their relative advantages. CT is particularly advocated because of its ability to better delineate the molar relationship to the inferior alveolar neurovascular bundle (IAN) [21, 22]. The bucco-lingual relationship of the inferior dental canal to the molar roots can be appreciated on axial slices, and the three-dimensional morphology of the canal and roots is demonstrable with 3-D CT or reformatted axial, coronal, and sagittal slices [143]. CT also permits detection of the intraradicular path of the neurovascular bundle, root angulation, and determination of the actual distance between the tooth and IAN canal [143, 170].

In clinical practice, there are other important considerations such as radiation dose exposure, cost, technicality demands, and relative significance to treatment outcome. If scientific evidence does not prove to be a practical advantage of an advance imaging technique, it may not worth the effort and investment; the simple techniques of conventional DPT should be preferred.

There is no substantial evidence in the literature to suggest that CT does better than DPT in the assessment of surgical difficulty of impacted third molar and detection of pathology associated with the tooth. On the other hand, the emphasis of CT has been on its relative importance in predicting injury to the IAN.

The radiographic signs on DPT predictive of injury to IAN are superimposition of the IAN canal and third molar, close relationship between IAN canal and third molar roots, loss of the cortical lines of the canal, darkening of the root, narrowing or diversion of the IAN canal where it crosses the third molar root, and a dark or bifid apex [146, 170]. With a CT scan, the relationship of the impacted molar to the IAN canal can be appreciated in more of a life form picture, bucco-lingual and apicocoronal [143, 146, 170]. Several prospective experimental studies have been done to assess the sensitivity and specificity of DPT in predicting IAN injury based on the fore stated criteria [21, 28, 161, 210]. The sensitivity is average, while the specificity is quite high [10].

This implies that whenever DPT suggests low risk, the predictions are most often correct, but when high risk is suggested, the predictions are less often true.

Only one study was found to compare the sensitivity and specificity of DPT with CT imaging for prediction of IAN injury [175]. The sample was composed of subjects referred for CT imaging secondary to detecting high-risk findings on DPT. The specificity and sensitivity were 70 and 63% vs. 93 and 77% for DPT and CT, respectively. The study indicated that prediction with CT is more likely to be accurate compared to DPT, and therefore, justifies request for CT when high-risk findings are noted on DPT. This will only become clinically important if the findings on CT will significantly alter the line of management such as abandoning wholesome extraction for coronectomy.

As of today, more investigations are still required to better understand and outline the parameters for effective use of CT imaging in the management of third molars [170]. The paucity of thorough randomized controlled clinical trials detracts from the strength of the current evidence.

8.2.3 Evaluation of Surgical Difficulty

The evaluation of the difficulty inherent in the surgical extraction of individual third molar is an important objective of preoperative assessment. This is particularly necessary in settings where a third molar removal may be carried out by less experienced surgeons and modification of treatment plan, technique, and versatility in the procedure becomes very important. Such is the case in teaching hospital settings where junior cadre residents may have to handle less difficult cases, while difficult cases are left for senior residents, chief resident, and attending specialists, or in general dental practices where the dentist is less versatile in third molar surgery and referral to specialist is indicated.

Although many efforts have gone into attempts to derive useful clinical indices for preoperative evaluation and prediction of surgical difficulty, none has produced a clear, accurate, and universally applicable tool for this purpose [5]. Some of the previous attempts are the WHARFE scoring system, Pell and Gregory's criteria, Pederson index, and Yuasa et al. index. These are all empirical criteria with limited accuracies. The WHARFE scores have not been clinically validated, while the Pell and Gregory's criteria [4, 78] and Pederson index [4, 59, 85, 87, 233] have been found to be unreliable. Unfortunately, very little has been done in the sense of evidence-based research to track down the best predictive factors for surgical difficulty on which a more accurate and universally applicable tool may be predicated [5].

Several parameters have been implicated in the literature; these traditionally included radiographic features of the impacted molars and the jaw. Recent evidences have implicated other variables such as demographic parameters and operative variables.

The spectrum include bony depth of impaction, angulation of impaction, space available for the impacted molar, root morphology and number, periodontal membrane space, proximity to IAN canal, bone density, etc., (Radiographic variables) [6, 197, 235]; age, sex, body weight, body mass index, body surface area, ethnicity, etc., (Demographic variables) [5, 6, 87]; and surgeon's experience, soft or hard tissue impactions, surgical technique, etc., (operative variables) [5, 24, 220].

Akadiri and Obiechina recently conducted a systematic review on this subject [5]. They did not find any randomized controlled trial on the subject. They identified those variables that have been consistently implicated in many prospective experimental studies as reliable predictors of difficulty. The variables so identified were age (demographic variable), surgeon, procedure type, number of teeth extracted (operative variables), and depth of impaction, angulation of impaction, and root morphology (radiographic variable). They enthused that a more accurate formula combining these factors may evolve in the near future.

Thus, as of now, no valid, comprehensive, universally applicable evidence-based index for predicting difficulty of surgical removal of impacted lower third molar is available. Individual surgeons use the known parameters to evaluate difficulty on a case-by-case basis, in which case disparity in judgments between different surgeons is likely. It is desirable that a clear, simple, accurate, and universally applicable index of prediction is developed, but more evidence is needed to synthesize this.

8.2.4 Prophylactic Use of Antibiotics

Opinions are still divided among oral surgeons as to the appropriateness and efficacy of routine antibiotic prescription in third molar surgery [52, 180, 182]. Recently published clinical trials only added to the confusion because of the contradicting results contained in them [186].

The reasons commonly adduced to justify the use of antibiotics in third molar surgery include [180, 237]: (1) therapeutic management of preexisting infection, (2) prevention of secondary infection in high-risk patients (e.g., immunocompromised, sickle cell disease), and (3) prophylaxis against postoperative infective and noninfective inflammatory complications in an otherwise healthy individual. While these first two reasons are not in dispute, the third reason has generated much controversies based on the following arguments [52, 97, 174]:

1. The risk of developing resistant strains is high
2. The potential for adverse events such as allergic reactions and anaphylaxis is considerable
3. There is an unwarranted exposure to the risk of drug toxicity.
4. There is unjustifiable disruption of the homeostatic balance of normal oral and enteral commensals

However, many oral surgeons still prescribe antibiotics routinely following third molar surgery in otherwise healthy patients [78]. Efforts to synthesize the best evidence through critical appraisal of published literature, especially systematic reviews and meta-analysis of RCT, have not produced a conclusive position on the debate, but certain facts for consideration can be delineated. The decision as to whether or not to prescribe, type, and timing of prescription can be made after thorough consideration of these facts.

1. The routine use of antibiotics is at variance with the general principle of antibiotic prophylaxis because the overall risk of infection following third molar surgery is low.

The commonly reported incidence of alveolar osteitis and surgical site infection following third molar surgery stands at 1–7% [42, 90]. With adequate compliance to the principle of asepsis, this rate could be even lower among healthy individuals without preoperative infection. Based on the guiding principles for prophylactic antibiotics, a procedure with low propensity for postoperative infection does not require prophylaxis [180, 237]. Therefore, the infection rate following third molar removal should not ordinarily warrant routine prophylaxis. However, another perspective has emerged favoring the use of antibiotics to alleviate postoperative inflammatory sequelae of third molar surgery [39, 98, 151]. This is further discussed in Sect. 7.2.5.

2. The noninfective inflammatory sequalae of third molar surgery are related to the extent of trauma and so are better treated with anti-inflammatory drugs and analgesics.

A critical review of literature including randomized clinical trials and prospective cohort studies [237] showed that there was no significant benefit derived from the use of antibiotics to reduce pain, swelling, and trismus. Although some authors [30, 39, 151] observed marginal benefits, they did not think it was sufficient for them to recommend routine antibiotics. In most cases where statistical differences were observed, the benefit was noticeable on day 7 or day 8 beyond when symptoms were virtually resolved in most patients, including the control or placebo groups [118, 144].

3. The risk of infection is relatively higher in partial or full bony impaction.

Two critical reviews of the literature including randomized controlled clinical trials and some prospective cohort studies [144, 196] indicated that extraction requiring moderate to high degree ostectomy presents higher risk of surgical site infection and alveolar osteitis. It was, therefore, recommended that antibiotics may be prescribed in such cases [144, 196]. What requires to be clarified about this observation is whether or not to complete the procedure before commencing antibiotics since the extent of trauma and degree of ostectomy are often determined intraoperatively or to employ proper prophylaxis at least 1 h prior to surgery based on radiographic estimation of the likely amount of bone removal, which is not always accurate.

4. Broad spectrum antibiotics, mainly penicillin (Amoxicillin, Co-amoxiclv), macrolides (Clindamycin), and narrow spectrum antianaerobicidal (Metronidazole, tinidazole) are appropriate and often adequate for prophylaxis in third molar surgery.

Penicillins, especially amoxicillin and co-amoxiclav, have been widely investigated in third molar surgery and their efficacy in the treatment of established preoperative and postoperative infection in oral surgery is well documented [52, 162, 186]. Another well-established

broad spectrum agent in third molar surgery is clindamycin [96, 182], while narrow spectrum antianaerobicidal imidazoles have also proven adequate probably because of the plethora of pathogenic anaerobes among the oral microflora [97, 118, 160]. Many other newer generation antibiotics may be equally effective; there may be no justification for their use since the simpler antibiotics (i.e., penicillins. Macrolides, and imidazoles) have proven adequate either as single agent or in combinations [226]. However, there is no evidence to justify the use of multiple agents for prophylaxis in third molar surgery.

5. The use of systemic antibiotics is supported by enough literature including randomized clinical trials.

The effectiveness of systemic antibiotics in oral surgery has been proven in many clinical trials [96, 118, 180, 186]. So far, there appears to be no significant difference in the effectiveness of oral and parenteral administration in a patient who is able to tolerate oral route based on available literature. The oral route is, therefore, recommendable except when compliance is doubtful.

Although the use of topical antiseptic and/or antibiotics is supported by some literature [95, 98, 169], there are not enough clinical trials or randomized prospective study to evaluate their relative benefits in comparison to systemic administration. Pieuch et al. [180] concluded that the outcome of topical tetracycline placed in the extraction socket was better for partial and full bony impaction compared to systemic administration. However, they did not disclose the systemic antimicrobial agent used or the regimen adopted.

6. Single bolus high-dose preoperative administration is often sufficient for prophylaxis and may be combined with 2–5 days postoperative regular dose regimen in high-risk patients.

Ren and Hans [186] performed the most rigorous systematic review of literature and meta-analysis of all relevant studies on the use of antibiotics in third molar surgery, including published and unpublished data in all languages. They concluded that single dose bolus antibiotic prophylaxis is sufficient in most cases to prevent alveolar osteitis and surgical site infection, especially where traumatic extraction is envisaged. For patients who have known risk for postoperative complications such as smokers, poor oral hygiene, old age, and severely traumatic extraction, additional 2–5 days of postoperative antibiotics is recommended. This might be the best evidence in the current literature.

8.2.5 Control of Postoperative Pain, Swelling, and Trismus

The postoperative period following the removal of an impacted mandibular third molar is frequently characterized by pain, swelling, and trismus [141, 205]. The symptoms are sometimes so severe, resulting in significant deterioration in patient's quality of life [48, 198]. While the occurrence is an inevitable physiologic response to trauma, the severity and consequences can be considerably mitigated. Several options have been postulated to achieve significant alleviation of these important postoperative sequelae of third molar surgery. These include variation of flap closure techniques, use of tube or gauze drains, facial ice pack therapy, use of anti-inflammatory drugs such as corticosteroids, nonsteroidal anti-inflammatory drugs (NSAIDs), and use of antibiotics. While some of these options have proven to be effective, the clinical efficacy of most is still to be established based on evidence. An appraisal of current literature would reveal the relative efficacy or otherwise of some of the options. Evidence-based answers to the following clinical questions might have been provided.

1. Does closure to permit secondary healing of the socket reduce the severity of pain, swelling, and trismus?

Conflicting opinions are expressed in the literature regarding the relative advantages of secondary healing over primary healing of third molar surgical extraction socket [173]. In secondary healing, the flaps are repositioned and/or sutured in a way to preserve the opening of the socket into the oral cavity [173]. This is achieved either by placing limited number of sutures to anchor the flap in position ensuring none across the socket, i.e., no hermetic closure [6, 24], or by removing a small chunk of mucosa flap distal to the second molar to keep the socket open for drainage while all other areas are closed [29, 64]. On the contrary, primary closure involves complete hermetic closure of the socket opening which leaves no room for drainage [29, 64, 173].

Some authors prefer primary closure, stating its better esthetic outcome as it results in healing without scarring [14, 100, 121, 129]. Antagonistic reports emphasize the problems associated with primary closure citing the greater degree of pain, swelling, and trismus in the immediate postoperative period [29, 64, 185]. A neutral opinion group also exists; they believe postoperative progress does not differ between patients who had primary closure and those who had secondary healing [45, 219].

Most of these opinions were either based on authors' experience or prospective comparative experimental studies often not randomized. Methodological differences such as the stringency of criteria for inclusions and evaluation, sample size determination and randomization, control groups, and blinding would account for most of the differences in observations and conclusions. Doing extensive literature search, we found no properly randomized controlled trial, systematic review, or meta-analysis of RCT to verify the clinical differences between these two modalities of closure. The best evidence is deducible from among the experimental studies and textbook teachings, some of which might have been premised on authors' experience. A closer appraisal of the available evidences showed that the older literature [14, 100, 121, 129] favor primary closure while secondary closure was overwhelmingly favored in the more recent literature [29, 64, 185].

A possible explanation to this is that emphasis on quality of life in third molar surgery only recently became an issue [48, 198]. The noninfective inflammatory sequelae of third molar surgery were hitherto accepted as inevitable consequences that patients had to cope with in the immediate postoperative period. These days, a lot of efforts are being put into deriving measures to reduce postoperative discomfort to the barest minimum. Undoubtedly, current evidence is in support of secondary healing. Quality controlled randomized trials are still required for comparison.

2. Does the use of drain offer relief from the noninfective inflammatory sequelae of third molar surgery?

The insertion of gauze or tube drain was advocated to provide drainage of inflammatory exudates and consequently reduce pain, swelling, and trismus [7, 185]. This hypothesis has been tested in some prospective experimental studies, but variable results have been reported [7, 44, 185]. Rakprasitkul and Pairuchvej reported efficacy in the control of pain, trismus, and swelling [185]; similarly in 1995, Ayad et al. [18] reported a statistically significant decrease in swelling, trismus, and pain in patients after use of a Penrose rubber drain. Cerqueira et al. [41] observed efficacy in the control of swelling only, and recorded no significant effect on pain and trismus. In fact, they noticed that pain in the first 24 h was indeed more severe in the drain group. Chukwuneke et al. [44] documented significant effect on swelling and trismus and no effect on pain. Other studies on tube drain either compared the effect of drain alone with drain in association with primary closure or with drain in association with secondary healing. It was found that the associated use of drain brought about greater relief of inflammatory discomfort in primary closure [185], while it had no additional advantage in secondary closure [29]. Further, comparisons of the effect of tube drain with corticosteroids have also been reported. The finding is contradictory; one study reported equal potency [171], while another study claimed better outcome with corticosteroids [236].

There is an obvious lack of strong evidence-based on properly controlled and blinded clinical trials of adequate sample size on the relative efficacy of tube drain in third molar surgery. Although claims of beneficial effect are consistently made in the literature, the comparative merits in relation to perioperative anti-inflammatory drugs are not established. Although the risk of adverse effect with drug use has been cited by antagonists to favor tube drain, this has not been reported where judicious patient selection and adherence to safe dosages have been employed. On the other hand, the use of drain requires an added effort: the surgeon has to be careful in inserting a drain into the buccal fold, to ensure it is not counterproductive, and the patient has to return one or more time for drain removal. Patients have complained of variable degree of irritation and discomfort associated with the presence of drain in the mouth and disturbance of healing and aggravation of pain during drain removal at the time when the surgical wound is often still tender. Prospective qualities of life studies are required to document patients' preferences.

3. What is the efficacy of facial ice pack therapy in reducing inflammatory sequelae of third molar surgery?

In some centers, facial ice pack is routinely used to relief inflammatory sequelae of dentoalveolar surgery [40, 50, 150]. The physiological basis for this therapy is assumed to be cold-mediated vasoconstriction resulting in decreased edema formation. While the efficacy of ice pack therapy has been established in certain inflammatory orthopedic conditions [54, 68, 199], no clear evidence of efficacy in third molar surgery is as yet documented. Investigation of this hypothesis is sparse in the world literature. Forsgren et al. [84] indicated that application of cold dressing does not influence postoperative edema. One randomized observer blind comparison of facial ice pack therapy with no ice therapy found no statistically significant difference between the two groups [225]. On the other hand, Filho et al. [81], in a similar study, reported efficacy of cryotherapy with facial ice pack in reducing pain and swelling, but not trismus. Mac Auley [145] performed a critical literature review concluding that ice therapy is effective in the control of postoperative inflammation in third molar surgery; repeated application at 10 min interval was found to be most effective. It appears from the current literature that cold therapy may be useful in alleviating postoperative discomforts following third molar surgery. How much of relief this offer is still to be quantified. More research is required to prove or discard the efficacy of cold therapy as antidote to pain, swelling, and trismus in third molar surgery, especially to know if any additional benefit in combination with anti-inflammatory drug therapy does exist.

4. Is perioperative corticosteroids useful in the control of postoperative inflammatory morbidity after third molar surgery?

Corticosteroids are potent anti-inflammatory agents [102, 103, 177]. Their use in oral surgery dates back to the early 1950s when Spies et al. [214] and Strean and Horton [218] administered hydrocortisone to prevent inflammation. Since then, several studies have demonstrated the effect of various preparations of corticosteroids on pain, swelling, and trismus following third molar surgery [74, 101, 155, 223]. However, the reported effect and duration of the effect vary depending on the agent used, dosages, timing, route of administration, and especially the settings and design of the various studies [20, 91, 101, 135, 148]. Although there have been several narrative reviews of the relevant literature [8, 88, 97, 126, 154, 196], these often lack objectivity and key characteristics such as sample size, designs of the studies reviewed, and validity of published results are often not addressed [126, 172].

Hence, evidences on several aspects of corticosteroids use in third molar surgery remain inconclusive.

The commonly used corticosteroids in third molar surgery experimental models are methyl prednisolone and dexamethasone in various preparations and dosages [8]. These have been particularly preferred because of their strong glucocorticoid and minimal mineralcorticoid effects [109, 163]. There is extensive evidence in proving the efficacy of these agents in alleviating the discomforts associated with the inflammatory sequelae of third molar surgery [8, 120, 126, 163, 167]. Some authors reported efficacy with respect to swelling alone [92], trismus alone [164], swelling and pain [38], or the three parameters [74, 91, 236]. One systematic review and meta-analysis exhaustively established the efficacy of corticosteroids in the control of swelling and trismus but was unable to conclude on pain due to insufficient data [147]. This is the highest evidence available in the current literature. The authors conducted a rigorous search of all published and unpublished data in all languages and selected studies based on stringent criteria including methodologic quality and validity of results. However, the article did not address some other areas where conflicting reports abound in the literature. These include issues related to differences in timing of administration, i.e., pre, intra, or postoperative; local vs. systemic administration; types or dose of corticosteroids relative to the outcomes; comparison of corticosteroids to NSAIDs; and comparison with combined corticosteroid – NSAIDs use. As yet, more standardized, quality, well-controlled clinical trials are required in these aspects.

An extensive review of the literature would highlight certain important consideration in respect of corticosteroid use in oral surgery. These include the need to be cautious in patients who have tuberculosis, peptic ulcer diseases, active viral or fungal infections (especially ocular herpes), active acne vulgaris, primary glaucoma, or patients with a history of acute psychoses or psychotic tendencies [103, 126, 147]. Also, an optimal dose should be chosen because suboptimal dose has not been effective [8, 126] and higher than optimal doses have added no significant advantage to outcomes, but the risk of adverse effect is increased [92, 101, 223]. The usual effective dosage range is 40–125 mg for methyl prednisolone and 4–12 mg for dexamethasone over a short duration; ranging from single preoperative dose to 1–3 days of regular dose postsurgery, depending on the route of administration [8, 122]. Such short-term use has not been associated with the known systemic side effects of steroids such as poor wound healing, infection, or adrenal suppression [20, 88]. The oral route has proven effective in many experimental studies; the need to commence administration 2–4 h prior to surgery was advocated to assure adequate plasma concentration before initiation of inflammation [8]. Intramuscular route, either locally (e.g., intramasseteric or into the medial pterygoid) or at distant sites (deltoid, gluteal), has similar efficacy [8, 28]. Submucosal injection and endoalveolar powder of dexamethazone in the vicinity of the operation site have also proven effective [91, 92]. Intravenous route is advised 10–30 min prior to surgery or intraoperatively if need was realized during surgery [8]. In spite of the proven efficacy, considering the potential side effects, corticosteroid is not advised for routine use; it is recommended for cases where significant amount of surgical trauma is anticipated or serendipitously encountered during surgery [8].

5. What is the analgesic drug of choice following third molar surgery?

The desire for the most potent analgesics appropriate following surgical removal of impacted third molars has been a motivation for numerous experimental studies comparing various types and dosages of analgesic drugs [202, 204]. Postoperative efficacy of simple analgesics (paracetamol) [47, 105, 209], NSAIDs (ibuprofen, diclofenac, piroxicam, tenoxicam) [60, 61, 62, 104, 108, 140, 189], COX-2 inhibitors (coxibs) [19, 55, 56], and weak and intermediate opiods (dihydrocodeine, tramadol) [155] has been tested using pain models involving third molar surgery. Among these are several clinical trials [50, 104, 140, 188, 189, 209, 238], systematic reviews, and meta-analysis of clinical trials [153, 157, 189, 235], which have helped to synthesize substantive evidence to guide analgesic prescription in the settings of third molar surgery.

Barden et al. [66] performed a rigorous meta-analysis of systematic reviews on analgesics efficacy in third molar surgery. Their work is arguably the best evidence on this subject so far in the current world literature. Stringent inclusion criteria were stated and were strictly adhered to. Several independent reviewers evaluated each report based on agreed consensus and appropriate statistics were employed. The lowest (best) NNTs (number needed to treat) were for NSAIDs and COX-2 inhibitors at standard or high doses. For these, NNTs could be as low as about two (meaning that two patients had to be treated with NSAID or COXIB for one of them to have an outcome of at least half pain relief that would not have occurred with placebo). Valdecoxib 20 and 40 mg, rofecoxib 50 mg, ibuprofen 400 mg, and diclofenac 50 and 100 mg all had NNTs below 2.4. For all of them, about 60–70% of patients had at least half pain relief with active treatment compared with about 10% with placebo.

Paracetamol 975/1,000 mg, aspirin 600/650 mg, and paracetamol 600/650 mg had NNTs of between four and five. Fewer than 40% of patients with paracetamol at these doses had at least half pain relief with active treatment. With dihydrocodeine 30 mg, only 16% of patients had at least half pain relief with active treatment in one small trial. As regard the risk of adverse effect, of the 15 drug and dose combinations assessed, only paracetamol 600/650 mg plus codeine 60 mg could be statistically distinguished from placebo. The NNT was 5.3 (4.1–7.4), indicating that five patients had to be treated with paracetamol 600/650 mg plus codeine 60 mg for one of them to have an adverse event that would not have occurred with placebo. For all other drugs and doses, there was no difference between analgesic and placebo. This evidence suggests that the nonaspirin NSAIDs and COX-2 inhibitors in regular doses are the most efficacious for pain control in third molar surgery and they are not likely to be associated with side effects if regular doses are adhered to in properly selected patients.

Aspirin has no proven superiority over paracetamol. In a study of comparative efficacy of aspirin and paracetamol, the two drugs were found to be equi-analgesic [49]. A quantitative systematic review of the efficacy of aspirin in postoperative pain management also supported the weak analgesic effect of aspirin [67]. On the contrary, some authors have argued that the formulation of aspirin has a significant effect on its analgesic potency and have demonstrated that soluble aspirin is more efficacious than paracetamol [203]. There is as yet no sufficient scientific evidence to substantiate this claim.

6. Does the preemptive analgesic effect of NSAIDs come to play in third molar surgery?

Even though preemptive analgesia has been demonstrated repeatedly in animal models of pain, the clinical evidence that support preemptive analgesia in human pain studies has been more variable [124, 131]. The best studied anti-inflammatory for preoperative use in third molar surgery is ibuprofen [60, 61, 140]. Most of these studies demonstrated significant analgesic effect when ibuprofen was used preoperatively as evidenced in delayed onset of postoperative pain and reduced quantity of analgesics in the immediate postoperative period. Other anti-inflammatory drugs have been studied for preemptive effect in fewer trials. Piroxicam [104], fenbufen [211], indomethacin [12], diflunisal [176, 208], flurbiprofen [61, 65], and valdecoxib [55] have also shown significant analgesic effect following preoperative use. However, there is no evidence about the relative efficacy of these drugs with respect to preemptive analgesic effect in third molar surgery.

On the contrary, three randomized controlled clinical trials with some NSAIDs [32, 207, 209] and one with paracetamol [94] showed no evidence of a preemptive effect. It has been suggested that every NSAID has a preemptive effect, but this is unlikely to be seen with conventional doses [114]. Therefore, any antinociceptive treatment should be extended into the postoperative period when generation of noxious stimuli from inflammatory process may be intense depending on the type of operation [114, 127].

There is a lack of systematic reviews of RCT on preemptive effect of NSAIDs in third molar surgery to enhance a consensus. Hence, preemptive use of NSAIDs is still not routinely practiced. Since it is now accepted that the policy of waiting for a patient to report severe pain before prescribing an analgesics produces discomfort and may reduce the efficacy of any subsequent treatment [58], preemptive use of NSAIDs may have a place.

A new horizon in the preemptive treatment of pain and inflammation in third molar surgery is emerging; preoperative corticosteroids and NSAIDs are being combined in clinical trials with reports that the combination produces analgesic and anti-inflammatory potency greater than the use of either drug [38, 164]. This evidence is still to be properly synthesized.

7. What is the usefulness of antibiotics in the control of postoperative inflammatory sequelae after third molar surgery?

Some authors [39, 98, 144, 180] concluded that antibiotics prevent noninfective inflammatory complications of third molar surgery, such as pain, swelling, and trismus. This impression has been contradicted by many subsequent studies [17, 182]. Although there is as yet no consensus on the routine use of systemic antibiotics after third molar surgery, a recent meta-analysis advised single preoperative bolus when a surgeon prefers to use antibiotics. Additional 2–5 days course was recommended in high-risk patients (Sect. 7.2.4). The suggestion that antibiotics reduce pain, swelling, and trismus would tend to justify routine use of antibiotics since these are inevitable outcomes of third molar surgery.

A critical appraisal of the methodology and results of some of those supportive studies revealed that the conclusion was often not justifiable [237]. Among these, two randomized double blind studies evaluated antibiotics vs. placebo in third molar surgical patients. Kaziro [118] did not observe a significant difference in pain, swelling, and trismus between metronidazole and placebo group until postoperative day 8. Macgregor and Addy observed a statistical difference at the lowest level that cannot justify recommendation for routine prescription. In a less stringent randomized study without blinding, Bystedt and Nord [39] noted that pain was significantly better on postoperative day 7. It is important to note that most symptoms of discomfort associated with third molar surgery are often resolved by 1 week after surgery [81, 151], so that these findings may not be enough to justify the use of antibiotics.

Contradictory reports were published by Poeschl et al. [182] and Ataoglu et al. [17] who did not find antibiotics to have significant effect on pain, swelling, and trismus. Following a review of the literature, Zeitler observed that antibiotics have no place in the control of noninfective inflammatory sequelae of third molar surgery [237]. Aseptic approach to the surgical site and careful surgical techniques to minimize trauma would seem to be the most appropriate mechanism to minimize inflammatory complications, such as pain, swelling, and trismus. Since there is a longitudinal relationship between extent of trauma and postsurgical inflammation, it would appear reasonable to use anti-inflammatory agents and analgesics to control pain, swelling, and trismus, instead of antibiotics.

position of the tooth, it may be necessary to remove distal, distolingual, or lingual bone [183, 229]. In such situation, buccal approach with lingual flap retraction or the lingual split technique with lingual flap elevation has been advocated [149, 165].

Encroaching on the lingual soft tissue exposes the lingual nerve to increased risk of injury [179, 187]. Protection of the lingual nerve using appropriately sized retractor is a measure advocated to prevent this complication [10, 183, 229]. Ironically, some literature reports affirmed that the use of lingual flap retractor tends to increase the incidence of temporary nerve damage without necessarily protecting against permanent injuries [179, 187].

An extensive literature review conducted by the AAOMS special task force on third molar surgery [48] found an average range of 0.0–0.5% incidence rate of permanent lingual nerve injury (>6 months) with use of lingual flap. This is comparable to the incidence commonly reported in cases without lingual flap elevation with or without lingual retraction. Only one systematic review of the literature was found on this subject matter. The review excluded a large number of studies based on certain strict inclusion criteria that border on methodological qualities of the studies. Meta-analysis of the eight included studies showed that the use of lingual flap retractor during third molar surgery was in fact associated with an increased incidence of temporary nerve damage and was neither protective nor detrimental with respect to the incidence of permanent nerve damage. However, it is noteworthy that the Howarth's periosteal elevator was used for retraction in all included studies, whereas some authors have indicated that size of the working end of this retractor is not wide enough to provide the desired protection [26, 149, 187] and that wider end retractor did better in a comparative experimental study [90]. This systematic review did not address some salient facts such as surgeon's experience and versatility with lingual flap retraction techniques and the influence of differently sized retractors.

8.2.6 Prevention of Lingual Nerve Injury

Most third molars can be removed by utilizing a purely buccal technique [86], in which it is unnecessary to encroach on the lingual soft tissues. However, in some rare circumstances, compelled by the patho-anatomic

8.3 Conclusion

Decision making in the management of impacted mandibular third molar is fraught with many controversies. Since the beginning of the nineteenth century till date, numerous studies have been geared toward resolving many of the controversies. Current evidences have tremendously helped in charting a course for standard practice in third molar surgery. Decision to remove or not can be guided by the knowledge that some level of periodontal pathology exists with every impacted third molar. Patients and their physicians can now make informed decision after proper evaluation of the risks and benefits. Proper preoperative radiographic evaluation is mandatory to assess difficulty and risk of complications. DPT is adequate but may be supplemented with CT where a high risk to IAN injury is suspected. Evidences are emerging to track down important factors predictive of difficulty, which now includes demographic, operative, and radiographic parameters. Also the era of antibiotic abuse is gradually ending as appropriate indications are now emerging. Current evidence suggests that single bolus prophylaxis may be used in most patients with partial to full bony impactions, but additional 3–5 days of regular dose may be restricted to high-risk patients such as smokers, poor oral hygiene, old age, and following very severe surgical trauma. Antibiotic prophylaxis is justified only as a preemptive measure against infection and probably dry socket, but not to alleviate posttraumatic pain, swelling, and trismus. The control of these inflammatory sequelae of third molar surgery can be appropriately accomplished with secondary flap closure techniques or with NSAIDs, COX-2 inhibitors and/or corticosteroids (40–125 mg methyl prednisolone, 8–12 mg dexamethasone), or with the use of tube drain. Buccal approach to removal largely avoids injury to lingual nerve, but where encroachment into the lingual tissues is indicated, the usefulness of lingual retractors to prevent damage is still questionable.

The management of impacted lower third molar has always been shrouded in controversies. It appears that with the evolution of the discipline of evidence-based dentistry, the veil is being removed, the facts are now converging, and the evidences are emerging.

8.4 Evidence-Based Decisions in Jaw Augmentation

8.4.1 Introduction

Patients with severe atrophy of the jaws due to after-effect of trauma, chronic periodontitis, and congenital missing teeth often suffer from problems with dentures and are poor candidates for endosseous implants [217]. The problems with dentures include insufficient retention, intolerance to loading by mucosa, pain, difficulties with eating and speech, loss of soft tissue support, and altered facial appearance [217]. Insufficient height and width of the alveolar segment also compromise the insertion of dental implants.

Since dental implants have been shown to provide a reliable basis for fixed and removable prostheses, reconstructive preprosthetic jaw augmentation has changed from surgery aimed to provide sufficient osseous and mucosal support for a conventional denture into surgery aimed to provide a sufficient bone volume to enable implants to be placed at the most optimal positions from a prosthetic point of view [217]. Jaw augmentation is generally accepted for the moderate to severely resorbed edentulous mandible and maxilla [80].

In the last three decades, the role of augmentation of the jaws prior to insertion of dental implants has been tested through brilliant animal experimental studies and later clinical human studies. Presently, jaw augmentation procedures have evolved from an experimental to a mature evidence-based discipline. Several clinical trials (randomized and nonrandomized trials) have shown that inadequate bone volume of the residual edentulous ridge can be adequately augmented prior to implant insertion.

Autogenous bone grafts are considered the "gold standard" in bone tissue replacement because they are immunologically inert and osteogenic [2, 3]. But, unpredictable resorption and structural collapse of the bone graft during remodeling has been a continuing problem. These processes of bone remodeling have a major influence on the clinical outcome in terms of volume maintenance and incorporation into the recipient site. The graft has been reported to decrease in volume to an extent of 50–70% during the first year after insertion due to remodeling [83]. Verhoeven et al. [227] also found that in the first year after bone grafting, resorption is significant and may continue for years. Cortical bone, for example, may lose up to 33% of its strength during incorporation and generally remodels over a 6–18-month period [73]. In a clinical study, Johansson et al. [112] reported that the volume of inlay (particulate grafts) and onlay (cortical) autogenous iliac bone grafts was reduced by an average of 49.5 and 47%, respectively, of the initial volume after 6 months. Fonseca et al. [83] reported that onlaying corticocancellous bone onto the mandibular buccal cortex for augmentation of the alveolar ridge is a poor method by which to change ridge morphological structure. Therefore, several methods have been advocated not only to enhance incorporation, but also to reduce resorption of autogenous graft and ultimately augment the volume of the jaws. These include guided bone regeneration (GBR) technique, perforation of recipient cortical bone, addition of bone substitute materials, and preservation of graft periosteum, rigid fixation, and inhibition of osteoclastic activities [192], and application of platelet-rich plasma [222]. Other methods that have been employed in jaw augmentation include alveolar distraction, ridge splitting technique, sinus lift, and Le Fort I osteotomy [79, 80, 89].

8.4.2 Osteogenesis, Osteoinduction, and Osteconduction

Osteogenesis is the synthesis of new bone cells by cells derived from either the graft or the host [222]. When correctly handled, cells from cortical and cancellous grafts can survive the transfer to the host site and form new bone that is critical in the initial phase of bone repair [73]. The properties of cancellous grafts, which consist of an intimate trabecular structure lined with osteoblasts and a large surface area, make them very attractive at sites where new bone formation is desired.

Osteoinduction is the process by which mesenchymal cells (MSCs) at and around the host site are recruited to differentiate into chondroblasts and osteoblasts [35, 73, 222]. Recruitment and differentiation are modulated by graft matrix-derived growth factors. These growth factors include BMP-2, -3, and -7, which are members of the TGF-β superfamily. Other factors include PDGF, IL, FGF, IGF, GCSF, and VEGF. Three phases of osteoinduction-chemotaxis, mitosis, and differentiation have been described. In response to a chemical gradient during chemotaxis, bone induction factors direct migration of cells to the area in which they are to be utilized. Following chemotaxis, these factors stimulate intense mitogenic and proliferative activity in these cells; the cells differentiate into cartilage and become revascularized by invading blood vessels to form new bone [35, 36, 222].

Osteoconduction is the process by which an ordered, spatial three-dimensional ingrowth of capillaries, perivascular tissue, and MSCs takes place from host site along the implanted graft [35, 36, 166]. This scaffold permits the formation of new bone along a predictable pattern determined by the biology of the graft and the mechanical environment of the host-graft interface. For bone grafting to be successful, osteogenetic activity and bone formation alone are insufficient [35, 36, 83, 166, 222]. New bone must be distributed evenly in the grafted volume and must unite with the local host bone. Failure results in discontinous bone formation without adequate mechanical strength to support function.

8.4.3 Healing of Autogenous Bone Graft

The term incorporation is used to describe the biologic interactions between graft materials and host site that result in bone formation, leading to adequate mechanical properties. After a bone graft is harvested and transplanted to a new region, it begins multiple biologic processes that occur as the graft becomes incorporated into its host bed [35, 36, 222]. Healing and incorporation involve the processes of inflammation, revascularization, osteoconduction, osteoinduction, osteogenesis, and remodeling. An important aspect in (nonvascularized) bone graft is that a substantial portion of the biologic activity originates from the host [222]. Most viable osteocytes within the graft itself die quickly after transplantation, rendering the graft comparatively inert vs. the host. Despite this, substantial biologic interactions occur between the graft and the host, and the graft has a fundamental role in determining its own fate [9, 222]. This biologic interplay between graft and host establishes the final result.

There are some fundamental differences in the healing of cancellous and cortical autografts. Autogenous cancellous bone graft healing is divided into early and late phase [9, 222]. Hematoma formation around the bone graft is the first event that occurs after graft transplantation, usually caused by bleeding from the surgical disruption of host soft tissues and the recipient bony bed. During this early phase, only a small minority of the cells within the bone graft are still viable, located at the graft's peripheral surface [222]. These surface cells survive due to early vascularization or by plasmatic imbibition [166]. Revascularization that may begin as early as 2 days after transplantation rapidly progresses. BMPs and other growth factors induce migration of osteoblast precursor cells to the graft. These stem cells differentiate into osteoblasts and new bone forms at the end of this phase. The late phase is a continuum, proceeding through osteoconduction and eventual graft incorporation [166, 222]. Active graft resorption with new capillary ingrowth continues. Mature osteoblasts line the edges of the dead trabeculae as osteoid is deposited around the necrotic core. Remodeling proceeds and the graft is eventually replaced with the live host bone at the end of the late phase. This occurs approximately 6 months after transplantation and is usually completed by 1 year [166].

In contrast, cortical bone graft revascularization proceeds slowly, and thus, incorporation is prolonged [166, 222]. Vascular invasion of cortical bone graft is thought to be limited due primarily to its dense lamellar structure that constrains vessels to invading the graft along preexisting Haversian and Volkmann's canals. While cancellous bone grafts proceed with initial osteoblastic activity, revascularization of cortical bone grafts proceeds with initial osteoclastic activity [35, 166, 222]. The course of revascularization begins at the graft periphery and progresses to the interior of the graft. In cancellous grafts, vessels invasion may begin within few hours posttransplantation, and the process is completed in a few days. In cortical grafts, the earliest vessels enter the graft at 6 days, and the process of revascularization may take months, often resulting in incomplete graft revascularization [35, 36]. It is quite probable that, as suggested by Kenzora et al. [119], the initial stimulus to repair is the same in the cortical and cancellous bone, but there is no space available for cell proliferation in the dense bone, and therefore, bone resorption will prevail initially after transplantation.

8.4.4 Membranous vs. Endochondral Bone Grafts

There are two basic types of bone with respect to embryologic formation, and some debate exists as to which is preferable for bone grafting. Membranous bones include the flat bones of the cranium, face, and mandible (the mandible has some endochondral component with Meckel's cartilage origin). These bones form by intramembranous ossification in which embryonic MSCs differentiate directly into osteoblasts that synthesize a collagenous osteoid [35, 36, 159, 222]. The osteoid then becomes hard bone after undergoing mineralization by calcium phosphate. Endochondral

bones are long bones of the skeleton (including iliac bone and rib), as well as the petrous, occipital, ethmoid, mastoid, and sphenoid. These bones form by endochondral ossification whereby cartilage growth occurs at an epiphyseal surface, which is then replaced by osteoid that eventually becomes mineralized [9]. Clinical practice and literature concur that bone grafts from calvarial and facial sites (membranous) have a superior volumetric maintenance and survival over grafts from rib, tibia, or iliac crest (endochondral) [9, 159, 222]. The better incorporation of mandibular bone in the maxillofacial region has been attributed to a similarity in protocollagen and a higher concentration of morphogenetic proteins and growth factors [79, 158]. However, the search for the explanation for the difference in behavior between the membranous and endochondral bone continues to be a subject of continuing research, speculation, and controversy.

8.4.5 Donor Site for Autogenous Bone Graft

Depending on the amount of bone needed for jaw augmentation, several intraoral and extraoral sites are suitable donor sites. The most common extraoral site for bone graft harvest is the iliac crest. A large amount of corticocancellous graft can be harvested from iliac crest, especially the posterior iliac crest [79, 80]. Calvarial bone is another suitable extraoral site. However, harvesting of iliac or calvarial bone causes major intra and postoperative discomfort to the patient [79]. Therefore, it may be preferable to harvest block graft from an intraoral donor site (chin, angle, and ramus) to treat limited portion of the jaws [158].

8.4.6 Guided Tissue Regeneration

The biological concept of GTR was developed to regenerate lost tissues by preventing undesired cells from migrating into the wound area and permitting entrance of desired cells only, using different kinds of barrier membranes [117]. This concept was later employed in bone regeneration (GBR). It has also been shown that by using such membranes, it is possible to create bone at sites where bone normally is not present [3, 117]. Membranes used for GTR are either resorbable (e.g., collagen) or nonresorbable (e.g., e-PTFE). Resorbable membranes resorb; therefore, a second surgery for removal of the membrane is not necessary. However, an advantage of a nonresorbable membrane is the length of time the membrane will remain in place, and thus, exclude invagination of the graft by soft tissues [3, 117].

In the clinical situation, however, the GTR technique does not always result in predictable bone fill of the area to be regenerated [115, 206]. Several factors such as barrier stability, size of barrier perforations, peripheral sealing between barrier and bone, blood supply, and access to bone forming cells have been pointed out to be critical for a successful outcome [142]. It has been reported that collapse of the barrier membrane into the treated bone defect compromises the formation of new bone, as it eliminates the space that is necessary for bone formation [3, 53, 127]. The use of membranous bone grafts as space-keepers, in combination with nonresorbable or resorbable membranes, not only reduces the resorption of grafts, but also results in complete integration of the bone grafts into the bone at recipient site, provided that the membrane is kept covered with tissue during healing [3]. Adeyemo et al. [3] reported that the combination of iliac bone grafting and GTR for augmentation of the lateral surface of sheep mandible resulted in integration of the bone graft into recipient site.

8.4.7 Bone Substitute Materials in Jaw Augmentation

Development of bone substitutes has been a major interest for a number of years in oral and maxillofacial surgery, due to the inherent problems associated with autogenous and allogeneic bone grafts. An ideal bone substitute should be biocompatible, and it should gradually be replaced by newly formed bone and preferably possess osteoinductive or osteoconductive properties [111]. In recent years, hydroxyapatite (HA) bone substitutes have been developed synthetically (e.g., calcium phosphate), derived from corals or algae (e.g., Pro Osten 500®, Interpore 500 HA/CC®, and Algipore®), or originated from natural bone mineral (e.g., Bio-Oss®, and Endobon). These bone substitutes are generally regarded as being biocompatible and osteoconductive, although reports concerning their biodegradability have

been inconclusive [99]. They have also been found to contain no impurities that would make them unsuitable for clinical use [111]. Due to their (bone substitutes) lack of osteoinductive effect, a combination of autogenous bone graft and bone substitute is a preferred method of jaw augmentation [15].

Bio-Oss® is one of the bone substitutes that have been extensively studied. Bio-Oss®, like any other porous mineral bone graft substitutes, is osteoconductive. In osteoconduction, the implanted material serves as a scaffold for ingrowth of capillaries, perivascular tissue, and osteoprogenitor cells from recipient bed [35, 111]. In addition, Bio-Oss® particles have the additional advantage of having a larger surface area than the ceramic-type implants, which make them more osteoconductive. Recent evidence also suggested that the material is also osteopromotive through bioactive factors like TGF-β and BMP-2 found in the minute protein residues in the material [221].

The fate of Bio-Oss® as a bone substitute during healing and incorporation has been a subject of controversy in the literature. Some authors have reported that there is extensive resorption of this material [125], while others [13, 111, 201] have shown that there is little or no resorption at all. However, several studies have reported that autogenous bone graft covered with Bio-Oss® resulted in remarkable increase in augmented surface of the mandible and the maxillary sinus [2, 3, 200]. Ewers [77] reported an excellent long-term result of sinus lift procedure with Algipore® and platelet-rich plasma. The procedure enhanced enough new bone in 6 months to allow implant osseointegration after 6 months with a high implant survival rate [77].

8.4.8 Sinus Lift Procedure

Sinus lift procedure has become an established augmentation procedure prior to implant restoration of the edentulous maxilla. Grafting the floor of the maxillary sinus has become the most common surgical intervention for increasing alveolar bone height prior to the placement of endosseous dental implants in the posterior maxilla [228]. The aims of sinus grafting are to reestablish not only adequate bone volume for implant placement, but also a favorable intermaxillary relationship to optimize the functional and aesthetic outcome of the final prosthetic rehabilitation [43]. Clinical, histologic, and histomorphometric analysis have established the role of sinus lifting as a reliable and efficacious preprosthetic augmentation for the resorbed edentulous maxilla [77, 80]. Based on accumulated clinical and histologic evidence in the literature, sinus lift procedure is regarded as the best clinical practice in preimplant augmentation surgery of the maxilla [27]. However, there are still yet unanswered questions regarding the best material for sinus augmentation. There are several reports on the use of autogenous cancellous graft alone or in combination with bone substitutes, or the use of bone substitutes with platelet-rich plasma [27, 57, 77, 80]. A systematic review of the literature showed survival rates for implants placed in grafts made of bone substitutes alone and grafts of composite material were slightly better than the survival rates for implants placed in 100% autogenous grafts [57].

8.4.9 The Role of Distraction Osteogenesis in Jaw Augmentation

Distraction osteogenesis (DO) is a technique of gradual bone lengthening, allowing natural healing mechanisms to regenerate new bone [217]. The results of DO of the alveolar segment of the anterior and posterior edentulous mandible have been evaluated in several studies [72, 152, 184]. The advantage of DO is that there is little or no bone resorption as typically occurs in bone graft reconstruction [133]. Another advantage is the concomitant proliferation of attached gingival, obviating the need for the soft tissue augmentation. Therefore, DO avoids donor site morbidity associated with both hard and soft tissue harvest [133]. The short-term clinical, radiographic, and histomorphologic results are very promising. Presently reports on alveolar DO in the literature are mainly case reports and case series; and these are considered low level evidence in clinical practice [72, 133, 152, 184]. There is however, some evidence for the assumption that, in the near future, DO can develop into a reliable tool for augmentation of the jaws.

8.4.10 Ridge Splitting and Inlay Technique in Jaw Augmentation

Ridge splitting and inlay techniques for the expansion and/or increase width/height of the jaws prior to dental

implant insertion are increasingly being used as jaw augmentation techniques, especially for posterior edentulous mandible [159]. Although the level of evidence for ridge splitting and inlay techniques remains cases series and case reports, the bone expansion achievable has been reported to allow successful dental implant osseointegration [79, 159, 234]. Inlay techniques has a great potential for bone graft incorporation, assuring a good blood supply with a low final resorption of the graft and high implant survival and success rates [79, 110, 234]. An inlay bone graft undergoes less resorption in comparison with an onlay graft [110], and therefore, augmentation with inlay bone graft techniques has been shown to be remarkable [110].

8.4.11 The Role of Platelet-Rich Plasma in Jaw Augmentation

Strategies to accelerate autogenous bone graft healing have recently included the use of platelet-rich plasma (PRP). PRP is a source of a myriad of growth factors found within the alpha-granules of platelets, including platelet-derived growth factor, transforming growth factor-$\beta1$ and -$\beta2$, vascular endothelial growth factor, platelet-derived endothelial growth factor, interleukin-1, basic fibroblast growth factor, and platelet activating factor-4 [37]. Among the growth factors found in PRP, platelet-derived growth factor, basic fibroblast growth factor, and transforming growth factor-$\beta1$ and -$\beta2$ are the most osteogenically active growth factors found within PRP [37]. PRP growth factors do not induce osteoprogenitor cell differentiation, as is seen with the bone morphogenetic proteins, but instead act through stimulation of chemotaxis, mitogenesis, and angiogenesis of surrounding cells, acting as a catalyst in the very early phases of bone remodeling [138].

A number of studies have examined the use of PRP in conjunction with mandibular graft, sinus lift procedures, early implant placement, and grafts to other sites. However, the results of these studies have been mixed. Phillipart et al. [178] reported on the use of PRP, rhTF, and tetracycline in conjunction with autologous bone in sinus floor augmentation in 18 patients. The authors suggested that this enhanced vascularization and osteoblast numbers, but no control were used in this study. Butterfield et al. [37] using histomorphometric analysis failed to find a direct stimulatory effect of PRP on healing of autogenous bone graft used for sinus augmentation in a rabbit model. A meta-analysis of studies looking at the use of PRP in conjunction with implants in humans concluded that there was a lack of scientific evidence to support the use of PRP in combination with bone grafts during augmentation procedures [195]. Another systematic review of the effect of PRP on bone regeneration found that evidence for beneficial effects of PRP on sinus lift procedure appeared to be weak [181], and that there are insufficient data to recommend the use of platelet-rich plasma in sinus graft surgery [75, 228].

Autogenous bone grafts are considered the "gold standard" in bone tissue replacement because of their osteogenic potential and immunological inactivity. Due to inherent resorption associated with autogenous bone grafts, other methods, alone or in combination with autogenous bone, have been employed in jaw augmentation. However, there are a few RCT comparing the efficacy of different treatment options. Bone grafting and bone regenerative procedures do hold promise for the rehabilitation of the edentulous jaws; however, future study designs with respect to reporting study outcomes with a higher level of evidence are required.

8.4.12 Le Fort I Osteotomy in Severely Resorbed Maxilla

The severely resorbed maxilla (Class VI) poses difficulties for the rehabilitation of the patient, from an aesthetic and biomechanical point of view [89]. The proximity of the maxillary sinus, the need for bone grafts, and the unfavorable maxillomandibular relationship (Class III) make reconstruction a challenge in these patients [89, 106]. In these cases, a combination of autogenous bone grafting, endosseous implant, and Le Fort I osteotomy has been employed in the restoration of dental occlusion and maxillomandibular discrepancies [80, 89, 106]. This approach provides implant stability and enhances the functional and aesthetic results. Le Fort I procedure in cases where there has been significant maxillary resorption offers the following advantages [80]:

1. It solves, in one surgical procedure, the bone deficiency and the discrepancy of the jaws.
2. It improves jaw relationships, simplifying prosthetic rehabilitation.
3. The grafts are placed in ideal or near ideal locations.
4. It improves facial aesthetics by inducing a younger appearance.

However, the level of evidence regarding these methods of jaw augmentation is still very low, because only case series and case reports are found in the literature.

8.4.13 Conclusions

Jaw augmentation procedures have evolved from an experimental to a mature evidence-based discipline.

References

1. Adeyemo WL (2006) Do pathologies associated with impacted lower third molars justify prophylactic removal? A critical review of literature. Oral Surg Oral Med Oral Pathol Oral Radiol Endod 102:448–452
2. Adeyemo WL (2006) Healing of onlay mandibular bone graft. A microscopy and immunohistochemical evaluation of different surgical techniques in sheep. University of Cologne, Germany
3. Adeyemo WL, Reuther T, Bloch W et al (2008) Healing of onlay mandibular bone grafts covered with collagen membrane or bovine bone substitutes: a microscopical and immunohistochemical Study in the Sheep. Int J Oral Maxillofac Surg 37:651–659
4. Akadiri OA, Fasola AO, Arotiba JT (2009) Evaluation of Pederson index as an instrument for predicting the difficulty of mandibular third molar surgery. Nig Postgrad Med J 16(2):105–108
5. Akadiri OA, Obiechina AE (2009) Assessment of difficulty in third molar surgery – a systematic review. J Oral Maxillofac Surg 67:771–774
6. Akadiri OA, Obiechina AE, Arotiba JT, Fasola AO (2008) Relative impact of patient characteristics and radiographic variables on the difficulty of removing impacted mandibular third molars. J Contemp Dent Pract 9:51–58
7. Akota I, Alvsaker B, Bjornland T (1998) The effect of locally applied gauze drains impregenated with chlortetracycline ointment in mandibular third molar surgery. Acta Odontol Scand 56:25–29
8. Alexander RE, Throndson RR (2000) A review of perioperative corticosteroid use in dentoalveolar surgery. Oral Surg Oral Med Oral Pathol Oral Radiol Endod 90:406–415
9. Alonso N, de Almeida OM, Jorgetti V et al (1995) Cranial versus iliac onlay bone grafts in the facial skeleton: a macroscopic and histomorphometric study. J Craniomaxillofac Surg 6:113–118
10. American Association of Oral and Maxillofacial surgeons (2007) White paper on third molar surgery. www.aaoms.org/docs/third_molar_white_paper.pdf. Accessed 12 Feb 2009
11. American Association of Oral Maxillofacial Surgeons (1994) Report of a workshop on the management of patients with third molar teeth. J Oral Maxillofac Surg 52:1102–1112

12. Amin MM, Laskin DM (1983) Prophylactic use of indomethacin for prevention of postsurgical complications after removal of impacted third molars. Oral Surg Oral Med Oral Path 55:448–451

13. Araujo MG, Sonohara M, Hayacibara R et al (2002) Lateral ridge augmentation by the use of grafts comprised of autologous bone or a biomaterial. An experiment in the dog. J Clin Periodontol 29:1122–1131

14. Archer WH (1975) Oral and maxillofacial surgery, 5th edn. WB Saunders, Philadelphia

15. Artzi Z, Kozlovsky A, Nemcovsky CE et al (2005) The amount of newly formed bone in sinus grafting procedures depends on tissue depth as well as the type and residual amount of the grafted material. J Clin Periodontol 32:193–199

16. Assael LE (2005) Editorial – indications for elective therapeutic third molar removal: the evidence is in. J Oral Maxillofac Surg 63:1691–1692

17. Ataoglu H, Oz GY, Candirli C et al (2008) Routine antibiotics prophylaxis is not necessary during operations to remove third molars. Br J Oral Maxillofac Surg 46:133–135

18. Ayad W, Johren P, Dieckmann J (1995) Results of a comparative prospective randomized study of surgical removal of mandibular wisdom teeth with and without rubber drainage. Fortschr Kiefer Gesichtschir 40:134–136

19. Barden J, Edwards JE, McQuay HJ et al (2002) Rofecoxib in acute postoperative pain: quantitative systematic review. BMC Anesthesiol 2:4. Online at http://www.biomedcentral.com/1471-2253/2/4

20. Beirne OR, Hollander B (1986) The effect of methylprednisolone on pain, trismus, and swelling after removal of third molars. Oral Surg Oral Med Oral Pathol 61:134–138

21. Bell GW (2004) Use of dental panoramic radiograph to predict the relation between mandibular third molar teeth and the inferior alveolar nerve. Radiological and surgical findings, and clinical outcomes. Br J Oral Maxillofac Surg 42:21–27

22. Bell GW, Rodgers JM, Grime RJ et al (2003) The accuracy of dental panoramic tomographs in determining the root morphology of mandibular third molar teeth before surgery. Oral Surg Oral Med Oral Pathol Oral Radiol Endod 95:119–125

23. Benediktsdóttir IS, Hintze H, Petersen JK et al (2003) Accuracy of digital and film panoramic radiographs for assessment of position and morphology of mandibular third molars and prevalence of dental anomalies and pathologies. Dentomaxillofac Radiol 32:109–115

24. Benediktsdottir IS, Wenzel A, Petersen JK et al (2004) Mandibulat third molar removal: risk indicators for extended operative time, pain and complications. Oral Surg Oral Med Oral Pathol Oral Radiol Endod 97:438–446

25. Bignamini AA (2003) Evidence-based medicine and practice guidelines: solution or problem? Part 1. Evidence-based medicine and evidence-based surgery. Asian J Oral Maxillofac Surg 15:7–13

26. Blackburn GW, Brambley PA (1989) Lingual nerve damage associated with the removal of lower third molars. Br Dent J 167:103–107

27. Blackburn TK, Cawood JI, Stoelinga PJW et al (2008) What is the quality of the evidence base for pre-implant surgery of the atrophic jaw? Int J Oral Maxillofac Surg 37:1073–1079

28. Blaeser BF, August MA, Donoff RB et al (2003) Panoramic radiographic risk factors for inferior alveolar nerve injury after third molar extraction. J Oral Maxillofac Surg 61:417–421

29. Brabander EC, Cattaneo G (1988) The effect of surgical drain together with secondary closure technique on postoperative trismus. Int J Oral Maxillofac Surg 17:119–121

30. Brickley MR, Kay E, Shephard J et al (1995) Decision analysis for lower third molar surgery. Med Decis Making 45:143–151

31. Brickley MR, Shepard JP (1996) An investigation of the rationality of lower third molar surgery based on USA NIH Criteria. Br Dent J 180:249–254

32. Bridgman JB, Gillgrass TG, Zacharias M (1996) The absence of any pre-emptive analgesic effect for non-steroidal anti-inflammatory drugs. Br J Oral Maxillofac Surg 34:428–431

33. Bruce RA, Fredrerickson GC, Small GS (1980) Age of patients and morbidity associated with mandibular third molar surgery. J Am Dent Assoc 101:240–245

34. Bui CH, Seldin EB, Dodson TB (2003) Types, frequency, and risk factors for complications after third molar extraction. J Oral Maxillofac Surg 61:1379–1389

35. Burchardt H (1983) The biology of bone graft repair. Clin Orthop 174:28–42

36. Burchardt H (1987) Biology of bone transplantation. Orthop Clin North Am 18:187–196

37. Butterfield KJ, Bennett J, Gronowitz G et al (2005) Effect of platelet-rich plasma with autogenous bone graft for maxillary sinus augmentation in a rabbit model. J Oral Maxillofac Surg 63:370–376

38. Buyukurrt MC, Gungormus M (2006) The effect of a single dose prednisolone with and without diclofenac on pain, trismus, and swelling after removal of mandibular third molars. J Oral Maxillofac Surg 64:1761–1766

39. Bystedt H, Nord CE (1980) Effect of antibiotic treatment on postoperative infection after surgical removal of mandibular third molars. Swed Dent J 4:27–38

40. Central Park Oral Surgery (2009) General post operative instruction. http://www.centralparkoralsurgery.com/dental-implants-nyc/doc/general_postop.pdf. Accessed 20 May 2009

41. Cerqueira PRF, Vasconcelos BC, Bessa-Nogueira RV (2004) Comparative effect of a tube drain in impacted lower third molar surgery. J Oral Maxilllofac Surg 62:57–61

42. Chiapasco M, Cicco LD, Marrone G (1993) Side effects and complications associated with third molar surgery. Oral Surg Oral Med Oral Pathol 76:412–420

43. Chiapasco M, Zaniboni M (2009) Methods to treat the edentulous posterior maxilla: implants with sinus grafting. J Oral Maxillofacial Surg 67:867–871

44. Chukwuneke FN, Oji C, Saheeb DB (2008) A comparative study of the effect of using a rubber drain on postoperative discomfort following lower third molar surgery. Int J Oral Maxillofac Surg 37:341–344

45. Clark HB Jr (1965) Practical oral surgery. Lea & Febiger, Philadephia

46. National Institute for Clinical Excellence (1997) Guidance on the extraction of wisdom teeth. Available at: http://www.nice.org.uk/pdf/wisdomteethguidance.pdf. Accessed 10 Feb 2009

47. Collins RA, Carroll SL, McQuay D et al (2000) Single dose paracetamol (acetaminophen), with and without codeine, for postoperative pain. In: The Cochrane Library (2000), Issue 4, Update Software, Oxford

48. Conrad SM, Blakey GH, Shugars DA et al (1999) Patients' perception of recovery after third molar surgery. J Oral Maxillofac Surg 57:1288–1294

49. Cooper SA (1981) Comparative analgesic efficacies of aspirin and acetaminophen. Arch Intern Med 141:282–285

50. Courage GR, Huebsch RF (1971) Cold therapy revisited. JADA 83:1070–1073

51. Curran AE, Damm DD, Drummond JF (2002) Pathologically significant pericoronal lesions in adults: histopathologic evaluation. J Oral Maxillofac 60:613–617

52. Curran JB, Kenneth S, Young AR (1974) An assessment of the use of prophylactic antibiotics in third molar surgery. Int J Oral Surg 3:1–4

53. Dahling C, Alberius P, Linde A (1991) Osteopromotion for cranioplasty. An experimental study in rats using a membrane technique. J Neurosurg 74:487–491

54. Daniel DM, Stone ML, Arendt DL (1994) The effect of cold therapy on pain, swelling and range of motion after anterior cruciate ligament reconstructive surgery. Arthroscopy 10:530–533

55. Daniels SE, Desjardins PJ, Talwalker S et al (2002) The analgesic efficacy of valdecoxib vs. oxycodone/acetaminophen after oral surgery. J Am Dent Assoc 33:611–621

56. Daniels SE, Talwalker S, Hubbard RC (2001) Pre-operative valdecoxib, a COX-2 specific inhibitor, provides effective and long lasting pain relief following oral surgery. In: Proceedings of American Society of Anesthesiologists Annual Meeting. New Orleans, LA

57. Del Fabbro M, Rosano G, Taschieri S (2008) Implant survival rate after maxillary sinus augmentation. Eur J Oral Sci 116:497–506

58. Desjardins PJ, Shu VS, Recker DP et al (2002) A single preoperative oral dose of valdecoxib, a new cyclooxygenase-2 specific inhibitor, relieves post-oral surgery or bunionectomy pain. Anesthesiology 97:565–573

59. Diniz-Freitas M, Lago-Mendez L, Gude-Sampedro F et al (2007) Pederson scale fails to predict how difficult it will be to extract lower third molars. Br J Oral Maxillofac Surg 45:23–26

60. Dionne RA, Campbell RA, Cooper SA (1983) Suppression of postoperative pain by preoperative administration of ibuprofen in comparison to placebo, acetaminophen, and acetaminophen plus codeine. J Clin Pharmacol 23:37–43

61. Dionne RA, Cooper SA (1978) Evaluation of preoperative ibuprofen for postoperative pain after removal of third molars. Oral Surg Oral Med Oral Path Oral Radiol Endod 45:851–856

62. Dionne RA, Sisk AL, Fox PC (1983) Suppression of postoperative pain by preoperative administration of flurbiprofen in comparison to acetaminophen and oxycodone plus acetaminophen. Curr Ther Res 34:15–29

63. Dodson TB (1997) Evidence-based medicine: its role in modern practice and teaching of dentistry. Oral Surg Oral Med Oral Pathol 83:192–197

64. Dubois DD, Pizer ME, Chinnis RJ (1982) Comparison of primary and secondary closure after removal of impacted third molars. J Oral Maxillofac Surg 11:630–634

65. Dupuis R, Lemay H, Bushnetter MC (1988) Preoperative flurbiprofen in oral surgery: a method of choice in controlling postoperative pain. Pharmacotherapy 8:193–200

66. Edwards BJ, JE McQuay HJ et al (2004) Relative efficacy of oral analgesics after third molar extraction. Br Dent J 197:407–411

67. Edwards JE, Oldman A, Smith L et al (1999) Oral aspirin in postoperative pain: a quantitative systematic review. Pain 81:289–297

68. Edwards DJ, Rimmer M, Keene GCR (1996) The use of cold therapy in the postoperative management of patients undergoing arthroscopic anterior cruciate ligament construction. Am J Sports Med 24:193–195

69. Elter JR, Cuomo CJ, Offenbacher S et al (2004) Third molars associated with periodontal pathology in the third national health and nutrition examination survey. J Oral Maxillofac Surg 62:440–445

70. Elter JR, Offenbacher S, White RP Jr et al (2005) Third molars associated with periodontal pathology in older Americans. J Oral Maxillofac Surg 63:179–184

71. Emmerson JD, Burdick E, Hoaglin DC et al (1990) An empirical study of possible relation of treatment differences to quality score in controlled random clinical trials. Control Clin Trials 11:339–352

72. Enislidis G, Fork N, Millesi-Schobel G et al (2005) Analysis of complications following alveolar distraction osteogenesis and implant placement in the partially edentulous mandible. Oral Surg Oral Med Oral Pathol Oral Radiol Endod 100:25–30

73. Enneking WF, Burchardt H, Puhl JJ et al (1975) Physical and biological aspects of repair in dog cortical-bone transplants. J Bone Joint Surg Am 57:237–252

74. Esen E, Tasar F, Akhan O (1999) Determination of the anti-inflammatory effects of methylprednisolone on the sequelae of third molar surgery. J Oral Maxillofac Surg 57: 1201–1206

75. Esposito M, Grusovin MG, Coulthard P et al (2006) The effect of various bone augmentation procedures for dental implants: a Cochrane systematic review of randomized controlled clinical trials. Int J Oral Maxillofac Implants 21:696–710

76. Evidence-based working group (1992) Evidence-based medicine; a new approach to teaching the practice of medicine. JAMA 17:2420–2425

77. Ewers R (2005) Maxilla sinus grafting with marine algae derived bone forming material: a clinical report of long-term results. J Oral Maxillofacial Surg 63:1712–1723

78. Falconer DT, Roberts EE (1992) Report of an audit into third molar exodontia. Br J Oral Maxillofac Surg 30:183–185

79. Felice P, Lezzi G, Lizio G et al (2009) Reconstruction of atrophied posterior mandible with inlay technique and mandibular ramus block graft for implant prosthetic rehabilitation. J Oral Maxillofac Surg 67:372–380

80. Ferri J, Dujoncquoy J-P, Carneiro JM et al (2008) Maxillary reconstruction to enable implant insertion: a retrospective study of 181 patients. Head Face Med 4:31

81. Filho JRL, Oliveira e Silva ED, Carmago IB et al (2005) The influence of cryotherapy on reduction of pain, swelling and trismus after third molar extraction. J Am Dent Assoc 136:774–778

82. Flick WG (1999) The third molar controversy: framing the controversy as a public health policy issue. J Oral Maxillofac Surg 57:438–444

83. Fonseca RJ, Clark PJ, Burkes EJ et al (1980) Revascularization and healing of onlay particulate autogenous grafts in primates. J Oral Surg 38:572–577

84. Forsgren H, Heimdahl A, Johanson B et al (1985) Effect of application of cold dressing on the postoperative course in oral surgery. Int J Oral Surg 14:223–228

85. Garcia AG, Sampedro FG, Ray JG et al (2000) Pell-Gregory classification is unreliable as a predictor of difficulty in removing impacted lower third molar. Br J Oral Maxillofac Surg 38:585–587

86. Gargallo-Albiol J, Buenechea-Imaz R, Gay-Escoda C (2000) Lingual nerve protection during surgical removal of lower third molars. J Oral Maxillofac Surg 29:268–271

87. Gbotolorun MO, Arotiba GT, Ladeinde AL (2007) Assessment of factors associated with surgical difficulty in impacted mandibular third molar extraction. J Oral Maxillofac Surg 65:1977–1983

88. Gersema L, Baker K (1993) Use of corticosteroids in oral surgery. J Oral Maxillofac Surg 50:270–277

89. Gil JN, Claus DP, Campos FEB et al (2008) Management of the severely resorbed maxilla using Le Fort I osteotomy. Int J Oral Maxillofac Surg 37:1153–1155

90. Goldberg MH, Nemarich AN, Marco WP (1985) Complications after mandibular third molar surgery. J Am Dent Assoc 111:277–279

91. Graziani F, D'Aiuto F, Arduino PG et al (2006) Perioperative dexamethasone reduces post-surgical sequelae of wisdom tooth removal. A split-mouth randomized double-masked clinical trial. Int J Oral Maxillofac Surg 35:241–246

92. Grossi GB, Maoriana C, Gerramone RA (2007) Effects of submucosal injection of dexamethasone on postoperative discomforts after third molar surgery: a prospective study. J Oral Maxillofac Surg 65:2218–2226

93. Gungormus M (2002) Pathologic status and changes in mandibular third molar position during orthodontic treatment. J Contemp Dent Pract 3:11–22

94. Gustafsson I, Nysytrom E, Quiding H (1983) Effect of preoperative Paracetamol on pain after oral surgery. Eur J Clin Pharmacol 24:63–65

95. Hall HD, Bildman BS, Hand CD (1971) Prevention of dry socket with local application of tetracycline. J Oral Surg 29:35–37

96. Halpern LR, Dodson TB (2007) Does prophylactic administration of systemic antibiotics prevent postoperative inflammatory complications after third molar surgery? J Oral Maxillofac Surg 65:177–185

97. Happonen RP, Backstrom AC, Ylipaavalniemi P (1990) Prophylactic use of phenoxymethylpenicillin and tinidazole in mandibular third molar surgery, a comparative placebo controlled clinical trial. Br J Oral Maxillofac Surg 28:12–15

98. Hellen S, Norderam A (1973) Prevention of postoperative symptoms by general antibiotics treatment and local badandage in removal of mandibular third molars. Int J Oral Maxillofac Surg 2:273–278

99. Holmes RE (1979) Bone regeneration with a coralline hydroxyapatite implant. Plast Reconstr Surg 63:626–633

100. Howe GL (1971) Minor oral surgery. Wright, Bristol, England, pp 62–66

101. Huffman GG (1977) Use of methylprednisolone sodium succinate to reduce postoperative oedema after removal of impacted third molars. J Oral Surg 35:198–199

102. Hupp JR (1998) Principles of surgery. In: Peterson LJ, Ellis E, Hupp JR, Tucker MR (eds) Contemporary oral and maxillofacial surgery, 3rd edn. Mosby, St Louis, p 56

103. Hupp JR (1998) Wound repair. In: Peterson LJ, Ellis E, Hupp JR, Tucker MR (eds) Contemporary oral and maxillofacial surgery, 3rd edn. Mosby, St Louis, pp 58–60

104. Hutchison GL, Crofts SL, Gray IG (1990) Preoperative piroxicam for postoperative analgesia in dental surgery. Br J Anaesth 65:500–503

105. Hyllested JS, Pedersen JL et al (2002) Comparative effect of paracetamol, NSAIDs or their combination in postoperative pain management: a qualitative review. Br J Anaesth 88:199–214

106. Isaksson S, Ekfeldt A, Alberius P et al (1993) Early results from reconstruction of severely atrophic (class VI) maxillas by immediate endosseous implants in conjunction with bone grafting and Le Fort I osteotomy. Int J Oral Maxillofac Surg 22:144–148

107. Jacks TM, White RP, Offenbacher S et al (2004) Progression of periodontitis in the third molar region in asymptomatic patients. J Oral Maxillofac Surg (suppl 1) 62:22–23

108. Jackson DL, Moore PA, Hargreaves KM (1989) Preoperative nonsteroidal anti- inflammatory medication for the prevention of postoperative dental pain. J Am Dent Assoc 119:641–647

109. Jackson DL, Moore PA, Roszkowski MT (2000) Management of acute postoperative pain. In: Fonseca RJ (ed) Oral and maxillofacial surgery. Saunders, London, pp 114–140

110. Jensen OT (2006) Alveolar segmental "Sandwich" osteotomies for posterior edentulous mandibular sites for dental implants. J Oral Maxillofacial Surg 64:471–475

111. Jensen SS, Aaboe M, Pinholt EM et al (1996) Tissue reaction and material characteristics of four bone substitutes. Int J Oral Maxillofac Implants 11:55–66

112. Johansson B, Grepe A, Wannfors K (2001) A clinical study of changes in volume of bone grafts in the atrophic maxilla. Dentomaxillofac Radiol 30:157–161

113. John JL (1979) Indication and contraindication for removal of impacted tooth. Dent Clin North Am 23:333–345

114. Joshi A, Parara E, McFarlane TV (2004) A double-blind randomised controlled clinical trial of the effect of preoperative ibuprofen, diclofenac, paracetamol with codeine and placebo tablets for relief of postoperative pain after removal of impacted third molars. Br J Oral Maxillofac Surg 42:299–306

115. Jovanovic SA, Spiekermann H, Richter EJ (1992) Bone regeneration around titanium dental implants in dehisced defect sites. Int J Oral Maxillofac Implants 7:233–245

116. Kahl B, Gerlach KL, Hilgers RD (1994) A long-term, follow up, radiographic evaluation of asymptomatic impacted third molars in orthodontically treated patients. Int J Oral Maxillofac Surg 23:279–285

117. Karring T, Nyman S, Gottlow J et al (1993) Development of biologic concept of guided tissue regeneration. An experimental study in rat. Clin Oral Implant Res 1:26–35

118. Kaziro GSN (1984) Metronidazole (Flagyl) and arnica Montana in the prevention of post surgical complications, a comparative placebo controlled clinical trial. Br J Oral Maxillofac Surg 22:42–49

119. Kenzora JE, Steele RE, Yosipovitch ZH et al (1978) Experimental osteonecrosis of the femoral head in adult rabbits. Clin Orthop 130:8–46

120. Key SJ, Hodder SC, Davies R et al (2003) Perioperative corticosteroid supplementation and dento-alveolar surgery. Dent Update 30:316–320

121. Killey HC, Kay LW (1971) The impacted wisdom tooth, 2nd edn. Churchill Livingstone, London

122. Kim K, Brar P, Jakubowski J (2008) The use of corticosteroids and nonsteroidal anti-inflammatory medication for the management of pain and inflammation after third molar surgery: A review of the literature. Oral Surg Oral Med Oral Pathol Oral Radiol Endod 107(5):630–640

123. Kingston R, Barry M, Tierney S et al (2001) Treatment of surgical patients is evidence-based. Eur J Surg 167: 324–330

124. Kissin I (2000) Preemptive analgesia. Anesthesiology 93:1138–1143

125. Klinge B, Alberius P, Isaksson S (1992) Osseous response to implanted natural bone material and synthetic hydroxyapaptite ceramic in the repair of experimental skull bone defects. J Oral Maxillofac Surg 50:241–249

126. Koerner KR (1987) Steroids in third molar surgery: a review. Gen Dent 35:459–463

127. Kostopoulos L, Karring T (1994) Guided bone regeneration in mandibular defects in rats using a bioresorbable polymer. Clin Oral Implants Res 5:66–74

128. Krimmel M, Reinart S (2000) Mandibular fracture after third molar removal. J Oral Maxillofac Surg 58: 1110–1112

129. Kruger GO (1974) Textbook of oral surgery. CV Mosby, St Louis, pp 77–95

130. Lai TY, Wong VW (2003) Is ophthalmology evidence based? A clinical audit of the emergency unit of a regional eye hospital. Br J Ophthalmol 87:385–390

131. Lascelles BDX (2000) Preemptive analgesia: an aid to postoperative pain control. J Pain Symptom Manage 1:93–95

132. Laskin DM (1971) Evaluation of the third molar problem. J AM Dent Assoc 82:824–827

133. Laster Z, Rachmiel A, Jensen OT (2005) Alveolar width distraction osteogenesis for early implant placement. J Oral Maxillofac Surg 63:1724–1730

134. Lau SL, Samman N (2007) Evidence-based practice in oral and maxillofacial surgery: audit of 1 training center. J Oral Maxillofac Surg 65:651–657

135. Leone M, Richard O, Antonini F et al (2007) Comparison of methylprednisolone and ketoprofen after multiple third molar extraction: a randomized controlled study. Oral Surg Oral Med Oral Pathol Oral Radiol Endod 103:e7–e9

136. Lida S, Nomura K, Okura M et al (2004) Influence of the incompletely erupted lower third molar on mandibular angle and condylar fractures. J Trauma 57:613–617

137. Liedholm R, Knutsson K, Lysell L et al (2000) The outcomes of mandibular third molar removal and non-removal: a study of patients' preferences using a multi- attribute method. Acta Odontol Scand 58:293–298

138. Linder BL, Chernoff A, Kaplan KL et al (1979) Release of PDGF from human platelets by arachidonic acid. Proct Natl Acad Sci USA 76:4107–4111

139. Lindqvist B, Thilander B (1982) Extraction of third molars in cases of anticipated crowding in the lower jaw. Am J Orthod 81:130–139

140. Lokken P, Olsen I, Bruaset I (1975) Bilateral surgical removal of impacted lower third molar teeth as a model for drug evaluation: a test with ibuprofen. Eur J Clin Pharm 8:209–216

141. Lopes V, Mumenya R, Feinmann C et al (1995) Third molar surgery: an audit of the indications for surgery, post-operative complaints and patient satisfaction. Br J Oral Maxillofac Surg 133:33–35

142. Lundgren D, Lundgren AK, Sennerby L et al (1995) Augmentation of intramembranous bone beyond the skeletal envelope using an occlusive titanium barrier. Clin Oral Implant Res 6:67–72

143. Macgregor AJ (1990) Reduction in morbidity in the surgery of the third molar removal. Dent Update 17:411–414

144. Macgregor AJ, Addy A (1980) Value of penicillin in the prevention of pain, swelling and trismus following the removal of ectopic mandibular third molar. Int J Oral Maxillofac Surg 9:166–169

145. Maegawa H, Sano K, Kitagawa Y et al (2003) Preoperative assessment of the relationship between the mandibular third molar and the mandibular canal by axial computed tomography with coronal and sagittal reconstruction. Oral Surg Oral Med Oral Pathol Oral Radiol Endod 96:639–646

146. Mahasantipiya PM, Savage NW, Monsour PR et al (2005) Narrowing of the inferior dental canal in relation to the lower third molars. Dentomaxillofac Radiol 34:154–163

147. Markiewicz MR, Ding EL, Dodson TB (2008) Corticosteroids reduce postoperative morbidity after third molar surgery: a systematic review and meta-analysis. J Oral Maxillofac Surg 66:1881–1894

148. Markovic A, Todorovic L (2007) Effectiveness of dexamethasone and low-power laser in minimizing edema after third molar surgery: a clinical trial. Int J Oral Maxillofac Surg 36:226–229

149. Mason DA (1988) Lingual nerve damage following third molar surgery. Int J Oral Maxillofac Surg 17:290–294

150. Oral and Maxillofacial Surgery, North Hawaii. Instruction before and after oral surgery. http://www.drjohnstover.com/oral-surgery-hawaii/before-after-oral-surgery.html. Accessed 20 May 2009

151. Mc Auley DC (2001) Ice therapy; how good is the evidence. Int J Sports Med 22:379–384

152. McAllister BS (2001) Histologic and radiographic evidence of vertical ridge augmentation utilizing distraction osteogenesis: 10 consecutively placed distractors. J Periodontol 72:1767–1779

153. McCormack K (1994) The spinal actions of nonsteroidal anti-inflammatory and analgesic effects. Drugs 47 (Suppl 5):28–45

154. Mehrabi M, Allen JM, Roser SM (2007) Therapeutic agents in perioperative third molar surgical procedures. Oral Maxillofac Surg Clin North Am 19:69–84

155. Micó-Llorens JM, Satorres-Nieto M, Gargallo-Albiol A et al (2006) Efficacy of methylprednisolone in controlling

complications after impacted lower third molar surgical extraction. Eur J Clin Pharmacol 62:693–698

156. Miloro M, Halkias LE, Sloane HW et al (1997) Assessment of the lingual nerve in the third molar region using magnetic resonance imaging. J Oral Maxillofac Surg 55: 134–137

157. Minami T, Nakano H, Kobayashi T et al (2001) Characterization of EP receptor subtypes responsible for prostaglandin E2-induced pain responses by use of EP1 and EP3 receptor knockout mice. Brit J Pharmacol 133:438–444

158. Misch CM (1997) Comparison of intraoral donor sites for onlay grafting prior to implant placement. Int J Oral Maxillofac Implants 51:767–776

159. Misch CM (2004) Implant site development using ridge splitting techniques. Oral Maxillofac Surg Clin North Am 16:65–74

160. Mitchell DA (1986) A controlled clinical trial of prophylactic tinidazole for chemoprophylaxis in third molar surgery. Br Dent J 160:284–286

161. Monaco G, Monteveechi M, Bonetti GA et al (2004) Reliability of panoramic radiography in evaluating the topographic relationship between the mandibular canal and impacted third molar. J Am Dent Assoc 135:312–318

162. Monaco G, Staffolani C, Gatto MR (1999) Antibiotic therapy in third molar surgery. Eur J Oral Sci 107:437–441

163. Montgomery MT, Hogg JP, Roberts DL et al (1990) The use of glucocorticosteroids to lessen the inflammatory sequelae following third molar surgery. J Oral Maxillofac Surg 48:179–187

164. Moore PA, Brar P, Smiga ER (2005) Pre-emptive rofecoxib and dexamethasone for prevention of pain and trismus following third molar surgery. Oral Surg Oral Med Oral Pathol Oral Radiol Endod 99:E1–E7

165. Moss C, Wake M (1999) Lingual access for third molar surgery: a 20 year retrospective audit. Br J Oral Maxillofac Surg 37:255–258

166. Mulliken JB, Kaba LB, Glowacki J (1985) Induced osteogenesis: the biological principle and clinical implications. J Surg Res 37:487–496

167. Mulrow CD (1987) The medical review article: state of the science. Ann Intern Med 106:485–488

168. National Institute of Health (1980) NIH consensus development conference for removal of third molars. J Oral Surg 38:235–236

169. Norderam A, Sydnes G, Odegaard J (1973) Neomycine-bacitracin cones in impacted third molar sockets. Int J Oral Surg 2:279–283

170. American Association of Oral Maxillofacial Surgeons (1993) The building of a specialty. Supplement to J Oral Maxillofac Surg. Rosemont IL

171. Ordulu M, Aktas I, Yalsin S et al (2006) Comparative study of the effect of tube drainage versus methylprednisolone after third molar surgery. Oral Sur Oral Med Oral Pathol Oral Radiol Endod 101:e96–e100

172. Oxman AD, Guyatt GH (1988) Guidelines for reading literature reviews. CMAJ 138:697–703

173. Pasqualini D, Cocero N, Castella L et al (2005) Primary and secondary closure of surgical wound after removal of impacted mandibular third molars: a comparative study. Int J Oral Maxillofac Surg 34:52–57

174. Paterson JA, Cardo VA, Stratigos GT (1970) An examination of antibiotics prophylaxis in oral and maxillofacial surgery. J Oral Surg 28:753–759

175. Pawelzik J, Cohnen M, Willers R et al (2002) A comparison of conventional panoramic radiographs with volumetric computed tomography images in the preoperative assessment of impacted mandibular third molars. J Oral Maxillofac Surg 60:979–984

176. Petersen JK (1978) The analgesic and anti-inflammatory efficacy of diflunisal and codeine after removal of impacted third molars. Curr Med Res Opin 5:525–535

177. Peterson LJ (1992) Principles of management of impacted teeth. Principles of oral and maxillofacial surgery, vol 1. JB Lippincott, Philadelphia, p 117

178. Phillipart P, Brasseur M, Hoyaux D et al (2003) Human recombinant tissue factor, platelet-rich plasma, and tetracycline induce a high-quality human bone graft: a 5-year study. Int J Oral Maxillofac Implants 18:411–416

179. Pichler JW, Beirne RO (2001) Lingual flap retraction and prevention of lingual nerve damage associated with third molar surgery: a systematic review of the literature. Oral Surg Oral Med Oral Pathol Oral Radiol Endod 91: 395–401

180. Pieuch JF, Arzadon J, Lieblich SE (1995) Prophylactic antibiotics for third molar surgery: a supportive opinion. J Oral Maxillofac Surg 53:53–60

181. Plachokova AS, Nikolidakis D, Mulder J et al (2008) Effect of platelet-rich plasma on bone regeneration in dentistry: a systematic review. Clin Oral Implants Res 19:539–545

182. Poeschl PW, Eckel D, Poeschl E (2004) Postoperative prophylactic antibiotic treatment in third molar surgery – a necessity? J Oral Maxillfac Surg 62:3–8

183. Pogrel MA, Golman KE (2004) Lingual flap retraction for third molar removal. J Oral Maxillofac Surg 62:1125–1130

184. Raghoebar GM, Liem RSB, Visssink A (2002) Vertical distraction of the severely resorbed edentulous mandible. A clinical, histological and electron microscopy study of 10 treated cases. Clin Oral Implants Res 13:558–556

185. Rakprasitkul S, Pairuchvej V (1997) Mandibular third molar surgery with primary closure and tube drain. Int J Oral Maxillofac Surg 26:187–190

186. Ren Y, Hans MS (2007) Effectiveness of antibiotic prophylaxis in third molar surgery: a metaanalysis of randomized controlled trials. J Oral maxillofac Surg 65:1909–1921

187. Robinson PP, Smith KG (1996) Lingual nerve damage during lower third removal: a comparison of two surgical methods. Br Dent J 180:456–461

188. Rosenquist JB, Nystrom E (1987) Long-acting analgesic or long-acting local anesthetic in controlling immediate postoperative pain after lower third molar surgery. Anesth Prog 34:6–9

189. Roszkowski MT, Swift JQ, Hargreaves KM (1997) Effect of NSAID administration on tissue levels of immunoreactive prostaglandin E2, leukotriene B4, and (s)- flurbiprofen following extraction of impacted third molars. Pain 73:339–345

190. RushtonVE HK, Worthington HV (1999) Factors influencing the selection of panoramic radiography in general dental practice. J Dent 27:565–571

191. Sacket DL, Rosenberg WM, Gray JA et al (1996) Evidence-based medicine: what it is and what it isn't. BMJ 312:71–72

192. Sahni M, Guenther HL, Fleisch H et al (1993) Bisphosphonates act on rat bone resorption through mediation of osteoblasts. J Clin Invest 91:2004–2011

193. Sampson WJ (1995) Current controversies in late anterior crowding. Ann Acad Med Singap 24:129–137

194. Sampson WJ, Richards LC, Leighton BC (1983) Third molars eruption patterns and mandibular dental arch crowding. Aust Orthod J 8:10–20

195. Sanchez AR, Sheridan PJ, Kupp LI (2003) Is platelet-rich plasma the perfect enhancement factor? A current review. Int J Oral Maxillofac Implants 18:93–103

196. Sands T, Pynn BR, Nenninger S (1993) Third molar surgery: current concepts and controversies. Oral Health 83:19–30

197. Santamaria J, Arteagoitia I (1997) Radiographic variables of clinical significance in the extraction of impacted mandibular third molars. Oral Surg Oral Med Oral Pathol Oral Radiol Endod 84:469–473

198. Savin J, Ogden GR (1997) Third molar surgery–a preliminary report on aspects affecting quality of life in the early postoperative period. Br J Oral Maxillofac Surg 35:246–253

199. Scarcella JB, Cohn BT (1995) The effect of cold therapy on the postoperative course of total hip and knee arthroplasty patients. Am J Orthop 24:847–852

200. Schlegel KA, Fichter G, Schultze-Mosgau S et al (2003) Histologic findings in sinus augmentation with autogenous bone chips versus a bovine bone substitute. Int J Oral Maxillofac Implants 18:53–58

201. Schlickewei W, Paul C (1991) Experimentelle Untersuchunggen zum Knochenersatz mit bovinem Apaptlt. Hefte Unfallheilk 216:59–63

202. Seymour RA, Blair GS, Wyatt FA (1983) Post-operative dental pain and analgesic efficacy, Part 1. Br J Oral Surg 21:290–297

203. Seymour RA, Hawkesford JE, Sykes J et al (2003) An inv into the comparative efficacy of soluble aspirin and soluble paracetamol in postoperative pain after third molar surgery. Br Dent J 194:353–357

204. Seymour RA, Meechan JG, Blair GS (1985) An investigation into post-operative pain after third molar surgery under local analgesia. Br J Oral Maxillofac Surg 23:410–418

205. Seymour RA, Walton JG (1984) Pain control after third molar surgery. Int J Oral Surg 13:457–385

206. Simion M, Trisi P, Piattelli A (1994) Vertical ridge augmentation using membrane technique associated with osseointegrated implants. Int J Periodontics Rest Dent 14:497–511

207. Sisk AL, Grover BJ (1990) A comparison of pre-operative and postoperative naproxen sodium for suppression of postoperative pain. J Oral Maxillofac Surg 48:674–678

208. Sisk AL, Mosley RO, Martin RP (1989) Comparison of preoperative and post- operative diflunisal for suppression of post-operative pain. J Oral Maxillofac Surg 47:464–468

209. Skjelbred J, Lokken P (1977) Acetylsalicylic acid vs. paracetamol, effects on post- operative course. Eur J Clin Pharmacol 12:257–269

210. Smith AC, Barry SE, Chiong AY et al (1997) Inferior alveolar nerve damage following the removal of mandibular third molar teeth. A prospective study using panoramic radiography. Aust Dent J 42:149–152

211. Smith AC, Brook IM (1990) Inhibition of tissue prostaglandin synthesis during third molar surgery: use of preoperative fenbufen. Br J Oral Maxillofac Surg 28:251–253

212. Solomon MJ, Mcloed RS (1993) Clinical studies in surgical journals – have we improved? Dis Colon Rectum 36:43–48

213. Solomon MJ, Mcloed RS (1998) Surgery and the randomized controlled trials: past, present and future. Med J Aust 169:380–383

214. Spies T, Dreizan S, Stone R et al (1952) A clinical appraisal of ACTH and cortisone as therapeutic agents in dental medicine. Oral Surg Oral Med Oral Pathol 5:25–40

215. Srinivas DT (2007) Age as a risk factor for third molars complications. J Oral Maxillofac Surg 65:1685–1692

216. Stanley HR, Alattar M, Collett WK et al (1988) Pathologic sequelae of 'neglected' impacted third molars. J Oral Pathol 17:113–117

217. Stellingsma C, Vissink A, Meijer HJA et al (2004) Implantology and the severely resorbed edentulous mandible. Crit Rev Oral Biol Med 15:240–248

218. Strean P, Horton C (1953) Hydrocortisone in dental practice. Dent Digest 59:8

219. Suddhasthira T, Chaiwat S, Sattapongsda P (1991) The comparison study of primary and secondary closure technique after removal of impacted mandibular third molars. Thai J Oral Maxillofac Surg 5:67–73

220. Susarla SM, Dodson TB (2004) Risk factors for third molars extraction difficulty. J Oral Maxillofac Surg 62:1363–1371

221. Taylor JC, Cuff SE, Leger JPL et al (2002) In vitro osteoclast resorption of bone substitute biomaterials used for implant site augmentation: a pilot study. Int J Oral Maxillofac Implants 17:321–330

222. Tong L, Buchman SR (2000) Facial bone grafts: contemporary science and thought. J Craniomaxillofac Trauma 6:31–41

223. Üstün Y, Erdogan O, Esen E et al (2003) Comparison of the effects of 2 doses of methylprednisolone on pain, swelling, and trismus after third molar surgery. Oral Surg Oral Med Oral Pathol Oral Radiol Endod 96:535–539

224. Van der Linden W, Cleaton-Jones Lownie M (1995) Diseases and lesions associated with third molars. Oral Surg Oral Med Oral Pathol 79:142–145

225. Van der Westhuijzen AJ, Becker PJ, Morkel J et al (2005) A randomized observer blind comparison of bilateral facial ice pack therapy with no ice therapy following third molar surgery. Int J Oral Maxillofac Surg 34:281–286

226. Venta I, Ylipaavalniemi P, Turtola L (2004) Clinical outcomes of third molars in adults followed during 18 years. J Oral Maxillofac Surg 62:182–185

227. Verhoeven JW, Ruijter J, Cune MS et al (2000) Onlay grafts in combination with endosseous implants in severe mandibular atrophy: one year results of a prospective, quantitative radiological study. Clin Oral Implants Res 11:583–594

228. Wallace SS, Froum SJ (2003) Effect of maxillary sinus augmentation on the survival of endosseous dental implants. A systematic review. Ann Periodontol 8:328–343

229. Walters H (1995) Reducing lingual damage in third molar surgery: a clinical audit of 1350 cases. Br Dent J 178:140–144

Evidence-Based Issues in Maxillofacial Trauma

9

Oladimeji Adeniyi Akadiri, Babatunde Olayemi Akinbami, and Abiodun Olubayo Fasola

Core Message

> Injuries to the maxillofacial region sometimes result in significant physical disfigurement and psychological debilitations. In spite of several techniques and technologies currently available for treatment, the residual long-term impact of maxillofacial injury on an individual is still considerable. Some maxillofacial injuries are particularly more challenging to manage and are often associated with suboptimal aesthetic and functional outcomes. Periodic appraisal of epidemiological and clinical evidences in maxillofacial traumatology is desirable in order to formulate measures to optimize both preventive and therapeutic outcomes.

9.1 Epidemiological Evidences in Maxillofacial Trauma

9.1.1 Introduction

Traditional epidemiological researches on maxillofacial trauma from different parts of the world were focused on mere descriptive statistics of prevalence, etiology, and pattern of maxillofacial injuries. However, recent studies involve extensive documentations to reflect regional variations and the influence of socio-economic, political, and cultural environment on the etiology, pattern, and management of maxillofacial injury. This new approach in epidemiological studies should enhance the development of appropriate country or region-specific preventive policies and capacity enhancement programs to minimize the occurrence as well as improve treatment and rehabilitation of victims. Here is an attempt to correlate some epidemiologic variables based on the best available evidence in the current world literature.

9.1.2 Socio-Demographics Characteristics in Relation to Etiology

The etiology of trauma generally includes road traffic crashes (RTC), interpersonal violence, sports, falls and domestic injuries, industrial and other work-related accidents, and animal assaults [105, 106,113]. Each of these represent a broad group of factors, for example, RTC include motor vehicles, motorcycles, bicycles, and pedestrian accidents; interpersonal violence includes physical assaults with or without the use of weapons;

O.A. Akadiri (✉)
B.O. Akinbami
Department of Oral and Maxillofacial Surgery,
College of Health Sciences, University of Port Hacourt,
Post Box 212, Choba, Port Harcourt, Rivers State, Nigeria
e-mail: oaakadiri@yahoo.com
e-mail: akinbamzy@yahoo.com

A.O. Fasola
Department of Oral and Maxillofacial Surgery,
College of Medicine, University of Ibadan,
PMB 5116, Ibadan, Oyo State, Nigeria
e-mail: aolubayofasola@yahoo.com

F. Chiappelli et al. (eds.), *Evidence-Based Practice: Toward Optimizing Clinical Outcomes*,
DOI: 10.1007/978-3-642-05025-1_9, © Springer-Verlag Berlin Heidelberg 2010

133

there are various types of sports, various types of high-risk works/industrial machines; and animal assaults range from bites to kicks and butts.

There are substantial epidemiological evidences based on large scale retrospective studies and observational cohort studies to support the fact that certain age groups, gender, religious, or cultural sects present higher risks for different etiological factors [55, 59, 63].

Young adults are particularly prone to injuries by RTC, sports, and interpersonal violence [6, 55, 59, 73, 113], while at the extremes of life people are prone to falls and other domestic accidents [34, 37, 54, 56, 107]. The common explanation is that young adults, particularly those within the age range of 18–35 years, get more actively involved in driving, productive sector of the economy, interpersonal violence, and sports. This category of individuals is also more involved in drug abuse and alcohol consumption, which have been found to predispose to higher prevalence of RTC and interpersonal violence [52, 67]. On the other hand, younger children are prone to falls because of their less developed locomotive and posture control systems, while the older children experience relatively higher incidence of trauma due to rough plays, fights, and sports [56]. At the other extreme, the elderly patients are prone to falls due to age-related changes in eyesight, muscle coordination, balance, and postural stability, which reduce an individual's ability to avoid environmental hazards [37].

The evidence in support of predominant male involvement in trauma is conclusive [55, 59, 61, 63, 113]. This is reported irrespective of the causative factors, but the relativity varies according to the etiological factors. For example, most studies reported 2.1–5:1 considering all etiological factors [3, 40, 55, 61, 113]. The commonly reported male to female ratio in RTC is within the range of 2–4.5:1 [49, 80], while in sports-related injury, it is 5.5–9:1 depending on the types of sports [6, 47, 73, 77, 90, 103]. The gender gap is 3.8–8.4:1 [52, 67] when the cause is interpersonal violence. However, the incidence of battery is considerable for women and children in some societies where kids and wives are often beaten up by parents and spouses, respectively [38, 59, 83, 94].

Some studies [59, 61, 81, 82, 95] have adduced the influence of cultural and religious practices on some etiological factors. For example, studies from the southern part of Nigeria have consistently identified RTC as the major cause of injury, while interpersonal violence has recently shut higher in the north eastern part of the country [82]. The prevalence of assaults-related injury in north eastern Nigeria has been attributed to the nomadic life style in the region, whereby animals are moved over several kilometers of land grazing without strict laws guiding their movement, thereby destroying cash crops [1, 81]. This frequently led to fights between farmers and cattle men, and various objects such as cutlasses/machetes, arrows, and wooden objects are used in inflicting injuries during fight [81, 82]. Kadkhodaie [59] and Klenk and Kovacs [61] also noted that interpersonal violence is relatively low in Islamic countries due to strict objection to alcohol consumption in the Muslim countries.

It is, however, noteworthy that change in etiological trends has been observed in some parts of the world. While RTC still predominates in many countries, the gender and age gap seem to be narrowing due to the increasing involvement of women in fending for the family and extended retirement age forced on the elderly by the harsh economic realities in some of those countries [1, 35, 61]. Elsewhere, interpersonal violence is gaining predominance, especially in many EU countries, Zimbabwe, Scandivanian, and North American States [16, 113].

9.1.3 Pattern of Injuries in Relation to Etiology

The patterns of maxillofacial injury vary according to the mechanism of injury, which is also determined mostly by the causative factor. Understanding the pattern and mechanism of injury is, therefore, crucial to the formulation of policies and development of appropriate preventive devices. High velocity injuries such as those associated with RTC and missile weapons often present the most severe damage involving multiple facial bones and other systems [40, 49, 87]. In a large scale prospective study involving 9,543 patients over 10 years, Gassner et al. [49] observed a 2.25-fold higher risk for severe maxillofacial injury among victim of RTC. Similarly, Kumoona [64] and Puzovic et al. [87] also observed complex soft tissue and hard tissue injuries following missile injuries to the oral and maxillofacial region. On the other hand, injury due to interpersonal violence often involves isolated facial bone fractures or soft tissue injury [52, 63]. The mandible and zygoma are most frequently fractured in such cases [29, 52, 55, 63, 67].

Injuries due to falls, either domestic falls or falls from heights or off a motorcycle or bicycle, often result in zygoma fractures or mandibular fractures, particularly symphysis, parasymphysis, and/or condyles; the incidence of severe midfacial fracture from falls is comparatively low [54, 89].

The pattern of sports-related injury is highly varied depending on the types of sports. Higher incidence of sports-related maxillofacial injury varies from place to place depending on the popularity of the sporting event, number of participants, and the risk involved. Soccer and rugby were most implicated in France [73], while a Japanese study [103] cites skiing and rugby with the higher rate of injury, followed by baseball and soccer. In a British report [47], most injuries were sustained during rugby, followed by bicycling and soccer. However, many sports-related facial fractures were associated with vehicular sports [39]. The other sports frequently responsible vary from place to place; skiing, basketball, tae kwon do, cycling, horse riding are implicated in some developed country, while boxing and hockey have been implicated in some developing countries [36] where most of the other sports are still to be popular. Generally, it has been noted that the incidence of sports-related maxillofacial injuries is increasing, but the severity is less compared to other causes [73, 77, 90]. Mostly, it involves soft tissue contusions and abrasions, more significant soft tissue injury is very rare [47, 90]. Fractures of the mandible involving mostly the angle and of the midface involving mostly the zygoma are the skeletal injury mostly reported in association with sports [73, 90, 103].

9.1.4 Regional Differences in Maxillofacial Trauma Epidemiology

Geographical differences in epidemiological variables in relation to maxillofacial trauma are well reported. These are partly the reflections of the different cultures, religion, civilization, governmental policies, general socio-economic development, and lifestyle of citizens.

Traditionally, the predominance of RTC as the major cause of trauma all over the world is well reported [55, 59, 82, 114]. However, while the trend remains the same in some underdeveloped and developing countries, some countries have reported a gradual change in trends, while a complete paradigm shift has been noted in many developed countries whereby interpersonal violence now dominates [16, 35, 59, 82, 113].

The influence of governance such as the introduction and enforcement of driving regulations, rules against drunk driving supported by appropriate investigative facility, and penalty for violation of speed limit has been shown to reduce the incidence of RTC in many western states [51, 86]. Other developmental measures such as better road construction and maintenance, vehicle roadworthiness assessment, and control on the issuance of driving licenses have also been shown to reduce RTC in many developed countries [61]. On the contrary, studies from the developing nations have continued to adduce the reasons of nonenforcement of driving rules, bad roads, and aging vehicles for the persistence of higher incidence of RTC [1, 37, 59, 61, 82, 113].

In the Middle East, particularly the Arabian countries, low level of alcohol consumption due to Islamic objection is cited as being responsible for the relative sparseness of interpersonal violence [59, 61]. Fewer female victims are also observed in these countries because their women are less involved in economic struggles to sustain the family [59, 61].

Literature on methods and outcomes of treatments revealed that in most developing countries of Africa and Asia the traditional methods of closed reduction with wire intermaxillary fixation are still the mainstay for the treatment of most maxillofacial fractures [1, 82, 94, 113]. Open reduction and internal fixation with interosseous wires are performed occasionally, while the use of mini and compression plates is seldom. Nonaffordability and nonavailability of materials and inadequate expertise are the common explanation for the retention of the old practice. Although the authors often assert that outcomes have been largely acceptable, no proper comparative studies with the use of plate osteosynthesis have been conducted among their patient populations. On the contrary, open reduction and internal fixation with miniplates and compression plates are employed for all but the simplest maxillofacial fractures in the developed world and part of Asia with obvious advantages [10, 13, 85]. Plate osteosynthesis is particularly indicated in some complex maxillofacial fractures without which the outcome will be suboptimal [10].

9.1.5 Controversial Cases in Maxillofacial Trauma

Particular attention is required to articulate the best evidence in support of treatment methods in cases of some maxillofacial injuries that are generally difficult to manage, and for which controversies exist about the optimal methods and principles of treatment. Among these are mandibular condyle fractures, naso-ethmoidal complex fractures, and zygomatico-orbital fractures.

The mandibular condyle is the weakest part of the mandible, and therefore, the most susceptible to fracture from a transmitted force [10, 29]. The peculiar anatomical and physiological constitution of the temporomandiblar joint and the delicate anatomical relations of the condyle to the base of skull make the condyle a very important structure in oral and maxillofacial traumatology [12]. Inappropriately treated mandibular condyle fracture will often have a deleterious long-term effect both in children and adult patients [10, 12].

The naso-ethmoidal complex fracture is regarded by some as the most difficult maxillofacial fracture to manage [27]. The delicate and complex bony articulation constituting the complex and its anatomical relation to vital structures imbibe a major significance in treatment considerations.

The zygomatico-orbital fracture is another technically difficult maxillofacial injury from management's point of view. Opinions differ as to the appropriate diagnostic techniques, guidelines for intervention, and methods of treatments [2].

A comprehensive discussion on these three complex injuries is beyond the scope of this book. However, we shall provide an elaborate discussion on the current evidences in the management of mandibular condyle fractures because of the peculiar consideration across the various age groups and the different types of fractures.

9.1.6 Conclusion

Available epidemiological information from various regions of the world and specific countries is useful for guiding policy makers, rescue teams, sports physicians, engineers, and clinicians to formulate preventive strategies targeted at various age groups, gender groups, work groups, and athletes, cultural and religious sects. The information can be used to guide the future funding of public health programs geared toward prevention of maxillofacial injuries. In addition, they may also be helpful in developing meaningful guidelines for training primary care providers in the management of maxillofacial injuries. Regional discrepancies in the quality of specialized maxillofacial trauma care in different parts of the world could be eliminated or reduced with the assistance of world funding bodies and health organizations through the provision of aids in training and equipment in the less privileged countries of the world.

9.2 Current Evidences in the Management of Mandibular Condyle Fractures

9.2.1 Introduction

Fractures of the mandibular condyle constitute about 19–52% of all fractures of the mandible. Much has been written in the literature on the diagnosis and treatment of these fractures, yet management decisions continue to be controversial [4–15]. The controversy is in part attributable to a misinterpretation of the literature from decades prior, a lack of uniformity of classification of the various anatomical components of the mandibular condyle, and a perceived potential to cause harm through the open method based in part on the surgeon's lack of a critical examination of the literature [5–9]. The major controversy is between conservative and surgical management. Surgeons who prefer closed approaches claim that equally good results are achievable with reduced morbidities as compared to open approaches [15–17, 19, 20].

However, clinical outcome following conservative treatment has been found to be below the expected with regard to achieving close to ideal occlusion, deviation of the mandible, ankylosis, and internal joint derangement [9–24]. Therefore, the pendulum seems to be swinging toward achieving accurate anatomical reduction of the segments via a surgical approach [18–25]. There are various surgical approaches to the condyle and surgeons who prefer this open procedure determine the best approach that suites the treatment of the fractured condyle with the mind of minimizing possible complications such as facial nerve paralysis, unsightly scar, excessive bleeding, and at the same time, achieving optimal results [11, 60, 100]. However, evidence-based medicine has provided a means by which views and opinions of different authorities have been put together in other to adopt a unified treatment objective and policies based on large data-based researches and documentation of experiences in the treatment of fractures of the condyle of the mandible [9–15].

9.2.2 Classification of Condylar Fractures

Condylar fractures are classified according to the anatomic location (intracapsular and extracapsular) and degree of displacement/dislocation of the articular head. Intracapsular fractures of the mandibular condyle are classified as type A, fractures through the medial condylar pole; type B, fractures through the lateral condylar pole with loss of vertical height of the mandibular ramus; type C and type M which are multiple fragments or comminuted fractures. The majority of mandibular condyle fractures involve the condylar neck, with few reports of intracapsular fractures. Sagittal or vertical fractures of the mandibular condyle and chip fractures of the medial part of the condylar head are rarely detected by conventional radiography and are more commonly detected by computed tomography (CT) scan [20, 71].

9.2.3 Factors that Determine Treatment Method

The final choice of treatment modality for each individual patient takes into account a number of factors, including age of patient, position of the condyle, location of the fracture, degree/direction of displacement, presence and state of dentition, age of the fracture, character of the patient, presence or absence of other associated injuries, foreign bodies, presence of other systemic medical conditions, history of previous joint disease, cosmetic impact of the surgery, desires of the patient, and ease of establishing adequate occlusion [9, 14].

9.2.4 Goal of Treatment

A patient with aesthetic form, stable occlusion, and normal function as the final result is the goal of treatment. It has been generally agreed that a successful treatment includes a pain-free joint with a normal range of movement and a mouth opening of more than 30 mm, good occlusion, and symmetry of the mandible [116].

9.2.5 The Areas of Controversy

There are three main issues of debate in the management of condylar fractures, which are:

(a) The method of treatment: open vs. closed; and age-related issues
(b) The approach to open treatment: extraoral, intraoral, or endoscopic
(c) Debates on fixation vs. no fixation and the types of fixation

9.2.6 The Method of Treatment: Open or Closed

Functional therapy (closed treatment) is adopted most frequently, since it permits early mobilization and adequate functional stimulation of condylar growth (in growing subjects) and bone remodeling (in all subjects). It is indicated in almost all condylar fractures that occur in childhood, and in intracapsular and extracapsular fractures that do not include serious condylar dislocation in adults [42, 46–48, 50, 93]. On the other hand, surgical treatment is indicated primarily for adults with moderately or grossly displaced fractures. It is also indicated for both children and adults with dislocation of the condylar head because of the benefits of direct visualization of the fragments for correct reduction and fixation enabling proper healing, early mobilization of the mandible that ensures normal joint function and action, and restoration of normal mouth and jaw function [8, 17, 24, 25, 45].

Treatment opinions based on age groups and pattern of fracture In children, the management of mandibular condylar fractures has long been a matter of controversy. If not treated appropriately, it may result in complications such as disturbance of mandibular growth and temporomandibular joint (TMJ) ankylosis. From the studies of Guven and keskin, Hovinga et al., and Lindahl and Hollende [42, 50, 69], nonsurgical treatment has been proved to be satisfactory in terms of the long-term results; there were no growth disturbances, malocclusion, or ankylosis observed with closed treatment. Beginning of remodeling was evident at postoperative 1.3 months, and remodeling of the condyle was good virtually in all the children. Dahlstrom et al. [21] in their 15 years follow-up study on condylar fractures treated by closed reduction also documented that there were no major growth disturbances among the children and the function of their masticatory system was good. There are no arguments against closed treatment in children except that open treatment is preferred for low level/subcondylar and dislocated fractures because of improved functional outcome associated with it [121]. There are very few large case series documenting the use of surgical methods for repair of fractured condyles in children [24], perhaps because many surgeons shy away from open treatment to avoid interference with mandibular growth. The evidences in support of closed treatment in children are overwhelming; [9, 14, 18] they concluded that closed/conservative treatment of most condylar fractures in growing children results in good functional results and proper remodeling of the condyle. This evidence has been adopted over the years.

Based on this evidence, fractures in growing children are generally treated closed, but unilateral open reduction and bone plating have given good result in few cases for subcondyle fractures [24, 28, 41]. However, this is not a sufficient reason to recommend open methods for treatment of high-level condyle fractures in children. The growth of the mandible continues throughout childhood and adolescence. Some authors claim that condylar cartilage is a primary growth center for the mandible and others support the functional matrix theory of Moss [76]. Although it is now universally accepted that the condyle plays an important part in mandibular growth [24, 26, 29, 42, 50], the influence of functional activities on the mandible is equally well established. Hence, in children, IMF is restricted to 14 days to facilitate early movement and to prevent ankylosis of TMJ, especially in high-level fractures [42, 50].

In teenagers/adolescents, few reports are available to make substantial evidence and enhance decision. However, surgeons agree that anatomic and functional restitution following closed treatment is not as good as in children, and that almost equal evidences are available in support of both treatment methods [11, 21, 23]. Therefore, where intervention is indicated, the choice of treatment in this age group should be selected depending on the preference of patient, class/level, and pattern of fracture, especially in the postpubertal teens [5, 10–14].

In adults, the decision to treat by closed or open method is dependent on the site and level of fracture, degree of displacement/dislocation, patients' choice, and medical status among others [8–15, 23, 79]. The concerted evidence in the treatment of specific fracture patterns in adults will be considered in the following discussion.

Isolated intracapsular fractures Common medical opinions strongly agree that isolated intracapsular fractures, in almost every instance, should be treated solely with physical therapy [9, 14, 21, 41, 46–48, 70, 72]. While these fractures can result in significant anatomic/radiologic changes in the appearance of the condyle itself, most patients with these fractures do well if properly rehabilitated. Late complications (e.g., degenerative joint disease) are possible, but again, with appropriate rehabilitation (in the absence of other fractures and generalized joint disease), these patients tend to do well. In the early rehabilitative phase, controlling the occlusion (usually by means of arch bars and elastics) while emphasizing return of normal range of motion is important. The patient should receive occlusion-guiding hardware and instructions in range of motion exercises immediately postinjury. The patient must be carefully monitored. Not surprisingly, younger patients seem to return more quickly to the premorbid state than do older patients, but even elderly patients, with appropriate rehabilitation, tend to do well with these injuries. The patients who encounter trouble are generally those in whom the fracture is undiagnosed and those who, for reasons of pain, do not immediately resume a normal range of mandibular motion. These patients then heal in anatomically incorrect and nonfunctional configurations. Once a mandibular malunion has occurred, mandibular motion, in some cases, cannot be reestablished without surgical intervention [46–48]. However, only a minority preferred open treatment of intracapsular condylar fractures as application of any form of fixation is usually impossible because of the lack of space and absence of enough support in the literature for open treatment [17]. It is, therefore, recommended that intracapsular fractures should be handled by closed methods [9, 14].

Isolated unilateral undisplaced condylar neck fracture From the various studies on this type of fracture, there were no symptoms observed except pain, and no structural or functional problems as such, so the consensus is for conservative or closed treatment [5, 9–15, 21, 26, 28, 29, 43]. Open treatments were not contemplated because of the possibilities of associated complications and morbidities. Some of those treated with IMF (closed method) could have done well with jaw exercises alone, but for the reluctance of the surgeons to leave their patients without active treatment, even when the occlusion was normal. There is no evidence in the literature to demonstrate any added benefits of IMF for this type of condylar fracture. The only justification is predicated on the assumption that patients are sometimes less likely to comply with instructions if they do not receive active treatment [44, 46, 53, 62, 65, 74, 75, 84].

Undisplaced condylar neck fracture with normal or abnormal occlusion As stated above, an isolated, undisplaced condylar neck can be managed conservatively. When combined with undisplaced mandibular body fracture, there is variable potential for distortion of occlusion. In such situation, a significant number of surgeons and authors support the use of closed method with 3–4 week period of IMF as the treatment of choice if normal occlusion, and up to about 5–6 weeks for adults when the occlusion is deranged, to allow for sufficient healing and remodeling [5, 9–15, 21]. It has been argued that when the period of IMF is less, there will be occlusal problems in the form of cross bite and deviation of the jaw to the affected side on protrusion [5, 8, 30, 31]. There is no evidence in support of open reduction in this situation. However, when the condylar fracture is associated with displaced mandibular body fracture, majority is in support of open reduction and rigid fixation (ORIF) of the body fracture and a variable period of IMF for the condyle [5, 9–15, 21]. Bilateral undisplaced condylar fractures were treated with a short period of IMF, whereas with contralateral displacement, a significant number used ORIF for the displaced condyle and a variable period of IMF [3, 5, 9–15, 29, 30, 32–41]. These treatment modalities yielded satisfactory results in most cases.

Minimally displaced unilateral condylar neck fracture associated with abnormal occlusion A vast majority used a period of IMF without surgical exposure for the treatment of this fracture and the functional and structural outcome was significantly successful. When combined with undisplaced mandibular body fracture, a period of IMF is the advocated treatment of choice, whereas when associated with displaced body fracture, ORIF of the body fracture and a period of IMF is the appropriate decision [3, 5, 9–15, 21, 26, 29, 30, 32–41].

Grossly displaced unilateral condylar neck fracture associated with abnormal occlusion There is no consensus on the ideal recommended treatment for patients with grossly displaced unilateral mandibular condyle fractures. Closed treatment has an ongoing popularity because it has yielded satisfactory results in most cases. It avoids the risk of damage to the facial nerve and is associated with no scarring. This popularity has been sustained because of the lack of large series with a long-term follow-up on open treatment [14, 15, 26, 28]. However, there is a growing evidence that in selected cases, where there is considerable shortening of the ascending ramus and/or significant displacement of the condylar fragment, open treatment provides a better outcome, otherwise the likelihood of TMJ dysfunction and functional disturbances is increased [3, 19, 20, 29–41, 53, 62, 84–92, 97].

Fracture-dislocation of unilateral condylar neck associated with abnormal occlusion A significant proportion of surgeons perform open treatment and more than half of these thought a period of IMF was necessary postoperatively. When combined with undisplaced mandibular body fracture, many used ORIF of the condyle and a period of IMF. When associated with a displaced body fracture, many used ORIF of the condyle and body. Functional deficits, occlusal disharmonies, and asymmetries/deformities were found on the radiographs in many of such cases treated with closed methods. The recommendation, therefore, is that fractured dislocated condyle must be opened [4, 7, 9–17, 19, 20, 24, 33, 46, 53, 65, 66, 74, 75].

Comminuted condyle fractures The consensus on the management of this type of fracture is closed method [9–15, 118–120]. To a large extent, open method will strip the periosteum of the minute bone fragments and result in avascular necrosis and resorption of the fragments with consequent asymmetry and deviation during excursions. There are no reports on the use of open methods for comminuted fractures; many surgeons avoid open repair of such fractures even in other sites of the jaw. Although supraperiosteal dissection is possible, it is more tedious to perform [24, 25].

Bilateral condyle neck fractures In bilateral condylar neck fractures, most surgeons openly treat at least one condyle when either one or both condyles were displaced or dislocated. This is in line with emerging evidence that smaller mouth opening and persistence of anterior open bite are associated with closed treatment [8, 14, 19, 20, 25, 28, 33, 44]. However, a few proportion opted for ORIF of both condyles, with a period of IMF in bilateral displaced fractures [57, 58, 65, 66, 74, 78, 79]. It must be noted that there is scanty evidence in the literature on the advantage of openly treating both sides over one side [92, 97, 101–103]. A Consensus Panel at Garoningen in Netherlands commented that "there is good evidence that displaced bilateral fractures would benefit from at least one side being treated open" [14]. Hence, the enthusiasm for open treatment of both sides could not be justified. If only one condyle is displaced, ORIF of the condyle with a period of IMF gives satisfactory results [104, 112–119].

Patients with no dentition Patients who are edentulous require special consideration. Preexisting dentures or gunning splints have been wired in and adapted for interarch elastics with satisfactory outcomes [21, 43, 74]. In most cases, an equally good outcome can be obtained with careful physical therapy that trains patients to open to a normal distance without deviation [21, 29, 41]. Some patients require preexisting dentures to be remade or relined. Often, the denture is broken in the same incident that caused the fracture. Some patients may be able to wear their preexisting prostheses during and after rehabilitation. In a nutshell, closed treatment is recommended based on the good functional and acceptable structural outcomes obtained in most studies involving different types of condylar fractures in these patients [43, 74, 79]. Open treatment is only advocated based on patient choice, ability to withstand general anesthesia, and as a relative indication in subcondylar fractures when splints are not available [8–15, 23, 26–29, 31, 32, 57, 58].

In some cases of bilateral fractures, construction of a splint is difficult, though not impossible. Situations exist in which a patient does not easily tolerate such an appliance. This may be another indication for opening at least one side [9–15, 96, 97, 102, 120, 121], especially if the patient is enfeebled and uncooperative and stable mandibular position cannot be maintained. However, in patients who are cooperative, and not medically compromised, even bilateral fractures should be managed with arch bars, elastics, physical therapy, close supervision, and follow-up [9–15, 26–29, 31, 32,

57, 75, 79]. Despite excellent reduction and fixation, the overall outcome of a patient treated with ORIF alone (i.e., without physical therapy) is likely to be compromised.

Subcondylar fractures The subcondylar fracture poses a different and more complicated set of questions. Most practitioners agree that most unilateral subcondylar fractures can be treated in a closed fashion [5, 8, 9, 15, 17, 41, 45, 62, 101]. This closed treatment implies control of the occlusion, aggressive physical therapy, and close follow-up. In bilateral subcondylar fractures the dilemma remains whether to manage it conservatively, perform open reduction and bone plating of one side only, or perform open reduction and bone plating of bilateral condyles. Those preferring closed reduction claim that functional recovery is to the same extent after both open and closed treatment and also morbidities associated with surgical treatment could be reduced. On the contrary, those that advocate for open reduction claim faster rate of improvement in mouth opening, maximal interincisal distance, and maximal excursions toward fractured side than patients treated with closed reduction [15, 17, 41, 45, 62, 108, 109, 111]. However, the age of the patient, the level of fracture, angle of displacement, dislocation of condylar head, and presence of other associated fractures are among the factors that influence decision.

Long-term follow-up of subcondylar fractures treated with occlusal guidance, physical therapy, and close supervision is important, but clinical records of such practice are not commonly found. Nevertheless, a few practitioners have records of over 40 or more years on some patients. Such records indicate that in young patients, over time, function and form are completely restored to normal with closed treatment, while in older patients, less remodeling and less correction of the radiologic picture may occur, but function is excellent and patients are free of pain [3, 28, 30, 33–41, 45, 84, 92].

Indications for open treatment in subcondylar fracture The landmark article by Kent and Zide [121] gives absolute and relative indications for open treatment of subcondylar fractures as follows:

Absolute indications:

1. Dislocation into the middle cranial fossa or external auditory canal
2. Lateral extracapsular displacement

3. Inability to obtain adequate occlusion
4. Open joint wound with foreign body or gross contamination

Relative indications:

1. A patient who has no dentition and where a splint is unavailable or when splinting is impossible because of alveolar ridge atrophy.
2. Bilateral or unilateral subcondylar fractures, when splinting is not recommended for medical reasons or where adequate physiotherapy is impossible.
3. Bilateral condylar fractures associated with comminuted midfacial fractures.
4. Bilateral subcondylar fractures with associated gnathologic problems, such as (a) retrognathia or prognathism, (b) open bite with periodontal problems or lack of posterior support, (c) loss of multiple teeth and later need for elaborate reconstruction, (d) bilateral condylar fractures with unstable occlusion due to orthodontics, and (e) unilateral condylar fracture with unstable fracture base.

The authors stated that the "relative indications are arguable and patients may be treated differently by each surgeon."

Hayward and Richard [45] developed an algorithm for indications of open reduction of condylar fractures based on the absolute and relative indications given by Zide and Kent (see below).

In summary, the evidence-based decisions for subcondylar fractures treatment depend on the fracture type and pattern as reflected in the indications. Some fractures will heal without much deficits with closed treatment and occlusal posterior bite planes; open reduction for either or both sides must be selected appropriately [9–15]. A patient with aesthetic form and normal function as the final result is the goal of treatment. The appearance of the radiograph is insignificant when these two goals have been met. Open method does not by itself guarantee that these goals will be met. In most cases, these can be met with closed method, meticulous postoperative physical therapy, and follow-up. Clinical judgment and consideration of other medical conditions must always influence the treatment choice for any particular patient. Therefore, treatment should be chosen based on patient choice, indication, and suitability for either procedure.

Bilateral condylar in association with midfacial fractures The patient who has both bilateral condylar fractures and midfacial fractures poses a challenge for the reconstructive surgeon. The surgeon, thus, takes into consideration the degree of comminution, the associated injuries, and the state of the dentition when determining whether to open one or both subcondylar fractures in such a patient. The decision is that ORIF on both sides can facilitate the care of the patient with an orthognathic problem that predates the fracture,

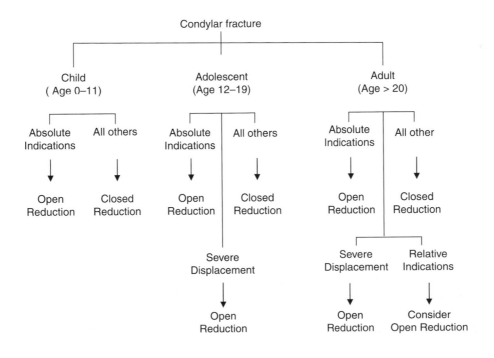

but splints should be constructed to facilitate the care of these patients as well [4, 7, 9–15, 23, 29, 45, 57]. If such patients are to be treated in an open fashion, models should be made and splints should be fabricated for intraoperative use. A millimeter of error at the fracture line may not be apparent to the operator, but a millimeter of error at the occlusion may be apparent to the patient.

Malunited condyle fractures There are but few articles on these fractures, but suggestions for management tend toward open treatment. Although there is yet no agreement on whether to create a new functional joint by doing sagittal split and/or external vertical ramus osteotomy or to refracture the malunion, the former option was consistently found to restore vertical ramus height and functions in patients compared to the latter [21, 29]. There were also good functional movements, occlusion, and sufficient bite force. It has also been argued that refracturing the malunion is technically difficult and may result in communition of the fragments [9–15, 21, 29]. Others have sectioned the upper fragment of the malformed condyle and restored with free nonvascularized bone graft. Associated donor site morbidities and unpredictable take of such grafts are important considerations [22].

9.2.7 The Approach to Open Treatment: Extraoral, Intraoral, or Endoscopy

There are various approaches in order to visualize and reduce the fractures of the condyles, these can be divided into two broad groups – extraoral and intraoral [11, 25, 60].

Extraoral approaches include preauricular, retroauricular, retromandibular, submandibular, and rhytidectomy (face-lift) incisions. These can also be used in different combinations [11, 25, 60].

Risdon described the submandibular approach; 4–5 cm skin incision, 2 cm below the angle of the mandible [60]. Access to the high condyle fractures with this approach is not as good as in preauricular and retromandibular approach, but the facial nerve, parotid gland, external carotid artery, and retromandibular vein are better avoided and kept out of the operation field. The scars are also more hidden in the

submandibular approach. However, most surgeons prefer retromandibular approach described by Hinds and Girotti [60] because of better direct access, shorter working distance from the incision to the condyle, excellent exposure even in the presence of marked edema, easy retrieval of the medially displaced condyle, and less conspicuous facial scar [10–14, 25, 29, 41, 44, 53, 60].

Silverman first described the open reduction and internal fixation of the condyle via intraoral route [60]. The major problem with this approach is access to the condylar fragments with consequent difficulty in manipulating and reducing the fragments. The merit is no obvious scars [44, 60]. Intraoral approach is usually by the mandibular vestibular incision with or without the use of an endoscope [11, 43, 100]. In any case, a transbuccal trocar is often necessary to aid the placement of some or all of the screws through plates on the reduced fragment [29, 41, 44, 60]. The use of an endoscope to assist with visualization of the fracture has become popular, and is commonly done in some centers. New instrumentation is frequently being developed.

In some cases, the use of the endoscope can add quite a bit to the length of the procedure, and therefore, to the anesthetic time and hospital charges without adding a great deal of advantage in terms of outcome [43, 100]. The evidence in support of its use elucidates the fact that it minimizes the incision needed and enhances visualization of small fragments. However, manipulation can be difficult and operation time increased especially with inexperienced surgeons [43, 68, 100]. As the equipment improves and operators' experience increases, operating times are expected to be reduced.

There are only few articles reporting outcomes with the use of endoscopes [43, 68, 100]. Hence, there is insufficient evidence to compare outcomes in terms of functional and aesthetic goals with properly performed and followed closed reduction, invasive intraoral, or extraoral approaches. In this regard, multidata based studies have to be conducted to answer the questions.

Generally speaking, most surgeons favor retromandibular approach, even though there are no conclusive evidences to suggest that outcome with one extraoral approach is better than the other or that extraoral approach is better than intraoral approach. In terms of scar perception, many patients prefer intraoral approach, even though access is better with the extraoral approach [11, 29, 41, 44, 60]. The approach used in each case would be determined by the surgeons' and patients' choice, amount of access obtainable, and the site of condyle fracture.

9.2.8 Debates on Fixation vs. No Fixation and the Types of Fixation

Whatever approach is chosen, once the fracture is exposed, it must be reduced. Whether the fracture must be fixated and how stable that fixation should be are other issues of controversy. Some surgeons believe that fixation is not always required. In studies that looked at a series of patients who had condyles significantly displaced out of the fossa and open reduction without fixation was done, the surgeons argued that significant malunion was prevented while avoiding rigidly fixating the condyles in a nonphysiologic position [8–15, 19, 21, 26, 32, 33, 41]. In essence, each of these markedly displaced fractures was converted to an undisplaced fracture and then treated as such, with occlusal control and physical therapy. If the fracture segment is unilateral and small enough, some surgeons advocate condylectomy [53, 74] instead of ORIF. The procedure simply removes the proximal segment altogether, while controlling the occlusion; the patient participates in extensive physical therapy afterward.

On the contrary, some others advocate mandatory fixation once a fracture is opened up and different methods of fixation have been discussed. Wire fixation and intramedullary pins have been used to stabilize condylar fractures [26, 32, 104, 110]. Again, occlusal control and physiotherapy remain crucial to successful outcomes.

In some cases, external fixators (e.g., Joe Hall Morris-type appliances) have been used with good success. Once again, occlusal control and physiotherapy are crucial to successful outcomes [68–71, 73, 74]. Finally, miniplates and screws are discussed. Argument exists as to whether these constitute rigid fixation or not [23–26, 32, 33]. The conclusion is that stable fixation, either semirigid with transosseous wires or external fixators or rigid with miniplates, is necessary once open treatment is performed to keep the segments in

physiologic position. Unstable fixation or fixation in a nonphysiologic position sets up the patient for pain, poor function, and degenerative joint disease [41, 53, 74, 91, 98, 99, 104, 110, 112, 120, 122, 123].

9.2.9 Physical Therapy Regimen

Of utmost importance for all patients, whether treated with closed or open techniques, is the general agreement that compliance with physical therapy regimens is highly essential [9–15]. These regimens do not require the patient to visit a rehabilitation center or to have any outside personal assistance (except for patients who are very young and/or some with physical or mental disabilities). Rather, physical therapy consists of a series of mouth opening exercises. There are commercially available devices such as the Therabite or EZ Flex jaw exercisers, which can be used by patients. An alternative and inexpensive method consists of a stack of tongue blades that can be increased in number each day [53, 74, 91, 98, 99]. Regardless of any device, during the first week post-treatment (i.e., non-IMF) or post-IMF, the patient should begin active movement of the jaws by attempting to open widely using their masticatory muscles. If sideward deviation is noted during this period, they are instructed to place a hand on the side of the face toward which the jaw deviates and apply gentle medial pressure as they open and close. By week 2, passive opening should begin with fingers, tongue blades, or exercise devices. Normal mandibular range of motion is 40 mm or more between the incisal edges of the anterior maxillary and mandibular teeth. In most patients, this distance should be achievable by week 2, if not sooner. Once the patient has reached the minimum goal of 40 mm, continued work in the straight opening plane is augmented with lateral and protrusive movements. The treatment is not complete until the patient has both a stable occlusion and normal function. Many care providers do not remove hardwares until both goals have been achieved; the removal thus serves as an additional motivational factor for some patients [19, 21, 26, 32, 33]. The result of an appropriate physical therapy regimen is a functional joint and masticatory system with little or no deformity [21, 26, 32].

9.2.10 Conclusion

The conclusive evidence based on collective reports of experiences documented in the literature can be itemized as follows:

1. Intracapsular fractures are best treated closed.
2. Fractures in children are best treated closed except when the fracture itself anatomically prohibits jaw function.
3. Most fractures in adults can be treated closed except in cases of gross displacements of the fragments and/or severe dislocations of the condylar head.
4. Physical therapy that is goal-directed and specific to each patient is integral to good patient care and is the primary factor influencing successful outcomes, whether the patient is treated open or closed.
5. When open reduction is indicated, the procedure must be performed well, with an appreciation for the patient's occlusal relationships, and it must be supported by an appropriate physical therapy and follow-up regimen.
6. The fractures that are openly reduced can be rigidly or semirigidly fixed in very stable physiologic position.

References

1. Adeyemo WL, Ladeinde AL, Ogunlewe MO et al (2005) Trends and characteristics of oral and maxillofacial injuries in Nigeria: a review of the literature. Head Face Med 1:7
2. Akadiri OA (2009) Zygomatico-orbital fractures: a case report. Nigerian J Orthop Trauma 8:37–40
3. Aksoy E, Ünlü E, Ömer S et al (2002) A retrospective study on epidemiology and treatment of maxillofacial fractures. J Craniofac Surg 13:772–775
4. Alkan A, Metin M, Muglali M et al (2007) Biomechanical comparison of plating techniques for fractures of the mandibular condyle. Br J of Oral Maxillofac Surg 45:145–149
5. Andersson J, Hallmer F, Eriksson L (2007) Unilateral mandibular condylar fractures: 31-year follow-up of non-surgical treatment. Int J Oral Maxillofac Surg 36:310–314
6. Antoun JS, Lee KH (2008) Sports-related maxillofacial fractures over an 11-year period. J Oral Maxillofac Surg 66:504–508
7. Asprino L, Consani S, De Moraes M (2006) A comparative biomechanical evaluation of mandibular condyle fracture plating techniques. J Oral Maxillofac Surg 64:452–456
8. Assael LA (2003) Open versus closed reduction of adult mandibular condyle fractures: an alternative interpretation of the evidence. J Oral Maxillofac Surg 61:1333–1339
9. Baker AW, McMahon J, Moss KF (1998) Current consensus on the management of fractures of the mandibular condyle. Int J Oral Maxillofac Surg 27:258–266
10. Bank P, Brown A (2001) Fractures of the facial skeleton. Wright, Oxford, Boston
11. Banks PA (1998) Pragmatic approach to the management of condylar fractures. Int J Oral Maxillofac Surg 27:244–246
12. Bhavsar D, Barkdull G, Berger J et al (2008) A novel surgical approach to subcondylar fractures of mandible. J Craniofac Surg 1:496–499
13. Bormann K-H, Wild S, Gellrich N-C et al (2009) Five-year retrospective study of mandibular fractures in Freiburg, Germany: incidence, etiology, treatment, and complications. J Oral Maxillofac Surg 67:1251–1255
14. Bos RR, Ward Booth RP, de Bont LG (1999) Mandibular condyle fractures: a consensus. Br J Oral Maxillofac Surg 37:87–89
15. Brandt MT, Haug RH (2003) Open versus closed reduction of adult mandibular condyle fractures: a review of the literature regarding the evolution of current thoughts on management. J Oral Maxillofac Surg 61:1324–1332
16. Brown DJ, Cowpe JG (1985) Pattern of maxillofacial trauma in two different cultures. J R Coll Surg Edinb 30:299–302
17. Chakraborty SK (2007) Subcondylar fracture: open reduction and bone plating. MJAFI 63:85–87
18. Choi J, Oh N, Kim IK (2005) A follow-up study of condyle fracture in children. Int J Oral Maxillofac Surg 34:851–858
19. Choi BH, Yi CK, Yoo JH (2001) Clinical evaluation of 3 types of plate osteosynthesis for fixation of condylar neck fractures. J Oral Maxillofac Surg 59:734–737
20. Choi BH, Yoo JH (1999) Open reduction of condylar neck fractures with exposure of the facial nerve. Oral Surg Oral Med Oral Pathol Oral Radiol Endod 88:292–296
21. Dahlstrom L, Kahnberg KE, Lindahl L (1989) 15 years follow-up on condylar fractures. Int J Oral Maxillofac Surg 8:18–23
22. Davis BR, Powell JE, Morrison AD (2005) Free-grafting of mandibular condyle fractures: clinical outcomes in 10 consecutive patients. Int J Oral Maxillofac Surg 34:871–876
23. De Riu G, Gamba U, Anghinoni M et al (2001) A comparison of open and closed treatment of condylar fractures: a change in philosophy. Int J Oral Maxillofac Surg 30:384–389
24. Deleyiannis FW, Vecchione L, Martin B et al (2006) Open reduction and internal fixation of dislocated condylar fractures in children: long-term clinical and radiologic outcomes. Ann Plast Surg 57:495–501
25. Devlin M, Hislop W, Carton A (2002) Open reduction and internal fixation of fractured mandibular condyles by a retromandibular approach: surgical morbidity and informed consent. Br J Oral Maxillofac 40:23–25
26. Eckelt U, Schneider M, Erasmus F et al (2006) Open versus closed treatment of fractures of the mandibular condylar process: a prospective randomized multi-centre study. J Craniomaxillofacial Surg 34:306–314
27. Egan KK, Kim DW, Byrne P et al (2009) Facial Trauma, Nasoethmoid Fractures. www.emedicine.com Accessed 06 May 2009
28. Ellis E (2000) Condylar process fractures of the mandible. Facial Plast Surg 16:193–205

29. Ellis E, Moos KF, El-Attar A (1985) Ten years of mandibular fractures: an analysis of 2, 137 cases. Oral Surg Oral Med Oral Pathol 59:120–129

30. Ellis E, Simon P, Throckmorton GS (2000) Occlusal results after open or closed treatment of fractures of the mandibular condylar process. J Oral Maxillofac Surg 58:260–268

31. Ellis E, Throckmorton G (2000) Facial symmetry after closed and open treatment of fractures of the mandibular condylar process. J Oral Maxillofac Surg 58:719–728

32. Ellis E, Throckmorton GS (2005) Treatment of mandibular condyle process fractures: biological considerations. J Oral Maxillofac Surg 63:115–134

33. Ellis E III, Throckmorton GS, Palmieri C (2000) Open treatment of condylar process fractures: assessment of adequacy of repositioning and maintenance of stability. J Oral Maxillofac Surg 58:27–34

34. Fasola AO, Denloye OO, Obiechina AE et al (2001) Facial bone fractures in Nigerian children. Afr J Med Med Sci 30:67–70

35. Fasola AO, Nyako EA, Obiechina AE et al (2003) Trends in the characteristics of maxillofacial fractures in Nigeria. J Oral Maxillofac Surg 61:1140–1143

36. Fasola AO, Obiechina AE, Arotiba JT (2000) Sports related maxillofacial fractures in 77 Nigerian patients. Afr J Med Med Sci 29:215–217

37. Fasola AO, Obiechina AE, Arotiba JT (2003) Incidence and pattern of maxillofacial fractures in the elderly. Int J Oral Maxillofac Surg 32:206–208

38. Fisher J, Kraus H, Lewis VL (1990) Assaulted women, maxillofacial injuries in rape and domestic violence. Plast Reconstr Surg 86:161–162

39. Garri JA, Perlyn CA, Johnson MG et al (1999) Patterns of maxillofacial injuries in powered watercraft collisions. Plast Reconstr Surg 104:922–927

40. Gassner R, Tuli T, Hachl O et al (2003) Cranio-maxillofacial trauma: a 10 year review of 9543 cases with 21 067 injuries. J Craniomaxillofac Surg 31:51–61

41. Goldman KE (2005) Fractures of the mandible: condylar and subcondylar. e Medicine World Medical Library 2:1–12

42. Guven O, Keskin A (2001) Remodelling following condylar fractures in children. J Craniomaxillofac Surg 29:232–237

43. Haug RH, Brandt MT (2003) Open versus closed reduction of adult mandibular condyle fractures: a review of the literature regarding the evolution of current thoughts on management. J Oral Maxillofac Surg 61:1324–1332

44. Haug RH, Brandt MT (2004) Traditional versus endoscope-assisted open reduction with rigid internal fixation (ORIF) of adult mandibular condyle fractures: a review of literature regarding current thoughts on management. J Oral Maxillofac Surg 62:1272–1279

45. Hayward JR, Richard FC (1993) Fractures of mandibular condyle. J Oral Maxillofac Surg 51:57–61

46. Hidding J, Wolf R, Pingel D (1992) Surgical versus non surgical treatment of fractures of the articular process of the mandible. J Craniomaxfac Surg 20:345–347

47. Hill CM, Burford K, Martin A et al (1998) A one-year review of maxillofacial sports injuries treated at an accident and emergency department. Br J Oral Maxillofac Surg 36:44–47

48. Hlawitschka M, Ecklet U (2002) Assessment of patients treated for intra-capsular fractures of the mandibular condyle by closed techniques. J Oral Maxillofac Surg 60:784–791

49. Holmes P-J, Koehler J, McGwin G et al (2004) Frequency of maxillofacial injuries in All-Terrain vehicle collisions. J Oral Maxillofac Surg 62:697–701

50. Hovinga J, Boering G, Stegenga B (1999) Long-term results of nonsurgical management of condylar fractures in children. Int J Oral Maxillofac Surg 28:429–440

51. Hussain OT, Nayyar MS, Brady FA et al (2006) Speeding and maxillofacial injuries: impact of the introduction of penalty points for speeding offences. Br J Oral Maxillofac Surg 44:15–19

52. Hutchison IL, Magennis I, Shepherd IJ et al (1998) The BAOMS United Kingdom survey of facial injuries part 1: aetiology and the association with alcohol consumption. Br J Oral Maxillofac Surg 36:3–13

53. Hyde N, Manisali M, Aghabeigi B et al (2002) The role of open reduction and internal fixation in unilateral fractures of the mandibular condyle: a prospective study. Br J Oral Maxillofac Surg 40:19–22

54. Iida S, Hassfeld S, Reuther T et al (2003) Maxillofacial fractures resulting from falls. J Craniomaxillofac Surg 31:278–283

55. Iida S, Kogo M, Sugiura T et al (2001) Retrospective analysis of 1502 patients with facial fractures. Int J Oral Maxillofac Surg 30:286–290

56. Iida S, Matsuya T (2002) Paediatric maxillofacial fractures: their aetiological characters and fracture patterns. J Craniomaxillofac Surg 30:237–241

57. Ishihama K, Iida S, Kimura T et al (2007) Comparison of surgical and nonsurgical treatment of bilateral condylar fractures based on maximal mouth opening. J Craniomaxillofac Surg 25:16–22

58. Joos U, Kleinheinz J (1998) Therapy of condylar neck fractures. Int J Oral Maxillofac Surg 27:247–254

59. Kadkhodaie MH (2006) Three-year review of facial fractures at a teaching hospital in northern Iran. Br J Oral Maxillofac Surg 44:229–231

60. Kempers KG, Quinn PD, Silverstein K (1999) Surgical approaches to mandibular condylar fractures: a review. J Craniomaxillofac Trauma 5:25–30

61. Klenk G, Kovacs A (2003) Etiology and patterns of facial fractures in the United Arab emirates. J Craniofac Surg 14:78 84

62. Konstantinovic VS, Dimitrijevic B (1992) Surgical versus conservative treatment of unilateral condylar process fractures: clinical and radiographic evaluation of 80 patients. J Oral Maxillofac Surg 50:349–352; discussion 52–53

63. Kotecha S, Scannell J, Monaghan A et al (2008) A four year retrospective study of 1,062 patients presenting with maxillofacial emergencies at a specialist paediatric hospital. Br J Oral Maxillofac Surg 46:293–296

64. Kummoona R (2008) Posttraumatic missile injuries of the orofacial region. J Craniofac Surg 19:300–305

65. Landes CA, Lipphardt R (2005) Prospective evaluation of a pragmatic treatment rationale: open reduction and internal fixation of displaced and dislocated condyle and condylar head fractures and closed reduction of non-displaced, non-dislocated fractures. Part I: condyle and subcondylar fractures. Int J Oral and Maxillofac Surgery 34:859–780

66. Landes CA, Lipphardt R (2006) Prospective evaluation of a pragmatic treatment rationale: open reduction and internal fixation of displaced and dislocated condyle and condylar head fractures and closed reduction of non-displaced, non-dislocated fractures. Part II: high condylar and condylar fractures. Int J Oral Maxillofac Surg 35:115–126

67. Laverick S, Patel N, Jones DC (2008) Maxillofacial trauma and the role of alcohol. Br J Oral Maxillofac Surg 46:542–546

68. Lee CSM, Young DM (2000) Cranial nerve VII region of the traumatized facial skeleton: optimizing fracture repair with the endoscope. J Craniomaxillofac Trauma 48:423

69. Lindahl L, Hollender L (1977) Condylar fractures of the mandible. A radiographic study of remodeling processes in the temporomandibular joint. Int J Oral Surg 6:153–165

70. Long X, Goss AN (2007) A sheep model of intracapsular condylar fracture. J Oral Maxillofac Surg 65:1102–1108

71. Loukota RA, Eckelt U, De Bont L et al (2005) Subclassification of fractures of the condylar process of the mandible. Br J Oral Maxillofac Surg 43:72–73

72. LR HM, Eckelt U (2005) Functional and radiological results of open and closed treatment if intracapsular (diacapitular) condylar fractures of the mandible. Int J Oral Maxillofac Surg 34:597–604

73. Maladière E, Bado F, Meninguad JP et al (2001) Aetiology and incidence of facial fractures sustained during sports: a prospective study of 140 patients. Int J Oral Maxillofac Surg 30:291–295

74. Marker P, Nielsen A, Lehmann BH (2000) Fractures of the mandibular condyle. Part 2: results of treatment of 348 patients. Br J Oral Maxillofac Surg 38:422–426

75. Mitchell DA (1997) A multicentre audit of unilateral fractures of the mandibular condyle. Br J Oral Maxillofac 35:230–236

76. Moss ML (1997) The functional matrix hypothesis revisited. The role of mechanotransduction. Am J Orthod Dentofacial Orthop 112:8–11

77. Mourouzis C, Koumoura F (2005) Sports-related maxillofacial fractures: a retrospective study of 125 patients. Int J Oral Maxillofac Surg 34:635–638

78. Newman L (1998) A clinical evaluation of the long-term outcome of patients treated for bilateral fracture of the mandibular condyles. Br J Oral Maxillofac Surg 36:176–179

79. Nussbaum ML, Laskin DM, Best AM (2008) Closed versus open reduction of mandibular condylar fractures in adults: a meta-analysis. J Oral Maxillofac Surg 66:1087–1092

80. Oginni FO, Ugboko VI, Ogundipe O et al (2006) Motorcycle-related maxillofacial injuries among Nigerian intracity road users. J Oral Maxillofac Surg 64:56–62

81. Olasoji HO (1999) Maxillofacial injuries due to assault in Maiduguri, Nigeria. Trop Doc 29:106–108

82. Olasoji HO, Tahir A, Arotiba GT (2002) Changing picture of facial fractures in northern Nigeria. Br J Oral Maxillofac Surg 40:140–143

83. Olasoji HO, Tahir A, Bukar A (2002) Jaw fractures in Nigerian children: an analysis of 102 cases. Cent Afr J Med 48:109–112

84. Palmieri C, Ellis E, Throckmorton G (1999) Mandibular motion after close and open treatment of unilateral mandibular condylar process fractures. J Oral Maxillofac Surg 57:764–775

85. Paza AO, Abuabara A, Passeri LA (2008) Analysis of 115 Mandibular angle fractures. J Oral Maxillofac Surg 66:73–76

86. Perkins CS, Layton SA (1988) The aetiology of maxillofacial injuries and the seat belt law. Br J Oral Maxillofac Surg 206:353–363

87. Puzovic D, Vitomir S, Konstantinovi KM (2004) Evaluation of maxillofacial weapon injuries: 15-year experience in Belgrade. J Craniofac Surg 15:543–546

88. Rallis G, Mourouzis C, Ainatzoglou M et al (2003) Plate osteosynthesis of condylar fractures: a retrospective study of 45 patients. Quintessence Int 34:45–49

89. Ramli R, Abdul Rahman R, Abdul Rahman N et al (2008) Pattern of maxillofacial injuries in motorcyclists in Malaysia. J Craniofac Surg 19:316–321

90. Roccia F, Diaspro A, Nasi A et al (2008) Management of sport-related maxillofacial injuries. J Craniofac Surg 19:377–382

91. Rowe NL, Kelley HC (1968) Fractures of the facial skeleton, 2nd edn. Churchill Livingstone, Edinburgh, pp 80–92

92. Rutges JPHJ, Kruizinga EHW, Rosenberg A et al (2007) Functional results after treatment of fractures of the mandibular condyle. Br J Oral Maxillofac Surg 45:30–34

93. Ryu SY, Hwang U, Yang KH (2004) Remodelling after conservative management of the mandibular condyle fracture in children. J Korean Assoc Oral Maxillofac Surg 30:49–55

94. Sakr K, Farag IA, Zeitoun IM (2006) Review of 509 mandibular fractures treated at the University Hospital, Alexandria, Egypt. Br J Oral Maxillofac Surg 44:107–111

95. Santler G, Karcher H, Ruda C et al (1999) Fractures of the condylar process: surgical versus nonsurgical treatment. J Oral Maxillofac Surg 57:392–397; discussion 97–98

96. Schön R, Roveda SIL, Carter B (2001) Mandibular fractures in Townsville, Australia: incidence, aetiology and treatment using the 2.0 AO/ASIF miniplate system. Br J Oral Maxillofac Surg 39:145–148

97. Silvennoinen U, Iizuka T, Pernu H et al (1995) Surgical treatment of condylar process fractures using axial anchor screw fixation: a preliminary follow-up study. J Oral Maxillofac Surg 53:884–893

98. Simsek S, Simsek B, Abubaker AO et al (2007) A comparative study of mandibular fractures in the United States and Turkey. Int J Oral Maxillofac Surg 36:395–397

99. Smets LM, Van Damme PA, Stoelinga PJ (2003) Non-surgical treatment of condylar fractures in adults: a retrospective analysis. J Craniomaxillofac Surg 31:162–167

100. SR LG (1999) Endoscope-assisted fixation of mandibular condylar process fractures. J Oral Maxillofac Surg 57:75–76

101. Stiesch-Scholz M, Schmidt S, Eckardt A (2005) Condylar motion after open and closed treatment of mandibular condylar fractures. J Oral Maxillofac Surg 63:1304–1309

102. Takenoshita Y, Ishibashi H, Oka M (1990) Comparison of functional recovery after nonsurgical and surgical treatment of condylar fractures. J Oral Maxillofac Surg 48:1191–1195

103. Talwar RM, Ellis E III, Throckmorton GS (1998) Adaptations of the masticatory system after bilateral fractures of the mandibular condylar process. J Oral Maxillofac Surg 56:430–439

104. Tanaka N, Hayashi S, Amagasa T et al (1996) Maxillofacial fractures sustained during sports. J Oral Maxillofac Surg 54:715–719

105. Tasanen A, Lamberg MA (1976) Transosseous wiring in the treatment of condylar fractures of the mandible. J Maxillofac Surg 14:200–211

106. Telfer MR, Jones GM, Shepherd IR (1991) Trends in the etiology of maxillofacial fractures in the United Kingdom (1977–1987). Br J Oral Maxillofac Surg 29:250

107. Terai H, Shimahara M (2004) Closed treatment of condylar fractures by intermaxillary fixation with thermoforming plates. Br J Oral Maxillofac Surg 42:61–63

108. Thomson WM, Stephenson S, Kieser JA (2003) Dental and maxillofacial injuries among older New Zealanders during the 1990s. Int J Oral Maxillofac Surg 32:201–205

109. Throckmorton GS, Ellis E (2000) Recovery of mandibular motion after closed and open treatment of unilateral mandibular condylar process fractures. Int J Oral Maxillofac Surg 29:421–427

110. Throckmorton GS, Ellis E, Hayasaki H (2003) Jaw kinematics during mastication following unilateral fractures of the mandibular condylar process. Am J Orthod Dentofac Orthop 124:695–707

111. Throckmorton GS, Ellis E, Hayasaki H (2004) Masticatory motion after surgical or nonsurgical treatment for unilateral fractures of the mandibular condylar process. J Oral Maxillofac Surg 62:127–138

112. Tominaga K, Habu M, Khanal A et al (2006) Biomechanical evaluation of different types of rigid internal fixation techniques for subcondylar fractures. J Oral Maxillofac Surg 64:1510–1515

113. Trost O, Kadlub N, Abu El-Naaj I et al (2007) Surgical management of mandibular condylar fractures in adults in France. Rev Stomatol Chir Maxillofac 108:183–188

114. Ugboko VI, Odusanya SA, Fagade OO (1998) Maxillofacial fractures in a semi-urban Nigerian teaching hospital. A review of 442 cases. Int J Oral Maxillofac Surg 27: 286–289

115. Van Beek GJ, Merkx CA (1999) Changes in the pattern of fractures of the maxillofacial skeleton. Int J Oral Maxillofac Surg 28:424–428

116. Villarreal PM, Monje F, Junquera LM et al (2004) Mandibular condyle fractures: determinants of treatment and outcome. J Oral Maxillofac Surg 62:155–163

117. Walker RV (1994) Condylar fractures: nonsurgical management. J Oral Maxillofac Surg 52:1185–1188

118. Widmark G, Bagenholm T, Kahnberg KE et al (1996) Open reduction of subcondylar fractures. A study of functional rehabilitation. Int J Oral Maxillofac Surg 25:107–111

119. Worsaae N, Thorn JJ (1994) Surgical versus nonsurgical treatment of unilateral dislocated low subcondylar fractures: a clinical study of 52 cases. J Oral Maxillofac Surg 52:353–360; discussion 60–61

120. Yang WG, Chen CT, Tsay PK et al (2002) Functional results of open versus closed reduction of mandibular condyle fractures: a systematic review of comparative studies of 107 unilateral mandibular condylar process fractures after open and closed treatment. J Trauma 52: 498–500

121. Zachariades N, Mezitis M, Mourouzis C et al (2006) Fractures of the mandibular condyle: a review of 466 cases. Literature review of reflections on treatment and proposals. J Craniomaxillofac Surg 34:421–432

122. Zide MF, Kent JN (1983) Indications for open reduction of mandibular condyle fractures. J Oral Maxillofac Surg 41:89–98

123. Zimmermann CE, Troulis MJ, Kaban LB (2005) Pediatric facial fractures: recent advances in prevention, diagnosis and management. Int J Oral Maxillofac Surg 34:823–833

Strengths and Limitations of the Evidence-Based Movement Aimed to Improve Clinical Outcomes in Dentistry and Oral Surgery

10

Pier Francesco Nocini, Giuseppe Verlato, Daniele De Santis, Andrea Frustaci, Giovanni De Manzoni, Antonio De Gemmis, Guglielmo Zanotti, Giovanni Rigoni, Alessandro Cucchi, Luciano Canton, Vincenzo Bondì and Eleonora Schembri

Core Message

> To lead dentistry in the third millennium, it is necessary to use the instruments developed by EBM when planning and evaluating research studies, but is impossible to produce sound knowledge without considering clinical expertise and quality of surgical procedures simultaneously.

P.F. Nocini (✉)
D. De Santis
A. Frustaci
A. De Gemmis
G. Zanotti
G. Rigoni
A. Cucchi
L. Canton
V. Bondì
E. Schembri
Department of Maxillo-facial Surgery and Dentistry, University of Verona, Piazzale L. A. Scuro 10, 37134 Verona, Italy
e-mail: pierfrancesco.nocini@univr.it

G. Verlato
Unit of Epidemiology and Medical Statistics, University of Verona, Strada le Grazie 8, 37134, Verona Italy

G. De Manzoni
1st Division of General Surgery, Borgo Trento Hospital, Piazzale Stefani 1, 37126, Verona, Italy

10.1 Introduction

Medicine is science when it is taught, but is art when it is performed

(Unknown)

EBM is a relatively new concept in medicine knowledge that requires a global approach. In this excerpt, we will try to make you focus your attention on a more specific field: the dental care point of view. But what is EBM? EBM tries to base medical care on the results of scientific studies, in particular to fill the gap between everyday practice and medical literature. The evaluation of the health care interventions takes advantage of the enormous progress in computer science, which has made available most of the medical literature on the Internet [33]. It is fundamental to establish what part of medical therapy can be rigorously evaluated by scientific methods and which are the best outcomes to assess the effectiveness of medical treatment [19]. EBM acknowledges that many aspects of medical care depend on individual factors, such as genetic traits, cultural factors, compliance to treatment, quality of life, which cannot be fully evaluated by quantitative methods. Thus, it is essential to take into account evidence coming from different investigations, that is, to perform a systematic review of all studies dealing with a particular disease and related treatments. By combining different disciplines, such as medicine, biology, engineering, and statistics, EBM tries to find the most effective treatment in order to obtain the ideal wellness in everyday practice [30, 31]. A great emphasis is

F. Chiappelli et al. (eds.), *Evidence-Based Practice: Toward Optimizing Clinical Outcomes*,
DOI: 10.1007/978-3-642-05025-1_10, © Springer-Verlag Berlin Heidelberg 2010

given to meta-analyses of clinical trials and risk-benefit analysis.

All "experts" consider two types of EBM: evidence-based guidelines (EBG), which is the practice of EBM at the institutional level including the production of guidelines to advise the best medical practice; and evidence-based individual decision (EBID), designed for the individual health care provider who, for instance, needs to relate with different patients (younger vs. older).

Lastly, evidence is not immediately transferable to routine clinical practice: the efficacy of a verified new treatment approach is limited to the patients' population studied in a certain clinical trial. In addition, treatment effectiveness reported from clinical studies may be higher than that achieved in routine clinical practice due also to the closer patient monitoring during trials, leading to higher compliance rates. There are contrasting reports about whether EBM is effective. The fact that EBM is divided into EBG and EBID may explain this conflict. It is hard to find evidence that EBID improves health care, whereas there is growing evidence of improvements in the efficacy of health care when EBM regarding guidelines is practiced at the organizational level [108]. One of the virtues of health care accreditation is that it offers an opportunity to assert the overall functioning of a hospital against the best of the currently available evidence and to assist the hospital to move toward a more effective application of EBM.

10.1.1 History and Evolution of Research: The Development of Evidence-Based Medicine (EBM)

The term "EBM" is relatively new. In fact, researchers from McMaster University began using the term during the 1990s [32]. EBM was defined as a systemic approach to analyze published results forming the base of clinical decision-making. Then in 1996, the term was more formally defined by Sackett et al. [79], who stated that EBM was *the conscientious and judicious use of current best evidence from clinical care research in the management of individual patients*. In addition, some authors find traces of EBM's origin in ancient Greece, others trace its roots to ancient Chinese medicine, but they consist in historical or anecdotal accounts of what may be loosely termed EBM. After this period, we could find the renaissance era of EBM, which

began roughly during the seventeenth century. During this era, personal journals were kept and textbooks soon became more prominent. This was followed by the 1900s, a period we term "the transitional era of EBM" (1900s–1970s). Knowledge during this era could be shared more easily in textbooks and eventually peer-reviewed journals [20, 25].

Lastly, although testing medical interventions for efficacy has existed since the time of Avicenna's "Canon of medicine" in the eleventh century, it was only in the twentieth century that this effort evolved to impact almost all fields of health care and policy [20].

Especially during the 1970s, we enter the modern era of EBM. Technology has had a large role in the advancement of EBM. Computers and database software have allowed compilation of large amounts of data. Professor Archie Cochrane, a Scottish epidemiologist, through his book "Effectiveness and Efficiency: Random Reflections on Health Services" (1972) and subsequent advocacy, caused increasing acceptance of the concepts behind EB practice. Cochrane's work was honored through the naming of centers of EB medical research (Cochrane Centers) and an international organization, the Cochrane Collaboration [29, 100].

Finally, the term "EB" was first used in 1990 by David Eddy and first inserted in the medical literature in 1992 in a paper by Guyatt et al. [39].

So EBM has been touted as an effective series of mechanisms not only for improving health care quality, but also for reducing medical errors precipitated in part by clinical practice variation. This new point of view favors the change as regard the efficacy of clinical therapy. Therefore, clinicians could use a set of increasingly accessible sources of data, evidence summaries, and guidelines that acknowledge the most current EBM thinking, perhaps the best in the GRADE system (a better literature filter), and in particular the role of values and preferences in decision-making. Medical and health policy training must continue to evolve, allowing clinicians and policy makers to successfully differentiate truly EB sources of information and interpretation of information from those that are not [7].

Following the birth of EBM, evidence-based dentistry (EBD) has developed some years later with the advent of the new millennium. In fact, we have to note that Dentistry over the last 100 years has been characterized by improved approaches to education and practice. Parallel to trends in the field of medicine as a whole, dentistry is moving toward EB practices. The goal of EBD is the assurance, through references to high-quality evidence data, that care provided is optimal for the patient and that treatment options are presented in a manner that allows for fully informed consent. The more we will move toward broad-based use of EBD in clinical practice, the more physicians will benefit through better and standardized clinical guidelines that will help in decision-making and quality of clinical results [36, 94].

One of the most important issues in deciding what kind of therapy is more indicated is to consider the balance between the potential risks and benefits of treatment. A framework for EB decision-making includes formulating the clinical question and then retrieving, appraising, and considering the applicability of the evidence to the single case. It is the duty of all health care providers to reduce patients' burden of treatment by selecting appropriate therapies and explaining possible unavoidable risks.

The purpose of this chapter is to assist physicians in locating and retrieving quality research reports and research evidence, which can be integrated into the clinical decision-making process, but in a more general view of how we cannot yet ignore the clinical expertise.

There is a certain philosophy that believes that medicine is a science and every question will get an answer, another view believes that medicine is actually an art, and the physician is the owner of this capability to create health through his knowledge, experience, and intuition.

Where is the truth? We do not know but probably it stands in the middle: we can help each other with some instruments. One of these is EBM.

As you will see there are not only a lot of strengths in EBM, but also limits that we cannot ignore.

10.2 Evaluating the Quality of Research

Today, there is a large amount of papers regarding specific topics for consultation in the scientific literature, so that it is becoming more and more difficult to choose those that have a real impact on clinical practice. Furthermore, some works had such an impact on the new treatments of patients that young scientists need to have a systematic approach in order to distinguish between landmark papers and other works with a different and often lower impact on clinical practice.

Therefore, it becomes essential in consulting scientific literature to find not only the works that answer a debatable question, but also to try to select among a large amount of data that are able to answer our questions in a scientific way and with a quality control assurance.

According to this point of view, EBM gave us an important help and is continuing to do this with the so-called Systematic Reviews.

A "systematic review" simply means the result of an organic review of most important works regarding a certain issue performed according to the rules of EB.

In particular, a systematic review can be distinguished from other types of analysis when the entire procedure is done together with the application of the following criteria:

1. The questions that we want to give an answer to must be expressed according to the so-called *PICO rule*, where PICO means the following four English words: *population, intervention, comparison, and outcome*. This methodology foresees the choice of a certain group of patients (population), who have to undergo a certain type of intervention (intervention), so that we can compare this approach with other different kind of interventions or with a placebo treatment (comparison) with the ultimate end point to study and try to interpret correctly the results finally obtained (outcome).

2. The obtained data will be reanalyzed (also with the aid of internet databases, paper reviews, or clinical expert opinions) and this critical reevaluation has the aim of giving a grade of scientific value. From this point of view, the studies will be classified according to a decreasing scale as follows:

   (a) Randomized and controlled clinical trials (RCTs)
   (b) Controlled trials not randomized (CTs)
   (c) Cohort studies
   (d) Case/control studies
   (e) Cross-sectional studies
   (f) Case report studies
   (g) Expert opinions

Scientific researchers are, therefore, evaluated with different systems, and the more useful and applied is the one by the *U.S. Preventive Service Task Force* that gives the so-called levels of scientific evidence in five different levels:

- Level I: is obtained with at least one controlled and randomized study supported by a valid statistical methodology.
- Level II-1: is obtained with controlled but not randomized trials.

- Level II-2: is obtained with cohort studies or with case/control studies, conducted preferably in more than one single Institution or Research Groups.
- Level II-3: is obtained from the observation and follow-up of consecutive series with or without an intervention (for instance, an exceptionally good result in a noncontrolled study is comprised in this level of evidence).
- Level III: is obtained from expert opinions based on their clinical experience, or with descriptive studies or with the summary of an expert panel.

From the analysis of data, we have to determine the validity of the study, which must be of two types:

(a) Internal, as it depends on the conceivability of the study and its rationale.
(b) External, as it regards the possibility to apply the obtained results to the overall population.

In particular, the methods in order to evaluate the quality of a study may look at:

1. Condition: it regards a certain pathological condition or physiological situation (for example pregnancy) where you want to test a certain surgical procedure or drug.
2. Study design: it regards the kind of study you want to perform. A single study may be an experimental study (randomized controlled trial, field trial, community intervention trial) or an observational study (cohort, case-control, cross-sectional, ecologic, case series etc.). An analysis of the current literature can be a meta-analysis, a review, or a systematic review. Most randomized trials are superiority trials, aiming at verifying whether a treatment is superior to another one; recently, equivalence or noninferiority trials have been introduced, aiming to verify whether a new treatment, less expensive or with fewer side effects, is equivalent or noninferior to the old treatment.
3. Authors and years: they comprise the names of the authors and the year of publication of the study.
4. Sample size: it should be large enough to achieve a sensible power in order to detect a minimal "clinical significant" difference.
5. Magnitude of the benefit: it represents the degree of the benefit, in terms of standard deviations (SD) of the results: it is high when it is more than 1 SD, intermediate when it is comprised between 0.5 and 0.9 SD and is low when it is comprised between 0.2 and 0.4 SD.
6. Measurement used to report results: it can largely affect the willingness to prescribe among family physicians. The most widely used are:

Relative risk or relative risk reduction.

Absolute risk reduction (ARR): it consists of the difference in percentages from the control group that reached a specific end point (control event rate) and the percentage of subjects in the test group that reached the same end point (test event rate).

Number needed to treat (NNT): it is the number of patients who need to be treated in order to prevent one additional bad outcome (death, major cardiovascular event, etc.); in other words, it is the number of patients who need to be treated for one to obtain a predefined benefit compared with a control in a clinical trial. It is defined as the inverse of the ARR. The ideal NNT is one, where everyone improves with treatment and no one improves with control. The higher the NNT, the less effective is the treatment. Indeed, an Italian study [12] showed that the willingness to prescribe was much higher when the results were reported as relative risk reduction (34.1%) and much lower when the number need to treat ($n = 71$) or the ARR (1.41%) was used.

1. Comments
2. Quality of the study: for instance, the Jadad Score [56] is widely used to evaluate clinical trials

The *Jadad Score* is an instrument that allows to evaluate the quality of different studies.

It gives a point ranging from 0 to 5 in evaluating seven items: the first five items indicate a good quality of the study; the last two indicate a poor quality of the study. For every positive study characteristic a point (+1) is assigned, while for every negative characteristic a point is deducted (−1) (Fig. 10.1).

Evaluation of randomized clinical trial (Jadad score)

It ranges from 0 (bad study) to 5 (optimal study)

+1) The study is randomized

+1) The method of randomization is described and is appropriate (e.g., casual numbers from tables or computer assisted)

+1) Description of reasons of loss to follow up

+1) The study is in double blind

+1) The method used to apply the blinding is described and it is appropriate

−1) The method used to apply the blinding is described and it is appropriate (e.g., placebo per os and drug by intravenous administration)

−1) The method of randomization is not correct (e.g., random allocation by date of birth or hospital number)

Fig. 10.1 The Jadad score

Positive characteristics are:

- Patients randomization: was the study described as randomized (this includes words such as randomly, random, and randomization)?
- Correct choice and description of the randomization method: was the method used to generate the sequence of randomization described and appropriate (table of random numbers, computer-generated, etc.)?
- Double blind clinical trial: was the study described as double blind?
- Correct and described performance of the blinding: was the method of double blinding described and appropriate (identical placebo, active placebo, dummy, etc.)?
- Predefined description of lost to follow-up: was there a description of withdrawals and dropouts?

Negative characteristics are:

- Not correct choice of the randomization method: deduct one point if the method used to generate the sequence of randomization was described and it was inappropriate (patients were allocated alternately, or according to date of birth, hospital number, etc.).
- Not correct blinding allocation: deduct one point if the study was described as double blind, but the method of blinding was inappropriate (e.g., comparison of tablet vs. injection without employing the double dummy technique).

Once we have understood the number and the importance of evaluation methods in clinical research, we have to move into meta-analysis which is the main part of EB movement.

10.3 Meta-Analysis as a New Approach in Clinical Research

Meta-analysis is a secondary instrument of research aimed to summarize data from various instruments of primary research, in particular from clinical studies.

Precisely, it consists of a series of mathematic-statistical methods designed to integrate the outcomes derived from clinical studies, with the goal of obtaining a unique quantitative evaluation index to draw conclusions stronger than those retrieved from every single study.

Meta-analysis has become popular in the medical research field where the available information is generally the result of various clinical researches, designed with similar protocols.

Some studies are often always limited when considered individually, either in the numerosity or in the definition of goals, in order to obtain crystalline conclusions, and above all, generalized statements in relation to the effect of the treatment. The possibility to gather results from various studies represents an interesting alternative approach that strengthens our knowledge on the effect of the treatment. Let us check some examples of meta-analysis in the medicine and dentistry fields.

10.3.1 Thrombolytic Therapy and Lidocaine in Myocardial Infarction

One of the main examples of the impact of meta-analysis is, for instance, the debate on the use of thrombolytic therapy in myocardial infarction. The large volume of published randomized, controlled trials has led, in fact, to a need for meta-analyses to track therapeutic advances in this field, in order to look at trends in efficacy and to determine whether this treatment appears to be significantly effective or deleterious. The investigators conducted the first RCT of thrombolytic therapy in the late 1950s, enrolling 23 patients and finding approximately half the number of deaths in treated patients as in control patients. With this very small sample size, the confidence interval (CI) was extremely wide. With the further advent of new trials in the 1970s and with the randomization number of over 2,500 patients, the CI no longer overlaps the line of no-effect, suggesting therefore that chance is no longer an explanation of the differences between treatment and control. By 1990, with the randomization of nearly 50,000 patients, the CI around the odd ratios of approximately 0.75 (an odds reduction of 0.25) are very narrow (Table 10.1).

As the evidence was accumulating that thrombolytic therapy was working, a considerable variability in expert opinion still existed. A consensus for administering thrombolytic therapy was not reached before 1990 (Table 10.2).

The opposite example regards the use of prophylactic lidocaine to prevent lethal ventricular arrhythmias in patients presenting with myocardial infarction.

Here the randomized trial evidence never supported therapy (Table 10.3), and in fact, suggested a possible increase in mortality. Nevertheless, some experts continue to recommend this practice until almost 1990 [67] (Table 10.4).

Table 10.1 RCTs on thrombolytic therapy

Years	Number of trials	Number of patients	p value
1960–1970	4	316	n.s.
1970–1980	19	5,451	<0.01
1980–1990	47	42,387	<0.00001

Table 10.2 Textbook/review recommendations on thrombolytic therapy

Years	Not mentioned	Experimental therapy	Routine/ specific
1960–1970	26	0	0
1970–1980	35	4	1
1980–1990	21	17	40

Table 10.3 RCTs on prophylactic lidocaine

Years	Number of Trials	Number of patients	p value
1960–1970	0	0	n.a.
1970–1980	12	1,986	n.s.
1980–1990	3	6,759	n.s.

Table 10.4 Textbook/review recommendations on prophylactic lidocaine

Years	Not mentioned	Experimental therapy	Routine/ specific
1960–1970	5	0	21
1970–1980	6	1	31
1980–1990	16	1	75

As regards myocardial infarction, fibrinolytic therapy would have been adopted and lidocaine would have been abandoned 10–15 years before if meta-analysis had been adequately recognized, allowing thousands of patients to benefit a more effective and secure therapy.

10.3.2 The Impact of Polyol-Containing Chewing-Gums on Dental Caries

Some meta-analyses have also been conducted in dentistry. Their role is to try to achieve some evidences from different studies executed in different centers in order to answer a common clinical question. Once a question is answered with a strong methodological base, it is time to stop searching in this context and to move on daily clinical practice. Our case deals with a recent meta-analysis conducted on the impact of sugar substitutes (called polyols) on dental caries [5].

It is important to affirm that dental caries in the United States is considered the most common chronic childhood disease and that more than 90% of children have experienced caries at some point in their lives [42, 75].

Many preventive programs (individual hygiene procedure and dental office procedure) have been developed and a reduction of overall caries burden could be more beneficial from a public health perspective [9].

Also, lots of studies have been executed on the effect of sugar substitutes known as "polyols" or "sugar alcohols" that are nonfermentable sugars commonly used in chewing-gum (xylitol, sorbitol, mannitol). Typical meta-analysis methods have been used to retrieve and evaluate the type and quality of studies. From a starting number of 231 eligible articles, 19 articles were finally selected for this meta-analysis. At the end of their analysis, they conclude that polyol-containing chewing-gum does reduce dental caries. Even if some gaps in literature are still present around dose-response relationship and the efficacy of different polyols, there are some consistent evidences to support the use of xylitol and sorbitol-containing chewing-gum as part of normal hygiene to prevent dental caries.

As we can see this is not only important for the individual patient, but also, and most importantly, for a possible reduction of these lesions in general population with lots of benefits for public health care services. Such kind of answer must be obtained only through the meta-analysis of well-designed and well-conducted studies.

Despite these positive examples, there are some concerns about the utility of meta-analysis regarding different points: there are few doubts about the fact that putting together results derived from different studies may give serious problems as regard the interpretation and methodological issues. As far as end points and study design are concerned, we will often have to analyze and interpret results obtained from numerous dissimilar studies. For instance, not all studies will be able to give the same input on the definition of treatment efficacy, while some will be underpowered due to the low number of treated patients or the loss of them during follow-up.

One of the most difficult issues is to try to give the correct importance to different results coming from similar studies that have identical end points but different conclusions.

Now we are going to accurately analyze the way meta-analyses are composed, and what is EB movement's basic process.

10.4 Randomized Clinical Trials (RCT) and Their Role in Medicine Progress

The strengths of EBM movement have been to try to give biology and medicine a more predictable approach, providing clear answers to open-ended questions.

In medicine and dentistry, learning and acquiring professional competences have been once based on experts' word (e.g., various specialists' personal experience, reference books, congress cultural exchanges). The non-systematic observations based on clinical experience were thought to be valid in order to form our knowledge on prognosis, diagnosis, and effectiveness of treatment.

The knowledge of the biological and physiological mechanisms, the good sense, and the clinical experience seemed to be sufficient in order to guide the specialist in clinical and the evaluation of new therapies or diagnostic techniques.

The field experts had to produce for consensus the guidelines for the treatment and the diagnosis of several pathologies.

With the advent of EBM, all has changed: the importance of the personal experience has been limited and it has been proposed that the decisions and the knowledge about diagnostic tests, prognosis, and treatments had to be based on all validated and statistically significant data derived from well-designed studies. The clinical experience was still fundamental; however, the clinical observation had to be made in a systematic, reproducible, and quantitative way (research methodology).

The knowledge of the biological mechanisms is necessary, but not sufficient to foretell the "best" clinical practice at our time in which new mechanisms of molecular biology always widen our knowledge on diseases on the basis of patients' characteristics. Formation and medical practice must not only be based, therefore, on the doctor's ability to retrieve the information on the best possible EB on the most important results of clinical research, but also on the ability to consult the medical literature and databases for dealing those cases that go far beyond clinical routine.

In particular, EBM's efforts focused on three fundamental points such as:

- Searching the information with the maximum efficiency.
- Interpreting the articles that bring back the information.
- Estimating validity.

Above all, for an efficient research of the information, EBM makes reference to research via scientific and computer science articles taking advantage of data collection, like Cochrane Collaboration, Embase, and Medline.

The main topic of EBM literature consists of therapy rather than diagnosis. The therapeutic procedures (drugs, surgical techniques, etc.) must always be estimated through RCTs, while the consequent meta-analyses quantitative and qualitative synthesis of multiple RCT.

These are RCTs, that is, extremely common scientific experiments performed on man in order to estimate the effectiveness of new instruments, drugs, or techniques, in respect of those used once in clinical practice, which represented the "gold standard." In RCTs, a comparison between gold standard and innovative therapy was studied to determine the most effective treatment.

RCTs are used in all scientific research fields; they are experimentations, in which the investigator proposes to the patient through an informed consent the possibility to be involved in a study to improve therapeutic results or to reduce the side effects of a specific treatment. Consequently, positive perturbations such as therapeutic, preventive, and rehabilitative interventions can be performed.

It is important to affirm that before any clinical trial is carried out, result of nonclinical investigations or previous human studies should be sufficient to indicate that the drug is acceptably safe for the proposed investigation in humans [55].

RCTs are carried out in dentistry as in any other medical specialty. In this case, RCTs are a guarantee of an advanced quality of result that will further be evaluated. They are structured in the same way, although the patients' recruitment phase and the collection of a high and statistically significant number of patients turn out to be more difficult.

RANDOMIZED CLINICAL TRIAL (RCT)

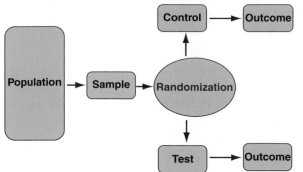

Fig. 10.2 Description of RCT design

The necessary number of RCT participants is determined through a statistic analysis before the beginning of the study based on the primary goal to reach and the quantification of a possible increase of the benefit in order to assure a statistic significance to the study.

The main characteristics of RCTs are (Fig. 10.2):

- There are two or more groups of study: Test group (new therapy) and Control group (placebo or gold standard therapy).
- Participants are randomly distributed in Test and Control groups in order to reduce the influence of known or unknown confusing factors.

This allows to increase the probability that the two groups are similar and that possible differences in study outcomes are due only to the type of procedure that has been attributed to the patient and not to known or unknown disease characteristics that they are canted in a group of treatment.

Other characteristics of RCT studies are perspective longitudinal design of the study, the necessity of an ethical committee approval, and beyond the necessity of having the patient's informed consent of as mentioned above.

RCT studies should be used in cases in which drug effectiveness, surgical techniques, screening interventions, sanitary education, and health care system organization are evaluated.

According to the degree of the staff's knowledge of participant distribution into Test and Control groups, it is possible to distinguish four RCT types:

- Open RCT: both the subjects and the clinicians know which group participants belong to.

- Single blind RCT: only the clinicians know which group participants belong to.
- Double blind RCT: only the staff involved in the randomization procedure know which group participants belong to through a code, but neither the clinicians who execute the procedure nor the patients know the type of treatment.
- Triple blind RCT: only the staff involved in the randomization procedure know which group participants belong to through a code, but neither the clinicians who execute the procedure, nor the patients nor those who analyze the outcomes know the type of treatment.

In the hierarchy of evidence that influences health care practice, RCTs are largely considered to be the top individual unit of research. They are considered the most reliable form of scientific evidence because they eliminate spurious causality and bias.

One example of a very important RCT is the one regarding the use of hormone replacement therapy (HRT) in postmenopausal women that was thought to reduce cardiovascular diseases, and indeed, was found not only to increase these issues, but also and more dramatically to increase the risk of breast cancer.

10.4.1 Hormone Replacement Therapy (HRT)

Despite decades of accumulated observational evidence, the balance of risks and benefits for hormone used in healthy postmenopausal women remained uncertain, and in common clinical practice, a wide use of such therapy was administered without any real EB data.

To assess the major health benefits and risks of the most commonly used combined hormone preparation in the United States, a randomized trial was finally performed. Overall health risks exceeded benefits from the use of combined estrogen plus progestin for an average 5.2-year follow-up among healthy postmenopausal US women as recently reported by Rossouw et al. [78] in their analysis of data from Women's Health Initiative randomized controlled trial.

Thus, in today's health care system, all the new procedures must have been previously estimated through RCTs to be approved and be applied in clinical practice. Such studies are used in order to determine not only the effects of a therapy, but also to detect and underline possible side effects.

10.4.2 RCT: What they Can Say and What they Cannot Say. Are Observational Studies Still Needed?

The onset of EB has generated many criticisms: too rigid, and not able to fit medical flexibility for the complexity of the subject as well as for cultural and ethical reasons.

One of Smith and Pell's famous articles clearly explained this EB question. A systematic review on the parachute effect in preventing death and major trauma related to gravitational challenge using EBM instruments was performed [88]. Obviously, there were no publications available in Medline, Embase, and Cochrane Library databases and the outcomes were considered insignificant; the authors ironically declared that the parachute was not safe enough to be widely used, since there were no RCTs present in Literature. In addition, the strongest advocates of EBM movement were invited to take part in a randomized, placebo-controlled, cross-over, double blind trial on the use of parachute. This would have for sure resulted in a disaster; other types of experimental studies exist for such purpose.

Scientific studies can be led as experiments or observations. In the first case, the researcher will establish the parameters of the study, while in the second case the researcher works only as an observer. Transversal or longitudinal studies determine the duration of the study. As regards, longitudinal studies can be carried out on the basis of previously existing data (retrospective studies) or data collected over time (prospective studies).

The so-called observational studies are based on the researcher's external observation of reality in which potentially harmful etiologic factors are investigated, such as bad habits (alcohol, smoke, etc.) and precarious environmental conditions (X ray, passive smoke, etc.). There is no sample randomization, but self-selection.

In EBM movement, observational studies have a minor evidence value and can be classified in:

1. *Study group or cohort* (or prospective). Two groups are confronted: the study group is exposed to treatment/causal agent, while the second group is that of control. Both groups are followed over time (prospective study) in order to detect the incidence of a pathology.

2. *Case/control study* (or retrospective). Two groups are controlled: one is affected by a pathology, while the other is not. Both groups are estimated on the base of the collected data in the past (retrospective or historical study) in order to discover an eventual causal agent of the pathology.

3. *Cross-sectional studies* (or of prevalence). The observation is limited to a determined period of time.

In this type of observational studies, drugs are prescribed according to the officially-registered commercial purpose. The patient's assignment to a specific therapeutic strategy is not decided in advance by an experimental protocol, but belongs to routine clinical practice. The decision to prescribe drugs does not depend on the patient's inclusion in the study. No additional diagnostic or monitoring procedure is applied to the patients, while epidemiological methods are used for the analysis of the collected data (in compliance with the Italian law: Law Decree 24 June 2003 no.11).

To be considered as observational studies, drugs must satisfy the following conditions:

1. The drug must be prescribed according to the officially-registered commercial purpose.
2. The prescription of the drug under investigation must be part of the routine clinical practice.
3. The decision to prescribe the drug to the subject must not depend on the patient's inclusion in the study (where possible).
4. The diagnostic and assessment procedures must correspond to the common practice (in compliance with the Italian Law: Gazzetta Ufficiale n.76 of – the 31/03/2008 AIFA – Determination 20 March 2008).

From this dissertation we clearly understand that observational studies guarantee a minor level of evidence. Therefore, are observational studies still necessary? Let us now see some examples both in medical and dental fields in order to answer this question.

10.4.2.1 Smoking

Can we perform a clinical controlled experimentation on active smoking subjecting two samples accurately selected and randomized to an intense and long-lasting exposure in order to estimate the pulmonary consequences?

It is clear that no study of this type could be performed since our ethics forbids it. How could we intentionally expose a patient to such risky and well-known carcinogenic factor?

For example, the studies linking smoking with lung cancer were bitterly criticized by "conventional" researchers who were not willing to accept evidence from studies where the exposure had not been randomized [74, 91].

10.4.2.2 Caries Lesions and *Mutans streptococci* Infection

Also, in dentistry, it seems difficult to be able, for example, to perform RCT on the correlation between caries and diet or daily habits; we cannot imagine a study in which a population is subjected to an intense and frequent carbohydrate daytime exposure and another population in which such exposure is simply absent, that is, ineffective from the caries point of view. Undoubtedly, we would worsen the oral health of the study group intentionally, obtaining outcomes not so different from those derived from longitudinal or retrospective observational studies [58].

It is therefore important to affirm that even if the reliability and the importance of RCTs as a model of research from a methodological point of view are undeniable, they are not universally applicable in medicine. Indeed this field requires a certain degree of flexibility in order to adapt to a myriad of not only biological, but also cultural and deontological variables, which are hardly compatible with such a rigid and unmodifiable method as RCTs.

Even though observational studies constitute a lower level of evidence for EBM purists, these studies should be promoted in surgery as a source of evidence along with the development of standards for meta-analyses of nonrandomized studies [107].

It has been shown that high-quality nonrandomized (observational) studies and high-quality RCTs can produce similar answers [8]. Despite the fact that clinical surgical research is mainly based on nonrandomized studies, there is no agreement on the methodological standards for such studies [28, 87].

Few attempts have been made to develop instruments allowing surgeons to evaluate published nonrandomized studies, and thus, quantify the strength of their results before applying their conclusions to "individual patients."

A systematic review [59] showed that study estimates of effectiveness may be valid in this case if confounding factors are controlled for, but a formal agreement on the standards of nonrandomized studies and meta-analyses of such studies is needed.

10.5 "Best Available Research Evidence" in the Field of Dentistry

EBD is an approach to oral health care that requires the judicious integration of systematic assessments of clinically relevant scientific evidence, relating to the patient's oral and medical condition and history, with the dentist's clinical expertise and the patient's treatment needs and preferences. EB care is now regarded as the "gold standard" in health care delivery worldwide [2].

But how can we reach this evidence in the dental arena?

Niederman [71] proposed in 1998 the following simple but simultaneously clear example:

"Professional or home bleaching can be a solution when aging is responsible for yellowed teeth."

- Problem: yellowed teeth due to aging...
- Procedure: ...professional bleaching...
- Comparison: ...or indicate a home bleaching...
- Result: ...to whiten teeth.

Once the problem has been defined, the solution must be searched in literature.

As already said, EBD is based on the information available online. As regards, there are some websites that deal with EBD. Among these, some databases can be used for retrieving information:

1. EviDents [48] is an EBD browser developed by the Forsyth Institute of Boston, in association with PubMed databases. This system is very practical since the clinician can formulate the problem and select the specific clinical field, the age range, Public Health studies, or Systematic reviews, to identify a solution. Furthermore, the clinician can focus his own research on diagnosis, Prognosis, treatment, and so on.
2. The US National Library of Medicine [65] allows an easier research thanks to RCT filters. The information is already selected and displays clinically relevant articles. PubMed is the most widely-used clinical basis worldwide. The website also offers a filter designed for the research of clinical study category, that is, systematic reviews [53].

3. The Cochrane Library: [104] Cochrane is an International Organization made of 50 staff groups (over 11,500 people) and dedicated to the systematic collection of research information on the effects of health care interventions in order to: (1) make this information rapidly and conveniently available to the largest number of people; (2) put this information in a more comprehensive perspective; and (3) carry out research on methodologies to improve systematic review. The Cochrane collaboration is committed: (1) to find the best way to make this information available; and (2) to do so in a way that helps those who have to make decision both for individuals and populations.

The Cochrane Library includes 3,625 systematic Cochrane revisions, and it is widely consulted all over the world, especially in English-speaking countries (Fig. 10.3). The Organization has officially created a group of study specialized in oral health in 1994 (managed by Prof. Shaw at Manchester University Hospital), which produces systematic reviews about diagnosis, prevention, and therapy of oral and maxillofacial diseases.

4. Best evidence [46].
5. Guidelines [105] where treatment protocols can be found.

There are also browsers specialized in meta-analysis:

1. Sum search [51]
2. TRIP (turning research into practice) database [54]

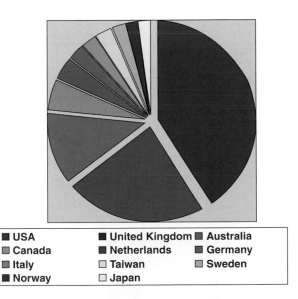

■ USA ■ United Kingdom ■ Australia
☐ Canada ■ Netherlands ■ Germany
☐ Italy ☐ Taiwan ☐ Sweden
■ Norway ☐ Japan

Fig. 10.3 Access on Cochrane database in 2008

3. EBM resources at Healthweb [47]
4. EBM metasite [50]

There are reviews that gather many studies considered relevant in terms of evidence.

• EBD [52]
• *Journal of EB dental practice*
• Peds critical care medicine [49]

The goal of all those websites is to produce and spread sound knowledge derived from gold standard research methodology that insures a high level of quantitative and qualitative clinical outcomes.

In developing appropriate treatment plans, dentists should combine the patient's treatment needs and preferences with the best available scientific evidence, in conjunction with the dentist's clinical expertise. To keep pace with other health professions in building a strong EB foundation, dentistry will require significant investments in clinical research and education to evaluate the best currently available evidence in dentistry and to identify new information needed to help dentists provide optimal care to patients [10].

10.5.1 How Evidence-Based Dentistry (EBD) Has Changed Clinical Practice

The American Dental Association defined EBD as an approach to oral health care that requires the judicious integration of systematic assessments of clinically relevant scientific evidence relating to patients' oral and medical condition and history, along with the dentists' clinical expertise and the patients' treatment needs and preferences [4].

Information derived from clinical trials is considered more reliable than information based on intuition, authority, or custom. There is a hierarchy when considering the levels of evidence (LOE). Systematic reviews of randomized controlled trials are considered to be at the highest level, whereas expert opinion is considered the lowest level of evidence [34]. This is only partially correct from our point of view.

Dentistry is a special field where the best evidence is not always applicable to the single patient. As the base of our work, we must align to protocols and guidelines for therapies and prognosis, but we also have to consider patient's preferences and values as well as costs and personal esthetic sense both for us and the patient.

This is important in order to prevent a phenomenon known as *physician-induced demand* [41, 70].

This may be exemplified by a case of a patient with four asymptomatic impacted third molars. Of the oral surgeons consulted, all of whom were working under a fee-for-service plan, 80% recommended the removal of all four teeth compared with 45% of general dentists working under a fee-for-service plan, and 27% of general dentists working under a capitation plan.

With the intention to turn over a new leaf, we go through the field of EBID and the decision itself has a great importance in everyday practice. A model for the factors influencing decisions in healthcare was described in 2000 by Chapman and Sonnenberg [17] and has been adapted to discuss decision-making in dentistry. The decision-making model describes two major components, the normative and the descriptive, which are involved in decision-making (Fig. 10.4).

The normative aspect of decision-making relies on quantitative information derived from systematic reviews and predictive models on the probabilities and uncertainties of treatment outcomes. Clinical outcomes, such as survival of a tooth or success of a restoration, are assessed on the basis of the utility they offer to the patient and their costs. Normative analyses

allow quantitative comparisons of alternative therapies and can identify optimal treatments for multiple attributes. The descriptive aspect in decision-making involves cognitive processes and biases of both providers and patients that translate the normative information into clinical action. Decision-making in health care occurs at three broad levels: the level of lawmakers and governmental regulators, the level of insurance plans that determine coverage and reimbursement for healthcare, and provider and patient's levels [34].

Thus, we enter in the field of EB practice. This term is defined as the conscientious, explicit, and judicious use of current best evidence in making decisions about the care of individual patients. It is currently defined as integration of best research evidence with clinical expertise and patient's needs.

This is the secret to obtain real answers. In our opinion best research evidence refers to clinically relevant research, especially from patient-centered clinical research. Clinical expertise is the ability to use clinical skills and experience to rapidly identify each patient's unique health state and diagnosis, individual risks and benefits of potential interventions, and personal values and expectations. Patient's values refer to unique preferences, concerns, and expectations that each patient brings to a clinical encounter and that must be integrated into clinical decisions if they are to serve the patient [37].

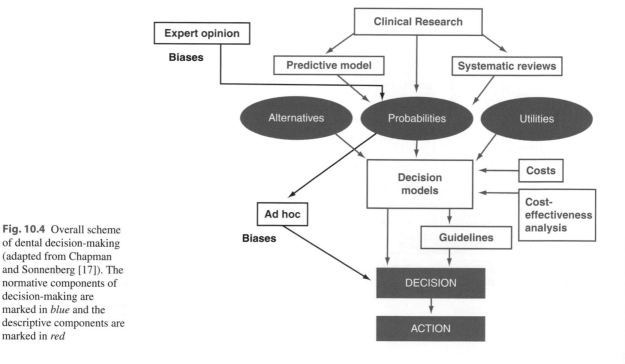

Fig. 10.4 Overall scheme of dental decision-making (adapted from Chapman and Sonnenberg [17]). The normative components of decision-making are marked in *blue* and the descriptive components are marked in *red*

The results of systematic reviews of databases referred to dental care have to be considered from this point of view.

10.6 Problems in Applying EBM to Surgery: Performing Surgical Procedure is Different from Administering Drugs

Even if EB movement has widely spread over the last years, some researchers do not agree to consider this scientific movement as entirely positive. As regard the fact that Holmes et al. compare EBM with fascism in their article is a clear demonstration. They affirm that EBM has had an evolution that corresponds to that of a microfascism: EBM has been colonized (territorialized) by an all-encompassing scientific research paradigm – that of postpositivism – but also and foremost in showing the process by which a dominant ideology comes to exclude alternative forms of knowledge, thereby acting as a *fascist* structure [43]. In fact, perhaps the comparison remains excessive since EBM has met considerable success in scientific research and literature. However, 96% of the articles do not satisfy the inclusion criteria of the EB research [95].

What is the meaning of this datum? Does it imply that only 4% of articles are significant because they are correctly executed? That 96% of studies conducted in medical research are not reliable?

Surgery (and dentistry) allows us to understand this methodological problem in the field of research and is always considered a qualitatively lower branch compared to medicine, for the humble origins of its tradition. Extraordinarily effective in its convenience, the ancestral art-surgery has always been limited to a subordinate role compared to medicine.

Also, while on the one hand, in all ancient civilizations the professional medical figure was represented by the noble priest, the astrologer, the philosopher or the esoteric magician, shaman, sorcerer, on the other hand, there was the surgeon. The latter belonged to some vulgar category even if he could treat some diseases and explain many of them. Many doctors do not like the idea of treating patients soiling one's hands (the word "surgery" comes from Greek words *cheir* (hand) and *ergon* (work), i.e., handiwork): a drug administration is more elegant than a surgical procedure. However, surgical procedures and drug administration are different.

What are these differences and how can they be associated with the EB method? Various articles in literature were run on this subject. In 1996, Horton compared surgical research to comic opera [44]. Experimental studies (RCTs or quasi-RCTs) that constitute the base of EBM are scarce in surgery even if surgeons are publishing them in increasing numbers [86]. In 1990 the surgical RCTs were the 7% of published articles, and most of them were retrospective or case series [89].

A more recent review showed that only 3.4% of all publications in the leading surgical journals are RCTs [101]. Thus, we have to affirm that surgical RCTs or meta-analysis remain scarce. Most available evidence in the field of surgery comes from "nonexperimental" studies (i.e., nonrandomized studies, case-control or cohort studies, and qualitative or narrative reviews, in contrast to quantitative reviews or meta-analyses), leading obviously to a lower level of evidence on the scale established in the original definition of EBM [85] (Fig. 10.5).

In addition, several studies according to multiple specialties were concordant to show that methodological issues such as the technique of randomization, unbiased assessment of endpoints, blinding, and prospective estimates of sample size were lacking in many trials [22, 38,93,102].

Because surgical intervention is not like a pill, surgical field has some difficulties that are unique.

Such difficulties related to RCTs in surgery are mainly the feasibility of randomization (ethical issues,

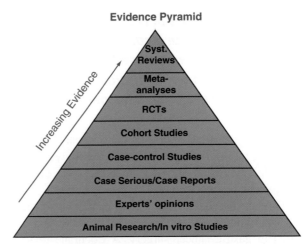

Fig. 10.5 Pyramid of evidence

emergency setting, palliative care), the learning curve, standardization of the procedure, and the problem of poor surgical performances and patients' and surgeons' equipoise [64].

Even though this problems could be overcome and more RCTs performed, 60% of surgical question could not be answered by an RCT [90].

In this view, we have to consider the difficulty based on clinical decision on RCT, most/above of all in the field of surgery. Most clinical decision in the "real world" remain based on clinical judgment and expertise, the results of nonrandomized studies, and even the influence of opinion leaders [106]. Randomized trials often include "reliable" hard data that can be used to interpret the results in a homogeneous population. In contrast, a "good clinician" uses other "soft" data that can be omitted in RCTs (severity of symptoms, severity of comorbidity, socioeconomic conditions) for clinical decisions about prognosis, diagnosis, or treatment. Such data are not always taken into account in EB practice guidelines [3].

In this view, we can affirm that nowadays, well-designed nonrandomized studies could be a good alternative to RCTs in such areas in which it is impossible to apply RCTs [85]. RCTs themselves must be improved developing education in clinical epidemiology, developing alternative methods of randomization, and encouraging whenever possible blinded observers, in particular in this field where the double blind is impossible to create.

Only in this way we can develop an EB surgery that will prove to be more than a passing fad [11].

10.6.1 An Example of Discrepancy Between Surgical Experience and Evidence-Based Review: Extension of Lymphadenectomy in Gastric Cancer Surgery

Up to now, EBM has appraised the surgical literature by taking into account the quality of the study design, while the quality of surgical procedures was largely overlooked.

This attitude has led to a failure, when extended (D2) and limited (D1) lymphadenectomies were compared in gastric cancer surgery. A Cochrane review [62, 63] concluded that "*randomized studies show no

evidence of overall survival benefit" after extended lymphadenectomy (D2), "*but possible benefit in T3 tumors. These results may be confounded by surgical learning curves and poor surgeon compliance.*"

These results were largely based on the Dutch [14, 15] and British [23, 24] clinical trials. These trials required great efforts and recruited a large number of patients, but, nevertheless, presented a rather low surgical quality, as outlined by the Cochrane reviewers themselves. Indeed, the trials were performed by surgeons without specialist training in extended lymphadenectomy, performing less than five interventions per year. The limited surgical experience yielded a very high postoperative mortality after extended lymphadenectomy (9.7% in the Dutch trial and 13.5% in the British trial), a high percentage of splenectomies (37 and 65%, respectively), and pancreatectomies (30 and 56%), and a low number of nodes retrieved (median of 17 nodes in the British trial).

In the Cochrane review, the Japanese literature was excluded for methodological reasons. As pointed out by two coauthors of the present chapter [26], this exclusion, although justified from a methodological point of view, hindered a lot the development of knowledge. Indeed, *at present the Japanese experience in gastric cancer is a kind of benchmark for surgeons throughout the world.* In Japan, the incidence of gastric cancer is particularly high, with about 100,000 new cases per year. Mortality after D2 dissection is less than 2% in the nationwide registry [35] and less than 1% in specialized institutions [81], and the median number of retrieved nodes is 54. In Japanese gastric cancer patients, overall 5-year survival has impressively increased during the last three decades, achieving the 74% [69], which is three-fourfolds higher than 5-year survival recorded in Italy in 1993-96 (20% in men and 23% in women) [6]. In European studies [14], Japanese surgeons are often invited to supervise surgical procedures. Indeed, *it is extremely difficult to ask Japanese surgeons, in whose series postoperative mortality is only 1–2%, to believe in randomized clinical trials, where postoperative mortality peaks to 10–14%, irrespectively of methodological quality of those studies* [98].

Unfortunately, while criteria to evaluate the quality of the study design (selection criteria, randomization, blindness, etc.) are well established, indexes of surgical quality have not been agreed upon [98]. To bridge this gap, some coauthors of the present chapter recently proposed the following indexes of surgical quality in gastric cancer surgery: number of retrieved nodes, avoidance of concomitant spleno-pancreasectomy, postoperative morbidity and mortality [98].

Meanwhile, the balance between D2 and D1 lymphadenectomy has changed in favor of D2. Indeed, a new randomized trial, performed in Taiwan [103], showed a mild but significant survival advantage after D2 with respect to D1; 5-year survival was 59.5 and 53.6%, respectively ($p = 0.041$). Moreover in the Dutch trial, 11-year survival was significantly higher after D2 than after D1 (39 vs. 31%), when excluding postoperative mortality [40].

A reevaluation of these trials was reported in a paper recently published in the New England Journal of Medicine, whose first author was Sasako, the Japanese surgeon who supervised the Dutch trial: *The excessive number of early deaths in these studies* (Dutch and British trial) *may have obscured any potential difference in long-term survival between patients undergoing D1 and D2 gastrectomy. The Dutch trial was conducted in 80 hospitals, including small community hospitals, by 11 surgeons who had little experience with D2 gastrectomy before the study. The limited experience of the surgeons made it difficult for them to learn how to perform the procedure safely and effectively, and the small volume of cases limited the ability of the hospitals to manage major surgical complications. By contrast, in a Taiwanese single-institution trial comparing D1 gastrectomy with D2 or more extensive gastrectomy, all the surgeons had performed at least 80 D2 procedures before participating in the study, and there were no deaths in either group* [82].

Hence, gastrectomy with D2 lymphadenectomy is the standard of care for advanced curable gastric cancer according to the Japanese Guideline [57].

10.6.2 Limitation of EBM in Dentistry and Oral Surgery

It is also important to bear in mind that dentistry does not often interact with ideal environments such as in scientific studies since it deals with reality and the patients' needs. It is also important to understand that the surgical and dental methodology can scarcely be adapted to randomized clinical researches. They have led to enormous benefits in medicine, have defined many lifesaving strategies, and corrected some important research mistakes [76].

Therefore, the parachute approach, as said before, can be the most suitable in situation of low resources, both in terms of money (poor setting situations, poor country health plans) and poorness of research data, which is a common problem in the field of surgery, oral surgery, and dentistry. First of all, we have to assert that randomized, double-blinded, and placebo-controlled trials are the only way not only to control the biased investigator, but also the placebo effects. Another source of bias in surgical trials is the blinding of patients and surgeons. Unfortunately, it is not always possible to blind all participants as effectively shown in the exemplary cited trial of Majeed et al. [60] where the same wound dressing was used for patients who underwent laparoscopic and small incision cholecystectomy. Especially, if the primary outcome criteria are not recurrence of disease or even death, but variable symptoms or quality of life measurements, a lack of blinding procedures may bias the results of these trials. This bias can be minimized by the assessment of the procedure outcome or by independent investigators. Furthermore, it remains difficult to standardize the tested surgical procedures: the latter continuously evolve and the complications decrease with the surgeons' improving skills. As such, the results vary with the individual surgeon because the participating operators vary in their surgical skill and experience. All participating surgeons should undergo appropriate training before the start of a randomized controlled trial to reach a certain minimum of standardization [13] (Fig. 10.6).

This example could explain how in all surgical fields it is very hard to base knowledge on data obtained through the Internet and databases (EBM methods) because of the complexity of this field where the result

Drugs	Surgical procedure
• Unchanging compound	• Evolves continuously
• Complications increase with use	• Complications decrease with use
• Results unrelated to physicians' skill	• Results vary with operator
• Crossover rare	• Crossover common
• Placebo usually available	• No placebo

Fig. 10.6 Differences between randomized trials for drugs and surgical procedures

is usually related with some emotional, individual, and uncountable aspects (such as experience, anxiety, technique preferences), which could anyway be involved in clinical outcome.

In such a specific field, both the surgeon's training and way of teaching are important. We think a strict collaboration between old surgeons and young surgeons could be useful. Richards' study enhances the introduction of this concept: he thought that the learning process must be considered separately for knowledge, critical appraisal skills, attitudes, and behavior. He considered two types of teaching models for assessing learning achievement: stand-alone teaching and clinical integrated teaching. His study showed that stand-alone teaching improved knowledge but not skills, attitudes, or behavior, while clinically integrated teaching improved knowledge, skills, attitudes, and behavior [77].

This study confirms that teaching of EBM should be moved from classrooms to clinical practice to achieve improvements in research and clinical outcomes.

10.7 Combining EBM with Clinical Expertise: The GRADE System

The limits of EBM in medical and surgical fields have led in the last few years to a step forward in methodological and statistical research.

In fact, the results derived from published RCTs are not anymore sufficient to produce knowledge mainly in the field of surgery that, as we have seen, suffers from an impossibility of results' standardization due to the dependence on the single surgeon's skill.

Statisticians and researchers have tried to overcome this issue constructing a new method with the aim of integrating expert's opinion, based on their long-lasting experience, with the accumulating data coming from RCTs on well-defined topics .

Here, experts (researchers, clinicians with experience, fame, and international credibility) are called to express themselves about focal point in terms of treatments or prognostic indexes and they have to produce *consensus report* answering the following questions:

1. Is the systematic review is exhaustive and precise?
2. Does new information appeared after the end of the preparation work exist?

3. Are interpretation and conclusion of reviewers shareable?
4. What researches are still needed in the field studied?
5. Are outcomes of systematic review useful for patients' treatment?

In particular, the answer to point five gives the idea of the practical utility of the results of the studies based on the level of evidence defined as follows by *U.S. Preventive Service Task Force* :

(a) Strong: studies of level I
(b) Moderate: studies of level II-1 or II-2 or extrapolation from level II-1
(c) Limited: studies of level II-3 or extrapolation from level II-1 or II-2
(d) Incomplete or insufficient: Not consistent or not conclusive studies of any levels, anecdotic evidence or level II

We would prefer just to cite exactly what is reported in the website of the GRADE collaboration..Hence, this part should be shortened, as follows. A group was created in the year 2000 *as an informal collaboration of experts with the aim of challenging the lack of the actual classification system in the sense of sanitary assistance addressing the shortcomings of present grading system in healthcare* (http://www.gradeworkinggroup.org) Therefore, in the last decade a new system to derive clinical recommendations from available scientific literature has been developed, by taking into account both scientific evidence and experts' opinion. This system is named GRADE, an acronym for Grading of Recommendations, Assessment, Development and Evaluation, and involves guideline developers, methodologists, and clinicians all over the world.

The GRADE system is based on the sequential assessment of:

1. Quality of evidence
2. Balance between benefits vs. risks, burden, and cost
3. Development and grading of a management recommendations

So the GRADE system utilizes both EBM and "experts" opinion.

This system has the main aim to overcome the classical limits of EB movement by integrating the information derived from studies with optimal statistical quality with experts' opinion that can add new experiences. In Fig. 10.5 is shown the pyramid of EBM modified according to the GRADE system. It is composed by LOE according to the study designs and critical appraisal of prevention, diagnosis, prognosis, therapy, and harm studies:

- Level A: Consistent Randomized Controlled Clinical Trial, cohort study, all or none, clinical decision rule validated in different populations.
- Level B: Consistent Retrospective Cohort, Exploratory Cohort, Ecological Study, Outcomes Research, case-control study; or extrapolations from level A studies.
- Level C: Case-series study or extrapolations from level B studies.
- Level D: Expert opinion without explicit critical appraisal, or based on physiology, bench research, or first principles.

The pyramid of EBM modified according to the GRADE System is slightly different from EBM classical pyramid (Fig. 10.7). In fact, even if the general superiority of experimental studies over observational studies is recognized, it is possible that an observational study is evaluated at a higher level, while on the contrary an experimental study is downgraded to a lower level.

Delphi process and Nominal (Expert) Group techniques are usually utilized for the organization of the work done by the experts group in order to draw conclusions able to add and produce new scientific knowledge.

The Delphi method was first developed at the RAND Institute as an alternative to the creation of complex computer models of the effects of Soviet weapons systems [96] than was used for the first time in medicine in the 1970s with some articles on this issue [18, 66].

The Delphi "method" helps to find solutions to complex problems by increasing the communication inside a group (or Panel), and on the same time, by limiting the power of each single individual. Participants to the Delphi panel are stimulated to produce new ideas which they consider more suitable to solve a given problem and these ideas are subsequently diffused among participants to the panel, so they can reconsider individually their ideas, without being obliged to rediscuss them in front of the group.

The reproposal of strategies that were suggested by the panelists continues until shared opinions are reached. So it is easier to reach a form of consensus on one or more issues to a given problem, and more importantly, this technique avoids the possibility that someone prevails simply because of its personality. Furthermore, this Delphi "process" helps to find solutions to difficult questions, also increasing the communication inside a group while contemporary limiting the influence power of single researchers. The ultimate aim of this technique is to obtain and summarize the opinions of more experts on a given debatable question.

In this Delphi technique, the members of the group communicate by mail, E-Mail, or phone.

In the Nominal (Expert) Group techniques, the members of the group join together but anonymous notes or similar systems are utilized.

In both cases in the first part of evaluation, the anonymity is guaranteed. Then, with the help of a coordinator, the opinion of the whole group is summarized by expressing the grade of concordance in a numerical way.

The main phases of Delphi process and nominal technique are as follows:

(a) A question is formulated (or a list of questions).
(b) Members gave an opinion without telling each other. The judgment may be: "agreement, disagreement, indifferent"; a priority order and a score system are to be assigned.
(c) The coordinator collects and syntheses the expressed ideas and informs the members of the group, also giving the score of the entire group and individual score in an anonymous way.
(d) Subsequently, there is a discussion (direct or indirect via mail) where the members of the group give an overall judgment.

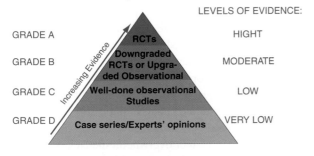

Evidence Pyramid modified

Fig. 10.7 The pyramid of EBM modified according to the GRADE system

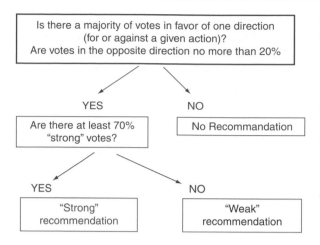

Fig. 10.8 Algorithm of the GRADE system

(e) The members of the group give a further opinion.

(f) The group rediscusses the different opinions and tries to arrive at an agreement. Eventual disagreement points are specified.

Therefore, the GRADE system utilizes either the EBM approach or the opinion of experts given by a democratic approach, for example, utilizing the "Delphi technique." The data accrued by this methodology can be synthesized with a recommendation graded as "strong" or "weak" depending on the cut-off arbitrarily set at 70% (Fig. 10.8).

GRADE is based on a well-defined stepwise process:

- The quality of evidence is classified as high, moderate, low, and very low, according to factors that include the study methodology, the consistency and precision of the results, and directness of the evidence.

- Recommendations are developed which can be either strong ("we recommend") or weak ("we suggest"), according to the balance of the benefits and downsides (harms, burden, and cost) after considering the quality of evidence.

"Strong recommendation" defines a decision that *most well-informed patients would accept. Weak recommendation indicates a decision generally not shared from the panel, which means that a majority of well-informed patients would accept it but a substantial proportion would not. Clinicians should consider its use according to particular circumstances.*

Furthermore, a "strong" recommendation cannot or should not be followed for an individual patient because

of that patient's preferences or clinical characteristics, which make the recommendation less applicable.

Thus, the GRADE system has several advantages:

1. The quality of evidence is graded with a transparent and rigorous methodology.
2. Benefits and harms of health care interventions are explicitly balanced.
3. Evaluation of the quality of evidence is separated from definition of the strength of the recommendation.
4. This separation allows to explicitly recognize that values and preferences, as well as clinical and social circumstances, play an important role in formulating practice recommendations.

The merit of GRADE is that it does not eliminate judgments or disagreements about evidence and recommendations, but rather makes them transparent. Moreover, it combines methodological rigor with interdisciplinary interspecialty participation.

The integration of data from systematic reviews and RCTs correctly set up and running with the opinion of experts that assess the same results seems to be the best technique to produce the most reliable and predictable knowledge in medical and surgical field with regard to diagnosis, prognosis, and treatment.

The system has been adopted by many health organizations and medical societies, including the World Health Organization, the American College of Physicians, the British Medical Journal, the National Institute for Clinical Excellence, the American Thoracic Society [83], and the Endocrine Society [92]. Moreover, it has been employed to develop guidelines in the field of allergy and asthma [16] and for the management of the following disorders: severe sepsis and septic shock [27], thyroid dysfunction during pregnancy and postpartum [1], hypoglycaemic disorders [21], corticosteroid insufficiency in critically ill adults [61], and nasal congestion [97].

Moreover, the GRADE system has been used to evaluate symptomatic slow-acting drugs in osteoarthritis [73], brachytherapy in cervix cancer [99], and indications for labor induction [68], and to investigate misdiagnosis in primary care [72] and define gastroesophageal reflux in the pediatric population [84].

Of course also an advanced methodology as the GRADE system cannot overwhelm the lack of studies with strong design and large sample size to produce reliable results [80].

Our experience of this practice is not widespread yet in the dental field; according to our experience, the limited number of these studies in literature is the perfect demonstration. A common effort to bring this useful method in the field of dentistry and oral surgery will certainly be needed in the future. It is hard to retrieve results derived from important studies in terms of number of patients and quality of clinical outcomes because it all depends on the operator.

Positive outcomes will be reached only through the experience of few experts able to manage training and clinical practice for the many.

10.8 Conclusions

We give evidences, you take clinical decisions
Presentation clinical evidence, Italian version [45]

The last 30 years have witnessed large oscillations in the methods to produce and convey clinical knowledge that we have called "Pendulum of knowledge" (Fig. 10.9).

We have gone from the era of Experts' opinion/Authority's Principle to the era of EBM and are now entering a new age where the two approaches are substantially mixed up through the GRADE system.

In the 1970s, clinical knowledge mainly resided in the brain of clinical experts, who had devoted their life to the care of individual patients. They had mainly learnt from their bedside experience under the guidance of their teachers, and likewise, passed their knowledge to their pupils using both verbal and nonverbal communications.

In that period exchanges between clinicians and researchers were limited, clinical knowledge was condensed in large textbooks, and there were linguistic barriers between countries. The progress in disease diagnosis and treatment was rather slow.

With the advent of English as an international "Esperanto" and World Wide Web, international communications have been magnified and the speed of clinical progress has incredibly increased, as witnessed by the sprout of thousands of specialized medical journals.

In the 1990s, there has been a useful reaction to the overpower of experts' opinion. EBM tried to base clinical practice on clear-cut evidence coming from clinical experiments (randomized clinical trials) and systematic observations. An effort was made to replace personal impressions with rigorous measurements, sparse observations with systematic collections of series, and observational studies with RCTs whenever feasible. This approach has further magnified the progress in medicine.

In the first decade of the third millennium, a new approach has appeared and gradually taken over, the GRADE system. EBM is still fundamental, but experts' opinion has been reevaluated.

To lead dentistry in the third millennium, it is necessary to take advantage of the rigorous methods produced by

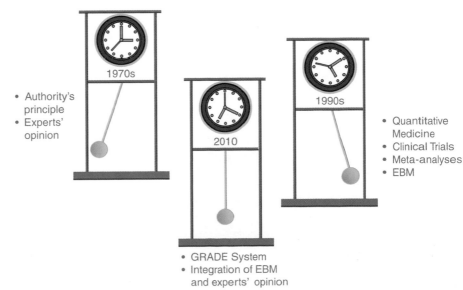

Evolution of Research Methodology

Fig. 10.9 "The Pendulum of knowledge"

EBM, especially when planning and evaluating research studies. However, it is impossible to produce sound knowledge without simultaneously considering clinical expertise and quality of surgical procedures.

In the last 5 years in the field of oral surgery, we have seen, perhaps for the first time in dental research, a new method involved in the design and operating procedure in implantology surgery.

The technology of CAD-CAM (computer aided design-computer aided manufacturing) applied to surgery led to the creation of a software (Nobel Biocare, Procera System, Gotheborg) capable of running the so-called computer-assisted surgery, which allows not only to three-dimensionally appreciate local anatomy and identify noble structures, but also to design and create a surgical template that will guide the insertion of implants. During the surgical procedure this template will provide information on angle, direction, depth of insertion, and distance from noble structures of the implant itself. This technology enables the standardization of surgical quality and the leveling of surgical skills for the first time, as it can be used by both skilled and novice operators. The possibility that surgical errors can be transferred to design phase on the computer must be kept in mind (Figs. 10.10–10.12).

This new technology can be useful during the study of implantology as it enables the achievement of the standardization of surgical quality criteria. Indeed, while in most trials where a new surgical technique is tested, the operator's hand remains a critical factor that can greatly influence the outcome, this new technique levels various manual skills and provide a unique opportunity to evaluate surgical techniques, without the confounding effect of different operators' expertise and training.

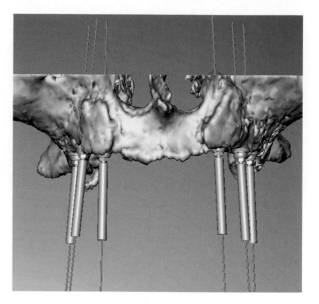

Fig. 10.11 3-D view derived from "Procera system," Nobel Biocare (with permission from Nobel Biocare AB, Agrate, Italy)

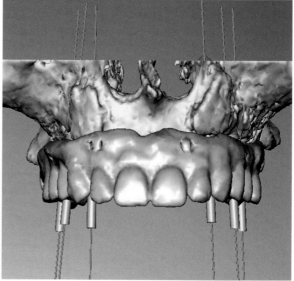

Fig. 10.12 3-D view derived from "Procera system," Nobel Biocare (with permission from Nobel Biocare AB, Agrate, Italy)

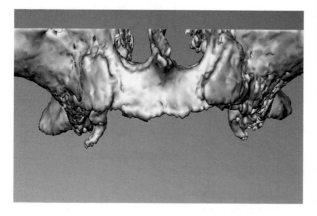

Fig. 10.10 3-D view derived from "Procera system," Nobel Biocare (with permission of Nobel Biocare AB, Agrate, Italy)

However, this technique is not yet widespread and we think it will help research in oral surgery from a methodological point of view by providing objectivity, which is still lacking. This is just an example, but it can help us understand the methodological backwardness of surgical research, for reasons that are intrinsic to the same subject; however, huge efforts have been made to improve the objectivity in assessing clinical results.

Then we can finally say that while criteria aimed to evaluate the quality of the study design (selection criteria, randomization, blindness, etc.) are well established, indexes of surgical quality have not been agreed upon. It would be extremely useful to establish, at an international level, quality criteria for any kind of surgery, including dentistry and oral surgery. Such indexes are urgently needed and their development should primarily involve dentists and oral surgeons, as well as other clinicians, statisticians, and patients' associations.

References

1. Abalovich M, Amino N, Barbour LA, Cobin RH, De Groot LJ, Glinoer D, Mandel SJ, Stagnaro-Green A (2007) Management of thyroid dysfunction during pregnancy and postpartum: an endocrine society clinical practice guideline. J Clin Endocrinol Metab 92(8):S1–S7
2. Adeyemo WL, Akinwande JA, Bamgbose BO (2007) Evidence-based dental practice: part I. Formulating clinical questions and searching for answers. Nig Q J Hosp Med 17(2):58–62
3. Aldrich R, Kemp L, Stewart Williams J et al (2003) Using socioeconomic evidence in clinical practice guidelines. BMJ 327:1283–1285
4. American Dental Association (2008) Evidence-based dentistry: glossary of terms. American Dental Association, Chicago, IL
5. Deshpande A, Jadad AR (2008) The impact of polyol-containing chewing gums on dental caries: a systematic review of original randomized controlled trials and observational studies. J Am Dent Assoc 139:1602–1614
6. Associazione Italiana Registri Tumori. http:// www.registri-tumori.it
7. Atkins D, Best D, Briss PA et al (2004) Grading quality of evidence and strength of recommendations. BMJ 328(7454):1490
8. Barton S (2000) Which clinical studies provide the best evidence? BMJ 321:255–256
9. Batchelor PA, Sheiham A (2006) The distribution of burden of dental caries in schoolchildren: a critique of the high risk caries prevention strategy for populations. BMC Oral Health 6(1):3
10. Bauer J, Chiappelli F, Spackman S, Prolo P, Stevenson R (2006) Evidence-based dentistry: fundamentals for the dentist. J Calif Dent Assoc 34(6):427–432
11. Black N (1999) Evidence-based surgery: a passing fad? World J Surg 23:789–793
12. Bobbio M, Demichelis B, Giustetto G (1994) Completeness of reporting trial results – effect on physicians willingness to prescribe. Lancet 343(8907):1209–1211
13. Bonchek LI (1997) Randomised trials of new procedures: problems and pitfalls. Heart 78:535–536
14. Bonenkamp JJ, Hermans J, Sasako M, van de Velde CJH, The Dutch Gastric Cancer Group (1999) Extended lymph node dissection for gastric cancer. New Engl J Med 340:908–914
15. Bonenkamp JJ, Songun I, Hermans J, Sasako M, Wevaart K, Plukker JTM, van Elk P, Obertop H, Gouma DJ, Taat CW, van Lanschot J, Meyer S, de Graaf PW, von Meyenfieldt MF, Tilanus H, van de Velde CJH (1995) Randomised comparison of morbidity after D1 and D2 dissection for gastric cancer in 996 Dutch patients. Lancet 345:745–748
16. Brozek JL, Akl EA, Alonso-Coello P, Lang D, Jaeschke R, Williams JW, Phillips B, Lelgemann M, Lethaby A, Bousquet J, Guyatt GH, Schuenemann HJ, The GRADE Working Group (2009) Grading quality of evidence and strength of recommendations in clinical practice guidelines. Allergy 64(5):669–677
17. Chapman GB, Sonnenberg FA (2000) Introduction. In: Chapman GB, Sonnenberg FA (eds) Decision making in healthcare: theory, psychology and application. Cambridge University, Cambridge, p 19
18. Clark LH, Cochran SW (1972) Needs of older Americans assessed by Delphi procedures. J Gerontol 27:275–278
19. Committee on the Use of Complementary and Alternative Medicine by the American Public (2005) The National Academies Press, Washington DC, 2005 Complementary and Alternative Medicine in the United States. National Academies Press
20. Craig Brater D, Daly WJ (2000) Clinical pharmacology in the middle ages: principles that presage the 21st century. Clin Pharmacol Ther 67(5):447–450
21. Cryer PE, Axelrod L, Grossman AB, Heller SR, Montori VM, Seaquist ER, Service FJ; Endocrine Society (2009) Evaluation and management of adult hypoglycemic disorders: an Endocrine Society Clinical Practice Guideline. J Clin Endocrinol Metab 94:709–728
22. Curry JI, Reeves B, Stringer MD (2003) Randomized controlled trials in pediatric surgery: could we do better? J Pediatr Surg 38:556–559
23. Cuschieri A, Weeden S, Fielding J, Bancewicz J, Craven J, Joypaul V, Sydes M, Fayers P, The Surgical Co-operative Group (1999) Patients survival after D1 and D2 resections for gastric cancer: long term results of the MRC surgical trial. Br J Cancer 79:1522–1530
24. Cuschieri A, Fayers P, Fielding J, Craven J, Bancewicz J, Joypaul V, Cook P (1996) Postoperative morbidity and mortality after D1 and D2 resections for gastric cancer: preliminary results of the MRC randomised controlled surgical trial. Lancet 347:995–999
25. Daly WJ, Craig Brater D (2000) Medieval contributions to the search for truth in clinical medicine. Perspect Biol Med 43(4):530–540
26. De Manzoni G, Verlato G (2005) Gastrectomy with extended lymphadenectomy for primary treatment of gastric cancer (letter). Br J Surg 92(6):784
27. Dellinger Phillip R, Levy Mitchell M, Carlet Jean M, Bion J, Parker MM, Jaeschke R, Reinhart K, Angus DC, Brun-Buisson C, Beale R, Calandra T, Dhainaut JF, Gerlach H, Harvey M, Marini JJ, Marshall J, Ranieri M, Ramsay G, Sevransky J, Thompson Taylor B, Townsend S, Vender JS, Zimmerman JL, Vincent JL (2008) Surviving Sepsis Campaign: International guidelines for management of severe sepsis and septic shock: 2008. Crit Care Med 36(1):296–327

28. Downs SH, Black N (1998) The feasibility of creating a checklist for the assessment of the methodological quality both of randomized and non-randomized studies of health care interventions. J Epidemiol Community Health 52:377–384

29. Eddy DM (1990) Practice policies: where do they come from? JAMA 263(9):1265, 1269, 1272

30. Eddy DM (2005) Evidence-based medicine: a unified approach. Health Affairs (Project Hope) 24(1):9–17

31. Monico EP, Moore CL, Calise (2005) The impact of Evidence-Based Medicine and evolving technology on the standard of care in Emergency Medicine. *The Internet Journal of Law, Healthcare and Ethics* Volume 3(2)

32. Elstein AS (2004) On the origins and development of evidence-based medicine and medical decision making. Inflamm Res 53(Suppl 2):S184–S189

33. Ezzo J, Bausell B, Moerman DE, Berman B, Hadhazy V (2001) Reviewing the reviews. How strong is the evidence? How clear are the conclusions? Int J Technol Assess Health Care 17(4):457–466

34. Flemmig TF, Beikler T (2009). Decision making in implant dentistry: an evidence-based and decision-analysis approach. Periodontol 2000 50:154-172

35. Fujii M, Sasaki J, Nakajima T (1999) State of the art in the treatment of gastric cancer: from the 71st Japanese Gastric Cancer Congress. Gastric Cancer 2:151–157

36. Gillette J, Matthews JD, Frantsve-Hawley J, Weyant RJ (2009) The benefits of evidence-based dentistry for the private dental office. Dent Clin North Am 53(1):33–45

37. (2005) Glossary of evidence-based terms. J Evid Based Dent 5(1):61–65

38. Grimes DA, Schulz KF (1996) Methodology citations and the quality of randomized controlled trials in obstetrics and gynecology. Am J Obstet Gynecol 174:1312–1315

39. Guyatt G, Cairns J, Churchill D et al (1992) Evidence-Based Medicine Working Group. Evidence-based medicine. A new approach to teaching the practice of medicine. JAMA 268:2420–2425

40. Hartgrink HH, van de Velde CJH, Putter H, Bonenkamp JJ, Kranenbarg EK, Songun I, Welvaart K, van Krieken JHJM, Meijer S, Plukker JTM, van Elk PJ, Obertop H, Gouma DJ, van Lanschot JJB, Taat CW, de Graaf PW, von Meyenfeldt MF, Tilanus H, Sasako M (2004) Extended lymph node dissection for gastric cancer: who may benefit? Final results of the randomized Dutch Gastric Cancer Group trial. J Clin Oncol 22:2041–2042

41. Hazelkorn HM, Macek MD (1994) Perception of the need for removal of impacted third molars by general dentists and oral and maxillofacial surgeons. J Oral Maxillofac Surg 52:681–686; discussion 686–687

42. Healthy People: 2010 (2008) www.healthypeople.gov/. Accessed 17 Sep 2008

43. Holmes D et al (2006) Deconstructing the evidence-based discourse in health sciences: truth, power and fascism. Int J Evid Based Health Care 4:180–186

44. Horton R (1996) Surgical research or comic opera: questions but few answers. Lancet 347:984

45. http://aifa.clinev.it/presentazione.php

46. http://ebm.bmj.com

47. http://healthweb.org/browse.cfm?subjectid=39

48. http://medinformatics.uthscsa.edu/EviDents

49. http://PedsCCM.wustl.edu/EBJournal_club.html

50. http://ray.leung.net/

51. http://sumsearch.uthscsa.edu/searchform4.htm

52. http://www.nature.com/ebd/index.html

53. http://www.ncbi.nlm.nih.gov:80/entrez/query/static/clinical.html

54. http://www.tripdatabase.com/

55. EMEA (European Medicines Agency) (1998) ICH Topic E 8, General Considerations for Clinical Trials, http://www.emea.eu.int, EMEA March 1998

56. Jadad AR, Moore RA, Carroll D et al (1996) Assessing the quality of reports of randomized clinical trials: is blinding necessary? Control Clin Trials 17(1):1–12

57. Japanese Gastric Cancer Association (2004) Gastric cancer treatment guideline, 2nd edn. Kanehara, Tokyo

58. Law V, Seow WK (2006) A longitudinal controlled study of factors associated with mutans streptococci infection and caries lesion initiation in children 21 to 72 months old. Pediatr Dent 28(1):58–65

59. MacLehose RR, Reeves BC, Harvey IM et al (2000) A systematic review of comparisons of effect sizes derived from randomized and nonrandomized studies. Health Technol Assess 4:1–154

60. Majeed AW, Troy G, Nicholl JP, Smythe A, Reed MW, Stoddard CJ, Peacock J, Johnson AG (1996) Randomised, prospective, single-blind comparison of laparoscopic versus small-incision cholecystectomy. Lancet 347:989–994

61. Marik PE, Pastores SM, Annane D, Meduri GU, Sprung CL, Arlt W, Keh D, Briegel J, Beishuizen A, Dimopoulou I, Tsagarakis S, Singer M, Chrousos GP, Zaloga G, Bokhari F, Vogeser M (2008) Recommendations for the diagnosis and management of corticosteroid insufficiency in critically ill adult patients: consensus statements from an international task force by the American College of Critical Care Medicine. Crit Care Med 36(6):1937–1949

62. McCulloch P, Niita ME, Kazi H, Gama-Rodrigues JJ (2005) Gastrectomy with extended lymphadenectomy for primary treatment of gastric cancer. Br J Surg 92:5–13

63. McCulloch P, Nita ME, Kazi H, Gama-Rodrigues J (2003) Extended versus limited lymph nodes dissection technique for adenocarcinoma of the stomach (Cochrane Review). In: The Cochrane Library, Issue 4. Wiley, Chichester, UK

64. McCulloch P, Taylor I, Sasako M et al (2002) Randomised trials in surgery: problems and possible solutions. BMJ 324:1448–1451

65. MEDLINE: www.ncbi.nlm.nih.gov/PubMed

66. Milholland A, Wheeler SG, Heieck JJ (1973) Medical assessment by a Delphi group opinion technique. N Engl J Med 188:1272–1275

67. Montori VM, Guyatt GH (2001) What is evidence-based medicine and why should it be practiced? Respir Care 46(11):1201–1211

68. Mozurkewich E, Chilimigras J, Koepke E, Keeton K, King VJ (2009) Indications for induction of labour: a best-evidence review. BJOG Int J Obstet Gynaecol 116(5):626–636

69. Nakajima T (2002) Gastric cancer treatment guidelines. Gastric Cancer 5:1–5

70. Nguyen NX, Derrick FW (1997) Physician behavioral response to a Medicare price reduction. Health Serv Res 32:283–298

71. Niederman R (1998) Evidence-based dentistry: what it is, and what does it have to do with practice? The methods of evidence-based dentistry. Quintessence Int 12:811–817

72. Olga K, Delaney Brendan C, Munro Craig W (2008) Diagnostic difficulty and error in primary care – a systematic review. Fam Pract 25(6):400–413

73. Olivier B, Nansa B, Delmas Pierre D, Rene R, Cyrus C, Jean-Yves R (2008) Evaluation of symptomatic slow-acting drugs in osteoarthritis using the GRADE system. BMC Musculoskelet Disord 9:165

74. Pearce N (2008) Point-counterpoint. Corporate influences on epidemiology Int J Epidemiol 37:46–53

75. Petersen PE (2003) The World Oral Health Report 2003: continuous improvement of oral health in the 21st century – the approach of the WHO Global Oral Health Programme. World Health Organization, Geneva

76. Potts M (2006) Parachute approach to evidence based medicine. BMJ 333:701–703

77. Richards D (2005) Integrating evidence-based teaching into clinical practice should improve outcomes. Evid Based Dent 6(2):47

78. Rossouw JE, Anderson GL, Rl P et al (2002) Risks and benefits of estrogen plus progestin in healthy postmenopausal women – principal results from the Women's Health Initiative randomized controlled trial. JAMA 288: 321–333

79. Sackett DL, Rosenberg WM, Gray JA, Haynes RB, Richardson WS (1996) Evidence based medicine: what it is and what it isn't. BMJ 312(7023):71–72

80. Salluh JI, Povoa P, Soares M, Castro-Faria-Neto HC, Bozza FA, Bozza PT (2008) The role of corticosteroids in severe community-acquired pneumonia: a systematic review. Crit Care 12(3):R76

81. Sano T, Sasako M, Yamamoto S, Nashimoto A, Kurita A, Hiratsuka M, Tsujinaka T, Kinoshita T, Arai K, Yamamura Y, Okajima K (2004) Gastric Cancer Surgery: morbidity and mortality results from a prospective randomized controlled trial comparing D2 and extended para-aortic lymphadenectomy – Japan Clinical Oncology Group Study 9501. J Clin Oncol 22:2767–2773

82. Sasako M, Sano T, Yamamoto S, Japan Clinical Oncology Group et al (2008) D2 lymphadenectomy alone or with para-aortic nodal dissection for gastric cancer. N Engl J Med 359(5):453–462

83. Schuenemann HJ, Jaeschke R, Cook DJ, Bria WF, El-Solh AA, Ernst A, Fahy BF, Gould MK, Horan KL, Krishnan JA, Manthous CA, Maurer JR, McNicholas WT, Oxman AD, Rubenfeld G, Turino GM, Guyatt G, The Group Authors Development AD (2006) An official ATS statement: grading the quality of evidence and strength of recommendations in ATS guidelines and recommendations. Am J Respir Crit Care Med 174(5):605–614

84. Sherman PM, Hassall E, Fagundes-Neto U, Gold BD, Kato S, Koletzko S, Orenstein S, Rudolph C, Vakil N, Vandenplas Y (2009) A global, evidence-based consensus on the definition of gastroesophageal reflux disease in the pediatric population. Am J Gastroenterol 104(5):1278–1295

85. Slim K (2005) Limits of evidence-based surgery. World J Surg 29:606–609

86. Slim K, Haugh M, Fagniez PL et al (2000) Ten-year audit of randomized trials in digestive surgery from Europe. Br J Surg 87:1472–1473

87. Slim K, Nini E, Forestier D et al (2003) Methodological index for nonrandomized studies (MINORS): development and validation of a new instrument. Aust N Z J Surg 73:712–716

88. Smith GC, Pell JP (2003) Parachute use to prevent death and major trauma related to gravitational challenge: systematic review of randomized controlled trials. BMJ 327: 1459–1461

89. Solomon MJ, McLeod RS (1993) Clinical studies in surgical journals: have we improved? Dis Colon Rectum 36:43–44

90. Solomon MJ, McLeod RS (1995) Should we be performing more randomized controlled trials evaluating surgical operations? Surgery 118:459–467

91. Stolley PD (1991) When genius errs: Fisher, R.A. and the lung cancer controversy. Am J Epidemiol 133:416–425

92. Swiglo BA, Murad MH, Schuenemann HJ, Kunz R, Vigersky RA, Guyatt GH, Montori VM (2008) A case for clarity, consistency, and helpfulness: state-of-the-art clinical practice guidelines in endocrinology using the grading of recommendations, assessment, development, and evaluation system. J Clin Endocrinol Metab 93(3):666–673

93. Thakur A, Wang EC, Chiu TT et al (2001) Methodology standards associated with quality reporting in clinical studies in pediatric surgery journals. J Pediatr Surg 36: 1160–1164

94. Thomas MV, Straus SE (2009) Evidence-based dentistry and the concept of harm. Dent Clin North Am 53(1):23–32

95. Traynor M (2002) The oil crisis, risk and evidence-based practice. Nurs Inq 9:162–169

96. Turoff M, Linstone HA (eds) (1975) The Delphi method techniques and applications. Addison-Wesley, Reading, MA

97. van Spronsen E, Ingels KJAO, Jansen AH, Graamans K, Fokkens WJ (2008) Evidence-based recommendations regarding the differential diagnosis and assessment of nasal congestion: using the new GRADE system. Allergy 63(7): 820–833

98. Verlato G, Roviello F, Marchet A, Giacopuzzi S, Marrelli D, Nitti D, de Manzoni G (2009) Indexes of surgical quality in gastric cancer surgery: experience of an Italian network. Ann Surg Oncol 16(3):594–602

99. Viani GA, Manta GB, Sefano EJ, de Fendi LI (2009) Brachytherapy for cervix cancer: low-dose rate or high-dose rate brachytherapy – a meta-analysis of clinical trials. J Exp Clin Cancer Res 28:47

100. Montori VM, Guyatt GH (2008) Progress in evidence-based medicine. JAMA 300(15):1814–1816

101. Wente MN, Seiler CM, Uhl W et al (2003) Perspectives of evidence-based surgery. Dig Surg 20:263–269

102. Wiebe S (2003) Randomized controlled trials of epilepsy surgery. Epilepsia 44(Suppl 17):38–43

103. Wu CW, Hsiung CA, Lo SS, Hsieh MC, Chen JH, Li AFY, Lui WY, Whang-Peng J (2006) Nodal dissection for patients with gastric cancer: a randomised controlled trial. Lancet Oncol 7(4):309–315

104. www.cochrane.org

105. www.guidelines.gov

106. Young JM, Hollands MJ, Ward J et al (2003) Role of opinion leaders in promoting evidence-based surgery. Arch Surg 138:785–791

107. Young JM, Solomon MJ (2003) Improving the evidence-base in surgery: evaluating surgical effectiveness. Aust N Z J Surg 73:507–510

108. Zielinski W, Goldstein M, König U (2001) Evidence-based medicine in internal guideline development in a general hospital--the Park-Clinic EbM-Project. Z Arztl Fortbild Qualitatssich 95:413-417

Evidence-Based Decision for Pharmacological Management of Alcoholic Liver Disease and Alcohol Dependence

Francesco Giuseppe Foschi, Fabio Caputo, Anna Chiara Dall'Aglio, Giorgio Zoli, Mauro Bernardi, Francesco Chiappellli, and Giuseppe Francesco Stefanini

Core Message

> ❭ It is important to note that the treatment modalities for alcoholic steato-hepatitis (ASH), acute alcoholic hepatitis (AAH), and alcoholic liver cirrhosis are insufficient. In particular, AAH is associated with a high mortality; glucocorticosteroids appear to be effective in patients with severe AAH, even though recent meta-analyses suggest that there is insufficient evidence to recommend or refute this therapy.

F.G. Foschi (✉)
A.C. Dall'Aglio
G.F. Stefanini
Dipartimento di Medicina Interna, Ospedale per gli Infermi,
Viale Stradone 9, 48018 Faenza, RA, Italy
e-mail: fg.foschi@ausl.ra.it
e-mail: chiaradall@gmail.com
e-mail: gf.stefanini@ausl.ra.it

F. Caputo
G. Zoli
Dipartimento di Med. Interna, Ospedale S. Annunziata
Vicini 2, 44042, Cento, FE, Italy
e-mail: f.caputo@dusl.fe.it
e-mail: g.tdi@ausl.fe.it

M. Bernardi
Dipartimento di Medicina Clinica, Università Via Massarenti 9,
40138, Bologna, BO, Italy
e-mail: mauro.bernardi@uniboat

F. Chiappelli
Divisions of Oral Biology and Medicine,
and Associated Clinical Specialties (Joint),
University of California at Los Angeles,
School of Dentistry, CHS 63-090,
Los Angeles, CA 90095-1668, USA
e-mail: fchiappelli@dentistry.ucla.edu

11.1 Introduction

Around 2 billion people worldwide drink alcoholic beverages and over 76 million people have alcohol use disorders. The World Health Organization estimates that the harmful use of alcohol causes about 2.3 million premature deaths per year worldwide (3.7% of global mortality) and it is responsible for 4.4% of the global burden of disease. Alcohol dependence is a very widespread disorder with prevalence estimates of 7–10% in most western countries. In the US, a prevalence of alcohol abuse and dependence of 8.5% has been reported, and similar figures have been observed in western countries [48].

Alcoholic liver disease (ALD) is a general term describing a spectrum of conditions ranging from alcoholic fatty liver to alcoholic hepatitis to cirrhosis; it is one of the main causes of morbidity and mortality in the Western world. The causal association between alcohol intake (in terms of quantity, duration and style of alcohol consumption) and the development of ALD has been well demonstrated [6]. Nevertheless, although 90–100% of heavy drinkers show evidence of fatty liver, only 10–35% develop alcoholic hepatitis and 8–20% develop cirrhosis [32]. It is presumed, therefore, that other factors, such as gender (female), ethnicity (hispanic), genetic background, and additional environmental influences, particularly chronic viral infection, play a role in the genesis of ALD [32].

Steatosis develops in many heavy drinkers, and it results from the redox imbalance generated by the metabolism of ethanol to acetate. Alcoholic steatosis completely reverses within several weeks of discontinuation of alcohol intake [33].

Alcoholic hepatitis is an acute or acute-on-chronic hepatic inflammatory response syndrome that occurs

F. Chiappelli et al. (eds.), *Evidence-Based Practice: Toward Optimizing Clinical Outcomes*,
DOI: 10.1007/978-3-642-05025-1_11, © Springer-Verlag Berlin Heidelberg 2010

in the setting of chronic alcohol abuse. It is a disease with a wide range of severity, from the asymptomatic patient with mild inflammation on liver biopsy to the severely ill patients with fever, cholestasis, coagulopathy, and leucocytosis. While in the majority of mild cases avoiding alcohol intake alone allows the clinical picture to resolve, severe alcoholic hepatitis carries a particularly poor prognosis, with 28-day mortality ranging from 30 to 50% [28].

In these high-risk patients, pharmacologic therapy can be an adjunct to supportive medical care in the attempt to improve short-term survival. Therefore, it is important to assess the severity of alcoholic hepatitis in order to identify patients who might benefit from aggressive intervention (*see below, Sect. 11.2.2*).

A number of validated scoring systems including the Maddrey discriminant function (DF), the model for end-stage liver disease score (MELD), and the Glasgow Alcoholic Hepatitis score are useful for this purpose.

- DF is calculated as total bilirubin (in mg/dL)+ 4.6×prothrombin time (in second prolonged); a DF score greater than 32 identify significant or severe alcoholic hepatitis and suggest to institute intensive treatment [28].
- MELD can be readily calculated (e.g., www.unos.org/meldcalculator); a score above 21 or 24 identifies patients with increased short-term mortality [20].
- The Glasgow Alcoholic Hepatitis score is a five-item scale containing four laboratory variables (bilirubin, blood urea nitrogen, prothrombin time, WBC count) along with patient age; patients with a score of nine or greater have an increased mortality [16].

The amount of alcohol consumption which places an individual at risk of developing alcoholic hepatitis is not known. However, in practice, most patients with alcoholic hepatitis drink more than 100 g/day, with 150–200 g/day being common. Like steatosis, once the acute phase is overcome, alcoholic hepatitis usually improves with abstinence [55].

On the contrary, when alcohol use continues, inflammation triggers fibrogenesis and, over times, collagen is deposited in a characteristic perivenular and pericellular distribution. Approximately, 40% of patients with this lesion will develop *cirrhosis* within 5 years [4].

Alcohol intake remains the most important cause of cirrhosis in the western world; the lower limit of alcohol use for the development of cirrhosis is in the range of 30–50 g of ethanol per day (12 oz [355 mL] of beer,

5 oz [125 mL] of wine, or 1.5 oz [45 mL] of spirits contains approximately 12–14 g of ethanol) [6].

Complications of cirrhosis that arise in patients with ALD should be sought and treated as done for any other type of cirrhosis; patients with end-stage liver disease should be considered for liver transplant (*see below*).

11.2 Pharmacological Management of Alcoholic Liver Disease

11.2.1 General Treatment

11.2.1.1 Abstinence

Abstinence remains the cornerstone of management of all forms of ALD, and its importance needs to be continually emphasized in the long-term management of these patients.

The prognosis of ALD is strictly related to abstinence. Abstinence plays an important role in the reversibility of steatosis, acute alcoholic hepatitis (AAH), lipid peroxidation, inflammation, and collagen deposition; even significant fibrosis may improve in patients who maintain sobriety [4].

Retrospective longitudinal observational studies have shown that "pure" alcoholic steatosis reverses completely with abstinence [53].

Abstinence improves survival in AAH; in the majority of mild cases, avoiding alcohol intake alone allows the clinical picture to resolve [32].

The 5-year survival of patients with clinically compensated alcoholic cirrhosis is about 90%, but declines to 70% if the patient continues to drink; in a patient with decompensated cirrhosis who continues drinking, the chance of living 5 years is 30% at best [4].

11.2.1.2 Nutritional Support

Malnourishment of patient with ALD is due to a combination of poor intake of nutrients, decreased intestinal assimilation (especially of fat and fat-soluble vitamins), and increased rate of catabolism. Protein-calorie deficiency could enhance the toxicity of alcohol through the influence of nutritional status on the integrity of the immune system and on the hepatic regeneration.

This is particularly true in the case of AAH: essentially, all of the patients with a DF > 32 are malnourished, and the degree of malnutrition correlates with survival. Mendenhall et al. evaluated 352 patients with alcoholic hepatitis for protein-calorie malnutrition, and found that the 30-day mortality was 2% in patients with mild malnutrition and 52% in those with severe malnutrition [35]. Consequently, multiple clinical trials evaluated nutritional therapy (enteral or parenteral) in alcoholic hepatitis, and it was the subject of a recent review; their predominant conclusion was that nutritional support results in an improvement of nutritional status and liver tests, but does not improve survival [52]. Some studies anyway suggested that nutritional therapy could also decrease the mortality of these patients. In particular, Cabrè et al. reported that total enteral nutrition was associated with an important reduction in the short-term mortality in patients with alcoholic cirrhosis [9]. More recently, the same group compared in a randomized study, the efficacy and safety of total enteral nutrition (2,000 kcal/day) and prednisolone (40 mg/day) in the treatment of severe AAH; mortality during treatment was similar in both groups, while mortality during follow-up was higher in steroids group (mainly because of infections) [10].

Thus, although nutritional supplements are reasonable for any severely malnourished patient, their efficacy in the management of AAH must be considered to be "unproven" [55].

The proposed recommendation for the American College of Gastroenterology is that patients with ALD should be kept well nourished, and nutritional supplements are indicated if dietary intake is insufficient; during hospitalization for acute decompensation of ALD, aggressive nutritional therapy should be instituted to ensure that the patient's nutritional requirements are being provided [32].

Nutritional support consists of 1.2–1.5 g of protein and an energy intake of 35–40 kcal/kg of ideal body weight per day; it is uncommon that the higher protein intake precipitates or worsens hepatic encephalophaty; due to the underlying malnutrition, patient with encephalopathy should be treated initially with lactulose, not protein restriction [12]. In the absence of hepatic encephalopathy or problems in the gastrointestinal tract, oral intake or naso-gastric feeding (in patients who do not voluntarily consume sufficient calories) should be given. If the gastointestinal tract cannot be used, total parenteral nutrition is necessary.

There are no published guidelines regarding the appropriate dosing of vitamin or mineral supplements in patients with alcoholic hepatitis; it has been recommended to provide B-vitamins (especially thiamine), folic acid, vitamin k at several times the minimum daily allowance; it is common to provide these intravenously for the first few days. Daily oral multimineral supplementation (without iron) should also be provided; in particular, zinc replacement (approximately 200 mg/day) should be considered, since most patients are deficient in zinc, and in animal models of ALD, zinc replacement prevents apoptosis and translocation of bacteria across the small intestines [21].

11.2.2 Pharmacological Treatment

Recent researches, which have elucidated the mechanisms of alcohol-induced liver injury, offer the prospect of advances in the management of ALD; anyway, till now none of the therapies proposed has been shown to improve consistently the course of alcoholic liver damage, and there is no FDA approved therapy for ALD.

Anyway, some of the following drugs, in particular corticosteroid and pentoxifylline (PTX), appear to be beneficial in the subgroup of patients with severe AAH.

11.2.2.1 Corticosteroids

The supposed mechanism of action of corticosteroids in ALD is the decreased transcription of proinflammatory cytokines such as tumor necrosis factor-α (TNF-α), the suppression of the formation of acetaldehyde adducts, and the inhibition of the production of collagen.

They have been evaluated in multiple randomized controlled trials and in at least three meta-analyses; the results are conflicting, with some reports suggesting a survival benefit while others fail to confirm any benefit. An analysis that combined and reanalyzed the primary data from three of the larger clinical trials of prednisolone vs. placebo, including only patients with a DF > 32, did show a survival benefit for corticosteroids [31]. A recent Cochrane meta-analysis that included 15 randomized trials did not find an improvement in overall survival with corticosteroids treatment; a subgroup analysis suggests possible beneficial effects in patients with either Maddrey score of at least 32 or hepatic encephalopathy, but this result requires confirmation in new trial [47].

Given the conflicting results, it is difficult to firmly recommend these agents; indications for starting corticosteroid therapy may include a DF>32, MELD>20, or the presence of hepatic hencephalopathy. Therapy is made with prednisolone, 40 mg/day for 28 days; standard contraindications include recent upper gastointestinal bleeding and uncontrolled infection [32]. Measuring the change in total bilirubin during the first week of treatment can predict outcome; one approach is to stop the treatment if the bilirubin is higher at day 7 than it was prior to starting cortiocosteroids [30]. Switching these patients to PTX did not appear to improve survival [27].

11.2.2.2 Pentoxifylline (PTX)

PTX is a nonselective phosphodiesterase inhibitor that increase the intracellular concentration of adenosine 3',5'-cyclic monophosphate (cAMP); increase in cAMP decrease the expression of cytokines such as TNF-α, IL-8, and others.

PTX has been proposed as an alternative of corticosteroids in the treatment of severe alcoholic hepatitis, especially in patients with contraindications for steroids, and in patients with early hepatorenal syndrome, who seems to especially benefit from this treatment. The proposed treatment is PTX at the dose of 400 mg 3 times per day for 28 days.

Akriviadis et al. [3] reported a randomized controlled trial involving 101 patients with severe alcoholic hepatitis (DF>32) who were treated with PTX (400 mg orally 3 times a day) vs. placebo for 4 weeks; mortality during the initial hospitalization was significantly higher for subjects receiving placebo than for those receiving PTX; improvement in survival with PTX was due to a reduction in the number of deaths from hepatorenal syndrome. There were no reported serious adverse events related to PTX use. A lot of other clinical trials both support [49] and refute [25] the effectiveness of PTX in the treatment of alcoholic hepatitis and cirrhosis. Recently, a randomized double-blind controlled study compared the efficacy of PTX and prednisolone in the treatment of severe AH; the results suggest a superiority of PTX in terms of reduced mortality, improved risk-benefit profile, and renoprotective effects [13]. No meta-analysis was present in the literature on PTX and ALD treatment.

In conclusion, PTX can be proposed as an alternative of corticosteroids in the treatment of severe alcoholic hepatitis, especially in patients with contraindications for steroids, and in patients with early hepatorenal syndrome, who seems to especially benefit from this treatment. The proposed treatment is oral somminsiration of PTX at the dose of 400 mg 3 times per day for 28 days. Anyway, even if the reported data are encouraging, other clinical trials are needed in order to validate this treatment.

11.2.2.3 Anti-TNF-α

TNF-α is a proinflammatory cytokine believed to contribute to the fever, anorexia, malnutrition, and liver injury (inflammation, apoptosis, etc.) that occurs in alcoholic hepatitis. Consequently, anti-TNF treatments (infliximab or etanercept) were tested in patients with advanced AH. Small and/or uncontrolled trials suggest that infliximab with or without prednisolone improves patient outcomes; however a perspective, randomized, blinded trial comparing prednisolone monotherapy against combination treatment with prednisolone plus infliximab (10 mg/kg at days 0, 14, and 28) was stopped early because of increased mortality in the second group of patients, related to the higher incidence of infections [37]. Also others studies, using smaller doses of infliximab, confirmed relatively high infection rates [54]. A randomized, placebo-controlled trial comparing etanercept with placebo shows that mortality was significantly higher in patients receiving etanercept; as with infliximab, more patients receiving etanercept developed infections and died from infections [8].

In conclusion, at the moment anti-TNF-α treatments should not be used in alcoholic hepatitis, except in carefully-designed clinical trials.

11.2.2.4 Propylthiuracil (PTU)

The rationale for the use of PTU in the treatment of ALD rests on the evidence that it can inhibit the hypermetabolic state so as to reduce hepatic oxygen consumption by hepatocytes, thus producing a benefit since the most severe alcohol-induced damage is often in the perivenular area (zone 3), thereby resembling ischemic injury.

One large trial reported that PTU improved 2-year survival in patients with ALD [40]. A meta-analysis of Cochrane on six randomized clinical trials including 710 patients demonstrated no significant effects of PTU vs. placebo on all-cause mortality, liver-related mortality, complications of the liver disease, and liver histology. Propylthiouracil was associated with a non-significant increased risk of nonserious adverse events and with the seldom occurrence of serious adverse events (leukopenia) [43]. Thus, PTU is not currently recommended as a treatment for ALD.

11.2.2.5 Antioxidant Treatment (*N*-Acetylcysteine, Coenzime Q, *S*-Adenosylmethioninine (SAMe), Silymarin, etc)

The rationale of this treatment is the presence of oxidative stress and the reduction in antioxidant capabilities in ALD.

Unfortunately, clinical trials have failed to demonstrate that antioxidant treatment, alone or with prednisolone, is beneficial in these patients [51]. Thus, although antioxidant treatment remains theoretical, it cannot be currently recommended in the absence of positive data from randomized controlled studies.

About SAMe in the treatment of ALDs, a Cochrane analysis identified nine randomized clinical trials. The methodological quality regarding randomization was generally low, but eight out of nine trials were placebo controlled. Only one trial including 123 patients with alcoholic cirrhosis used adequate methodology and reported clearly on all-cause mortality and liver transplantation. So, the analysis found no significant effects of SAMe on all-cause mortality, liver-related mortality, and liver transplantation or complications; SAMe was not significantly associated with nonserious adverse events. The study did not find evidence supporting or refuting the use of SAMe for patients with ALDs [45].

11.2.2.6 Anabolic Steroids

Since anabolic steroids (i.e., oxandrolone and testosterone) increase muscle mass in healthy men, their use in alcoholic hepatitis was proposed in the attempt to increase the incorporation of nutrients into muscle mass of these often malnourished patients.

Despite this theoretical benefit, only one study demonstrated improved survival at 6 months in patients receiving oxandrolone [34], while all the other studies did not confirm this data. The systematic review of Cochrane, selecting five randomized clinical trials randomizing 499 patients, has not shown any significant beneficial effects of anabolic-androgenic steroids on any clinically important outcomes (mortality, liver-related mortality, liver complications, and histology) of patients with ALD [46]. Thus, given a lack of convincing data, anabolic steroids cannot be recommended for routine use in the treatment of alcoholic hepatitis.

11.2.2.7 Colchicine

It is an inhibitor of collagen synthesis, and its use in the therapy of ALD was proposed because of its anti-inflammatory and antifibrotic action. Results of trials regarding the use of colchicine are conflicting: it is of no benefit in alcoholic hepatitis, but Kershenobich et al. suggest that it can improve the survival rate of long-term treated cirrhotic patients [22]. However, a Cochrane meta-analysis, including 15 randomized clinical trials in which 1,714 patients were randomized, demonstrated no significant effect of colchicine on mortality, liver-related mortality, liver biochemistry, liver histology, and alcohol consumption; conversely, the drug was associated with a significantly increased risk of adverse events [44].

11.2.2.8 Miscellaneous

Other treatment, such as insulin–glucagon (pro-growth), polyunsaturated phosphatidylcholine (antioxidant, TNF-α modulator, antifibrotic), and vitamin E, have been proposed for the treatment of ALD, but none of them have shown a convincing benefit [26, 56].

11.2.3 Liver Transplantation

Alcoholic cirrhosis is the second most important indication for ortotopic liver transplantation (OLT) after viral hepatitis in industrialized countries [18, 29]. Despite abstinence is an effective treatment that can improve cirrhosis in some patients, there is no parameter to predict which patients will have a good response to the abstinence; so, OLT remains the best therapeutic option in end-stage liver disease [12]. However, a definite period of 3 months seems to be adequate to separate those alcoholics who will have irreversible liver failure from those who will demonstrate recovery of their liver function [27, 57].

Survival for an OLT patient with cirrhosis related to alcohol does not show any difference with respect to other causes of end-stage liver disease with the condition to maintain the abstinence [36]. Patients receiving liver transplantation for ALD have a higher incidence of some malignancies, especially those arising from the aero-digestive tract, which appear to be related to the prolonged use of alcohol and tobacco before and after OLT. This underlines the utility of an extensive work-up before listing to exclude the presence of an occult tumor [7].

Relapse of alcohol intake have a detrimental effect on survival [23] and when considering the ethical aspects of living organ donation, in the limited availability of cadaveric liver, it is clearly reasonable to exclude recipient candidates who have risk factors for alcohol relapse. There are, however, few reports in literature of graft loss for patients that return to the previous pattern of alcohol abuse after OLT [38].

Unfortunately, at the moment, parameters that individualize the patients who will maintain the sobriety from those who will relapse overdrinking are not available; so many transplant centers require a period of abstinence of at least 6 months to appraise the real maintenance of the abstinence.

The Berlin Group demonstrates a significantly low relapse of alcohol abuse in those patients who were abstinent for >6 months prior to transplantation, and another recent study demonstrates that pre-transplant sobriety of less than 6 months was associated with an increased risk of recurrent alcohol consumption [41]. Two studies suggest that 6 months of abstinence alone is an inadequate predictor of relapse [15, 17]. True predictive abstinence may in fact take up to 5 years [36]. A meta-analysis of risk factors for relapse to alcohol, including 54 selected studies, demonstrates a mild but statistically significant predictive value of abstinence less than 6 months, but the author suggests a caution for the exit bias in the selection of the patients [14]. In conclusion, although 6 months of abstinence is a widely accepted standard, attaining 6 months of abstinence is by itself a poor predictor of relapse post-OLT [23].

Alcohol dependence (not alcohol abuse), serious lack of social support, pattern of nonadherence toward taking medications or attending scheduled appointments, and psychotic or personality disorders were identified in some studies as factors related to higher risk of recidivism of alcohol consumption and it is advisable for the transplant committees to very cautiously list these patients [23].

Pharmacologic approach to reduce the risk of relapse both before and after liver transplantation are needed; naltrexone (NTX) doesn't demonstrate utility for this hepatotoxic effect, but baclofen, that has demonstrated an anticraving effect in patients with alcoholic cirrhosis, could have a future role in this setting.

11.3 Pharmacological Management of Alcohol Dependence

About 50% of alcohol-dependent patients develop clinically relevant symptoms of alcohol withdrawal syndrome (AWS). Since risks of seizures and delirium rise with medical problems, a physical examination is essential for patients with AWS. Doses of multivitamins, including thiamine (about 100 mg/day) can be beneficial also to prevent the rare Wernicke–Korsakoff syndromes, which are much less likely to be seen in general-practice settings. Taking into account that for patients with alcohol dependence, abstinence is the primary goal, controlled clinical trials provided compelling evidence that a variety of compounds can be safe and effective medications for treating AWS, alcohol dependence, or both. However, in order to identify those drugs which have demonstrated evidence-based data for healthcare decision making, the most useful tool is the Cochrane Central Register of Controlled Trials (*The Cochrane Library*). At this moment, available data from the Cochrane Library regard three drugs for which it is possible to draw consistent indications for the pharmacological management of alcohol dependence: specifically, benzodizepines (BDZs) and anticonvulsants for the treatment of alcohol AWS and NTX for helping patients in reducing relapses in heavy drinking and maintaining sobriety.

11.3.1 Treatment of AWS

11.3.1.1 BDZs

A Cochrane review published in 2005 has investigated the effectiveness and safety of BDZs in the treatment of AWS in 57 trials, with a total of 4.051 subjects enrolled. BDZs when compared to placebo offer a large benefit against the onset of seizures, a complication of AWS ($p > 0.01$), while BDZs have a variable profile when compared with anticonvulsants. Two long-acting BDZs such as diazepam (5–20 mg every 4–6 h) and chlordiazepoxide (50–100 mg every 4–6 h), and two short-acting BDZs such as lorazepam (2–4 mg every 6 h) and oxazepam (15–30 mg every 6–8 h) are the most commonly used BDZs for the treatment of AWS. Lorazepam and oxazepam are strongly suggested in patients with advanced liver disease. After the first 3 days of treatment, independent of the type of BDZs employed, a dose tapering has to be planned with a daily decrease of 15–20% from day 4 to day 7 [39].

It should remain that in severe cirrhosis BDZ are controindicated since they can precipitate portosistemic encephalopathy.

11.3.1.2 Anticonvulsant

A Cochrane Review published in 2005 has investigated the effectiveness and safety of anticonvulsants in the treatment of AWS in 48 studies, involving 3,610 people. The anticonvulsants have not shown a statistically significant difference when compared to placebo both in treating AWS and in preventing the onset of seizures. In addition, the anticonvulsants have not evidenced any differences when compared to other drugs in reducing AWS symptoms too. The onset of seizures tended to be less common in the anticonvulsant-group than BDZs without reaching, however, a statistically significant difference. Thus, it is not possible to draw definite conclusions about the effectiveness and safety of anticonvulsants in the treatment of AWS, because of the heterogeneity of the trials both in interventions and the assessment of outcomes. There are limited data comparing anticonvulsants vs. placebo and no clear differences are between anticonvulsants and other drugs in the rates of therapeutic success. Data on safety

outcomes are sparse and fragmented. There is a need for larger, well-designed studies in this field [42].

11.3.2 Treatment for the Maintenance of Alcohol Abstinence

11.3.2.1 Opioid Antagonists

The effect of opioid antagonists, NTX and nalmefene is likely related to the blockade of alcohol-induced release of dopamine in the nucleus accumbens, which reduces the positive reinforcing and pleasurable effects of alcohol and, hence, the craving for alcohol. A Cochrane review published in 2005 has investigated the effectiveness and safety of these two drugs in reducing relapses and in maintaining alcohol abstinence in 29 clinical trials (two of NMF, all others of NTX). In comparison to placebo, a short-term treatment of NTX significantly decreased the relapse and decreased the return to drink alcohol. While a medium-term treatment of NTX gave no benefit for relapse prevention, it was found to be beneficial in delaying the time to first drink and reducing the craving for alcohol. A medium-term treatment of NTX was superior to acamprosate (ACP) in reducing relapses, standard drinks, and craving. The review findings support that short-term treatment with NTX decreases 36% of the number of alcohol relapses and, likely, reduces 13% of the probability to return to drink alcohol. The treatment with NTX can lower 28% of the risk of drop-out rate in alcohol-dependent patients. So far, the evidence has supported that NTX should be accepted as a short-term treatment for alcoholism. Strategies to improve adherence to NTX treatment (i.e., psychosocial interventions and management of adverse effects) should be concomitantly given. We have not yet known how long alcoholics who respond to NTX treatment should continue the treatment with this drug. NTX is given at 50–100 mg/day (or 150 mg 3 times a week), and it can also be given as an intramuscular dose of 380 mg once a month, which, although more expensive, optimizes compliance and has shown some promising results. NTX's side-effects include increased liver function tests, possible interference with pain control, and a potential blunting of mood. Nalmefene has too little evidence to support its clinical use [50].

11.3.3 Nonevidence-Based Drugs: Currently Approved for the Treatment of Alcohol Dependence

Even though the Cochrane Central Register of Controlled Trials have not provided evidence-based data regarding other drugs such as disulfiram, gamma-hydroxybutyric acid (GHB), and ACP, protocols of these three drugs are currently in progress; moreover, several clinical data have demonstrated their efficacy in the treatment of alcohol addiction so that they have been approved with this indication. For these reasons, it is warranted to mention the main features of these three compounds.

11.3.3.1 Disulfiram

Disulfiram is an aldehyde dehydrogenase (ALDH) blocker so that after the ingestion of alcoholic beverages by a patient who regularly uses this drug, the acetaldehyde blood level increases dramatically producing from moderate to severe side-effects characterized by nausea, vomiting, diarrhea, rapid heart rate, and changes in blood pressure, which, often, need hospitalization of the patient. Several weeks are needed after the discontinuation of disulfiram for ALDH to return to normal function. In order to ensure patient's compliance, it is best to give disulfiram under the observation of a referred familiar member to whom the administration of the drug has to be entrusted. The efficacy of this ALDH inhibitor is controversial, because the anticipation of adverse effects after drinking could contribute to the outcome even with placebo. At the same time, disulfiram has both relatively benign side-effects (i.e., a bad taste, sedation, a rash, and temporary impotence) and rarer, but more severe, sequelae (i.e., neuropathies, depression, psychotic symptoms, an increase in liver function tests, and severe hepatitis). In one study, the risk of fatal disulfiram-related hepatitis was 1 in every 25,000 patients per year, with as many as 1 in 200 patients per year having adverse drug reactions. It should be used with caution in the treatment of patients with liver disease. More than 500 mg/day of disulfiram are needed for maximum inhibition of ALDH, but this dose would produce unacceptable side-effects so that it is suggested to begin with 400 mg/day for the first 7 days, then 250 mg/day as usual maintenance dose [24].

11.3.3.2 Gamma-Hydroxybutyric Acid (GHB)

GHB is a short-chain fatty acid structurally similar to the inhibitory neurotransmitter γ-amino-butyric acid (GABA) that exerts an ethanol-mimicking effect on the central nervous system, by acting on its own receptor and on the $GABA_B$ receptor. In some European countries, this medication is currently used for the treatment of alcohol dependence with encouraging results. Indeed, clinical trials have demonstrated that GHB is able to suppress symptoms of AWS and favor the maintenance of abstinence from alcohol. GHB has also proved to be more efficient than NTX ($p > 0.02$) in maintaining sustained abstinence from alcohol. In addition, as far as combined treatments are concerned, the combination of GHB with NTX is more effective than either drug alone in maintaining alcohol abstinence and, likely, in avoiding craving for GHB. As a whole, these studies have shown that episodes of craving for GHB are a very limited phenomenon (about 10–15%) in pure alcoholics; rare episodes of sedation due to GHB abuse have been reported, no cases of intoxication, coma or deaths have occurred and a withdrawal syndrome has not been observed when this drug was discontinued. In addition, due to its short half-life (2–4 h), it is also safe in patients with decompensated liver disease with ascites effusion, while in those patients with a clinical condition of liver encephalopathy this drug is not indicated. GHB should be indicated in alcoholics who do not present a poly-drug dependence; its dosage should not exceed 50–100 mg/kg fractioned into three to six daily administrations, strict medical surveillance has to be planned, and, in order to avoid episodes of abuse of GHB, a family member to be entrusted with the drug should be designated [1, 11].

11.3.3.3 ACP

It is structurally similar to GABA, but with actions that inhibit the N-methyl-D-aspartic acid–glutamate receptor hyperactivity that occurs during protracted AWS. Most trials report that this drug delays the time to relapse, decreases the number of drinks per drinking day, or helps to maintain abstinence, with a rate of improved outcome similar to NTX. Side-effects include gastrointestinal upset and diarrhea, which rarely cause patients to stop the use of the drug. Combined NTX and ACP might be slightly better than either drug alone, although not all studies agree. The therapeutic dose of ACP is 666 mg 3 times per day [5].

11.3.4 Nonevidence-Based Drugs: Not Approved for the Treatment of Alcohol Dependence: The Near Future

11.3.4.1 Topiramate

Topiramate facilitates inhibitory $GABA_A$-mediated currents at nonbenzodiazepine sites on the $GABA_A$ receptor. Few studies on the effects of topiramate on ethanol consumption in animals have been published. Clinical studies have shown that topiramate (from 200 to 300 mg/day), compared with placebo, improved drinking outcomes, decreased craving, and improved the quality of life of alcohol-dependent individuals who received 12 or 14 weekly brief behavioral compliance enhancement treatment. The most common adverse effects are paresthesia, anorexia, difficulty with memory or concentration, and taste perversion. Taken together, these clinical studies provide strong evidence that topiramate may be a promising medication for the treatment of alcohol dependence [19].

11.3.4.2 Baclofen

Animal studies have demonstrated that the $GABA_B$ receptor agonist, baclofen, causes decreases in voluntary ethanol intake. Clinical trials have shown that baclofen reduced alcohol craving and intake, and improved abstinence in alcohol-dependent patients. In addition, due to its very low levels of liver metabolism (about 15%), baclofen has been recently tested in the treatment of alcohol-dependent subjects affected by cirrhosis. Eighty-four patients were randomized to receive baclofen (10 mg t.i.d.) or placebo for 12 consecutive weeks. Results of this trial showed a significantly higher number of patients who achieved and maintained abstinence throughout the experimental period in the baclofen group compared to the placebo group. In these studies, the treatment with baclofen improved significantly drinking outcomes, state anxiety scores, and craving measures; this drug generally was well tolerated and had no apparent abuse liability;

adverse events, none of which were serious, consisted of nausea, vertigo, transient sleepiness, and abdominal pain. These findings suggest a potential role for baclofen in treating alcohol-dependent individuals. Additional studies of larger sample size and longer duration would help to establish the efficacy of baclofen in the treatment of alcohol-dependent individuals [2].

References

1. Addolorato G, Leggio L, Ferrulli A, Caputo F, Gasbarrini A (2009) The therapeutic potential of gamma-hydroxybutyric acid for alcohol dependence: balancing the risks and benefits. A focus on clinical data. Expert Opin Investig Drugs 18:675–686
2. Addolorato G, Leggio L, Ferrulli A, Cardone S, Vonghia L, Mirijello A, Abenavoli L, D'Angelo C, Caputo F, Zambon A, Haber PS, Gasbarrini G (2007) Effectiveness and safety of baclofen for maintenance of alcohol abstinence in alcohol-dependent patients with liver cirrhosis: randomised, double-blind controlled study. Lancet 370:1915–1922
3. Akriviadis E, Botla R, Briggs W et al (2000) Pentoxifylline improves short-term survival in severe acute alcoholic hepatitis: a double-blind, placebo controlled trial. Gastroenterology 119:1637–1648
4. Alexander JF, Lichner MW, Galambos JT (1971) Natural history of alcoholic hepatitis. The long-term prognosis. Am J Gastroenterol 56:515–525
5. Anton RF, O'Malley SS, Ciraulo DA, Cisler RA, Couper D, Donovan DM, Gastfriend DR, Hosking JD, Johnson BA, LoCastro JS, Longabaugh R, Mason BJ, Mattson ME, Miller WR, Pettinati HM, Randall CL, Swift R, Weiss RD, Williams LD, Zweben A, COMBINE Study Research Group (2006) Combined pharmacotherapies and behavioral interventions for alcohol dependence: the COMBINE study: a randomized controlled trial. JAMA 295:2003–2017
6. Becker Deis U, Soresen TI et al (1996) Prediction of risk of liver disease by alcohol intake, sex, and age: a prospective population study. Hepatology 23:1025–1029
7. Bellamy CO, DiMartini AM, Ruppert K et al (2001) Liver transplantation for alcoholic cirrhosis: long term follow-up and impact of disease recurrence. Transplantation 72:619–626
8. Boetticher NC, Peine CJ, Kwo P et al (2008) A randomized, double-blinded, placebo-controlled multicenter trial of etanercept in the treatment of alcoholic hepatitis. Gastroenterology 135:1953–1960
9. Cabrè E, Gonzalez Huix F, Abad-Lacruz A et al (1990) Effect of total enteral nutrition on the short-term outcome of severely malnourished cirrhotics. A randomized controlled trial. Gastroenterology 98:715–720
10. Cabrè E, Rodriguez Iglesias P, Caballeria J et al (2000) On behalf of the spanish group for the Study of Alcoholic Hepatitis. Short- and long-term outcome of severe alcohol-induced hepatitis treated with steroids or enteral nutrition: a multicenter randomized trial. Hepatology 32:36–42

11. Caputo F, Addolorato G, Stoppo M, Francini S, Vignoli T, Lorenzini F, Del Re A, Comaschi C, Andreone P, Trevisani F, Bernardi M (2007) Comparing and combining gamma-hydroxybutyric acid (GHB) and naltrexone in maintaining abstinence from alcohol: an open randomised comparative study. Eur Neuropsychopharmacol 17:781–789

12. Cohen SM, Ahn J (2009) Diagnosis and Management of Alcoholic Hepatitis. Aliment Pharmacol Ther 30(1):3–13

13. De BK, Gangopadhyay S, Dutta D et al (2009) Pentoxifylline versus prednisolone for severe alcoholic hepatitis: a randomized controlled trial. World J Gastroenterol 15: 1613–1619

14. Dew MA, DiMartini AF, Steel J, De Vito Dabbs A, Myaskovsky L, Unruh M, Greenhouse J (2008) Meta-analysis of risk for relapse to substance use after transplantation of the liver or other solid organs. Liver Transpl 14(2):159–172

15. DiMartini A, Day N, Dew MA et al (2006) Alcohol consumption patterns and predictors of use following liver transplantation for alcoholic liver disease. Liver Transpl 12:813–820

16. Forrest EH, Evans CD, Stewart S et al (2005) Analysis of factors predictive of mortality in alcoholic hepatitis and derivation and validation of the Glasgow alcoholic hepatitis score. Gut 54:1174–1179

17. Foster PF, Fabrega F, Karademir S et al (1997) Prediction of abstinence from ethanol in alcoholic recipients following liver transplantation. Hepatology 25:1469–1477

18. Gedaly R, McHugh PP, Johnston TD, Jeon H, Koch A, Clifford TM, Ranjan D (2008) Predictors of relapse to alcohol and illicit drugs after liver transplantation for alcoholic liver disease. Transplantation 86(8):1090–1095

19. Johnson BA, Rosenthal N, Capece JA, Wiegand F, Mao L, Beyers K, McKay A, Ait-Daoud N, Anton RF, Ciraulo DA, Kranzler HR, Mann K, O'Malley SS, Swift RM, Topiramate for Alcoholism Advisory Board, Topiramate for Alcoholism Study Group (2007) Topiramate for treating alcohol dependence: a randomized controlled trial. JAMA 298:1641–1651

20. Kamath PS, Kim WR (2007) Advanced Liver Disease Study Group. The model for end-stage liver disease (MELD). Hepatology 45:797–805

21. Kang YJ, Zhou Z (2005) Zinc prevention and treatment of alcoholic liver disease. Mol Aspects Med 26:391–404

22. Kershenobich D, Vargas F, Garcia-Tsao G et al (1988) Colchicine in the treatment of cirrhosis of the liver. N Eng J Med 318:1709–1713

23. Kotlyar DS, Burke A, Campbell MS, Weinrieb RM (2008) A critical review of candidacy for orthotopic liver transplantation in alcoholic liver disease. Am J Gastroenterol 103(3):734–743

24. Laaksonen E, Koski-Jännes A, Salaspuro M, Ahtinen H, Alho H (2008) A randomized, multicentre, open-label, comparative trial of disulfiram, naltrexone and acamprosate in the treatment of alcohol dependence. Alcohol Alcohol 43:53–61

25. Lebrec D, Thabut D, Oberti F et al (2007) Pentoxifylline for the treatment of patients with advanced cirrhosis. A randomized, placebo-controlled, double-blind trial (Abstract). Hepatology 46(Suppl 1):249A

26. Lieber CS, Weiss DG, Groszman R, et al, The veterans Affairs Cooperative Study 391 Group. II (2003) Veterans Affairs cooperative study of polyenylphosphatidylcholine in alcoholic liver disease. Alcohol Clin Exp Res 27:1765–1772

27. Louvet A, Diaz E, Dharancy S et al (2008) Early switch to pentoxifylline in patients with severe alcoholic hepatitis is inefficient in non-responders to corticosteroids. J Hepatol 48:465–470

28. Maddrey WC, Boinott JK, Bedine MS et al (1978) Corticosteroid therapy of alcoholic hepatitis. Gastroenterology 75:193–199

29. Mandayam S, Jamal MM, Morgan TR (2004) Epidemiology of alcoholic liver disease. Semin Liver Dis 24:217–232

30. Mathurin P, Abdelnour M, Ramond MJ et al (2003) Early change in bilirubin levels is an important prognostic factor in severe alcoholic hepatitis treated with prednisolone. Hepatology 38:1363–1369

31. Mathurin P, Mendenhall CL, Carithers RL Jr et al (2002) Corticosteroids improve short-term survival in patients with severe alcoholic hepatitis (AH): individual data analysis of the last three randomized placebo controlled double blind trials of corticosteroids in severe AH. J Hepatol 36: 480–487

32. McCullogh AJ, O'Connor JF (1998) Alcoholic liver disease: proposed recommendations for the American College of Gastroenterology. Am J Gastroenterol 93:2022–2036

33. McSween RNM, Burt AD (1986) Histological spectrum of alcoholic liver disease. Semin Liver Dis 3:221–232

34. Mendenhall CL, Anderson S, Garcia-Pont P et al (1984) Short-term and long-term survival in patients with alcoholic hepatitis treated with oxandrolone and prednisolone. N Eng J Med 311:1464–1470

35. Mendenhall CL, Tosch T, Weesner RE et al (1986) VA cooperative study on alcoholic hepatitis. II. Prognostic significance of protein-calorie malnutrition. Am J Clin Nutr 43: 213–218

36. Murray KF, Carithers RL Jr, AASLD (2005) AASLD practice guidelines: Evaluation of the patient for liver transplantation. Hepatology 41(6):1407–1432

37. Naveau S, Chollet-Martin S, Dharancy S et al (2004) A double blind randomized controlled trial of infliximab associated with prednisolone in acute alcoholic hepatitis. Hepatology 39:1390–1397

38. Neuberger J, Schulz KH, Day C et al (2002) Transplantation for alcoholic liver disease. J Hepatol 36:130–137

39. Ntais C, Pakos E, Kyzas P, Ioannidis JP (2005) Benzodiazepines for alcohol withdrawal. Cochrane Database Syst Rev 20(3):CD005063

40. Orrego H, Blake JE, Blendis LM et al (1987) Long-term treatment of alcoholic liver disease with propylthiouracil. N Eng J Med 317:1421–1427

41. Pfitzmann R, Schwenzer J, Rayes N et al (2007) Long-term survival and predictors of relapse after orthotopic liver transplantation for alcoholic liver disease. Liver Transpl 13:197–205

42. Polycarpou A, Papanikolaou P, Ioannidis JP, Contopoulos-Ioannidis DG (2005) Anticonvulsants for alcohol withdrawal. Cochrane Database Syst Rev 20(3):CD005064

43. Rambaldi A, Gluud C (2001) Meta-analysis of propylthiouracil for alcoholic liver disease-a Cochrane Hepato-Biliary Group review. Liver 21:398–404

44. Rambaldi A, Gluud C (2001) Colchicine for alcoholic and non-alcoholic liver fibrosis and cirrhosis. Cochrane Database Syst Rev 3:CD002148

45. Rambaldi A, Gluud C (2006) S-adenosyl-L-methionine for alcoholic liver disease. Cochrane Database Syst Rev 19(2): CD002235

46. Rambaldi A, Gluud C (2006) Anabolic-androgenic steroids for alcoholic liver disease. Cochrane Database Syst Rev (Online) 4:CD003045

47. Rambaldi A, Saconato HH, Christensen E et al (2008) Systematic review: glucocorticosteroids for alcoholic hepatitis-a Cochrane Hepatobiliary Group systematic review with meta-analyses and trial sequential analyses of randomized clinical trials. Aliment Pharmacol Ther 27:1167–1178

48. Schuckit MA (2009) Alcohol use disorders. Lancet 373:492–501

49. Sidhu S, Singla M, Bhatia K (2006) Pentoxifylline reduces disease severity and prevents renal impairment in severe acute alcoholic hepatitis: a double blind, placebo controlled trial (Abstract). Hepatology 44(Suppl 1):373A

50. Srisurapanont M, Jarusuraisin N (2005) Opioid antagonists for alcohol dependence. Cochrane Database Syst Rev 25(1):CD001867

51. Stewart S, Prince M, Bassendine M et al (2007) A randomized trial of antioxidant therapy alone or with corticosteroids in acute alcoholic hepatitis. J Hepatol 47:277–283

52. Sticel F, Hoen B, Schuppan D et al (2003) Nutritional therapy in alcoholic liver disease. Aliment Pharmacol Ther 18:357–373

53. Teli MR, Day CP, Burt AD et al (1995) Determinants of progression to cirrhosis or fibrosis in pure alcoholic fatty liver. Lancet 346:987–990

54. Tilg H, Jalan R, Kaser A et al (2003) Anti-tumor necrosis factor-alpha monoclonal antibody therapy in severe alcoholic hepatitis. J Hepatol 38:419–425

55. Tome S, Lucey MR (2004) Review article: current management of alcoholic liver disease. Aliment Pharmacol Ther 19:707–714

56. Trinchet JC, Balkau B, Poupon RE et al (1992) Treatment of severe alcoholic hepatitis by infusion of insulin and glucagon: a multicenter sequential trial. Hepatology 15:76–81

57. Veldt BJ, Laine F, Guillygomarc'h A et al (2002) Indication of liver transplantation in severe alcoholic liver cirrhosis: quantitative evaluation and optimal timing. J Hepatol 36:93–98

Temporomandibular Joint Disorders, a Bibliometric Evidence-Based Approach to Analysis

12

Ricardo Viana Bessa-Nogueira, Janaina Andrade Lima Salmos-Brito, Belmiro Cavalcanti do Egito Vasconcelos, and Richard Niederman

Core Message

> The results discussed in this study indicate that in spite of the widespread impact of TMJD and the multitude of potential interventions, clinicians have expended sparse attention to identify knowledge gaps in the TMJD literature. Our analysis suggests the following as potential topics for new high quality studies: TMJ internal derangement, TMJ ankylosis surgical treatment, TMJ electromyography, and surgical treatment of condylar fractures.

12.1 Background

Temporomandibular joint disorders (TMJD) is a collective term used to describe a group of signs and symptoms involving the temporomandibular joints (TMJ), masticatory muscles, and associated facial structures [6]. Approximately, 60–70% of the general

R.V. Bessa-Nogueira (✉)
J.A.L. Salmos-Brito
B.C. do Egito Vasconcelos
Dental School, University of Pernambuco,
Avenida General Newton Cavalcanti n 1650,
54753-020, Camaragibe – Pernambuco, Brazil
e-mail: ricardobessa@msn.com
e-mail: janainasalmos@hotmail.com
e-mail: belmiro@pesquisador.cnpq.br

R. Niederman
The Forsyth Institute 140 Fenway,
Boston, MA, 02115, USA
e-mail: rniederman@forsyth.org

population has at least one sign of a temporomandibular disorder. Painful joints are typically the central complaint, and chronic, persistent pain is the greatest challenge in a segment of TMJD population [6, 8, 9]. Further, this pain is frequently associated with pain in regions outside the facial area and can include recurrent headaches and neck pain [6, 9, 30]. Patients afflicted with severe signs and symptoms can experience significant reductions in the quality of life, affecting both personal life and work, and everyday activities such as eating, talking, yawning, and laughing [6, 9, 30, 33].

Clinicians and researchers do not fully understand the resistance and susceptibility factors for TMJD [16]. Therefore, several widely diverging concepts exist [15, 16]. In addition, the often weak association between pain and observable tissue pathology has prompted researchers and clinicians to use a multidisciplinary symptom-oriented approach for studying and treating TMJD [19, 20, 30, 34].

Given the wide array of diagnostics and controversy, two approaches to therapy have evolved: nonsurgical and surgical. The nonsurgical approach includes, for example, acupuncture, physiotherapy, pharmacotherapy, and occlusal splint therapy [6, 12]. The Surgical therapy ranges from temporomandibular joint arthrocentesis and arthroscopy to the more complex open joint surgical procedures such as arthrotomy [3, 7]. Many patients can be managed nonsurgically [6, 30, 32], and surgical decision is typically based on the evaluation of the patient's response to previous nonsurgical care, his/her mandibular form and function, and the effect of the condition on his/her quality of life [6, 7, 33].

As might be expected, considerable controversy exists about the most effective treatment. For example, reports claim success rates of 40–70% [6] for nonsurgical treatment and as high as 83% [6] for surgical treatment. To examine this controversy, our previous work identified systematic reviews comparing surgical and nonsurgical TMJD treatment and evaluated their methodological quality and the evidence grade within the systematic reviews [1]. The studies queried four databases, included multiple languages, the years 1966–2007, and three appraisal instruments to identify and evaluate the current best evidence. The search strategy identified 211 reports, of which two were systematic reviews. The results indicated that in spite of the widespread impact of TMJD, and the multitude of potential interventions, clinicians have expended sparse attention to systematically implementing and evaluating clinical trial methodology that would improve the validity and reliability of outcome measures.

To better understand the TMJD knowledge base, we used OmniViz™ (BioWisdom Ltd, Cambridge, UK) to integrate text, numeric, and categorical information and visually represent this information. The goal of this analysis was (1) to generate a distribution and visual map of TMJD literature, (2) to categorize and locate high quality studies, and (3) to suggest possible topics for new clinical trials and systematic reviews.

12.2 Methods: Search Strategy and OmniViz™ Galaxy View Creation

A search strategy (Fig. 12.1) was developed using the PubMed service (www.ncbi.nlm.nih.gov/pubmed) and EviDents search engine (http://medinformatics. uthscsa.edu/EviDents/) to identify all TMJD literature that were indexed in MEDLINE database and published, in any language, between the years 1998 and 2008 (up to December).

All the information retrieved from the search strategy was saved and imported into OmniViz™ for analysis. Thus, a new database with nine components (publication type, author, title, affiliation, reference, abstract, medical subject headings or MeSH terms, PubMed unique identifier or PMID, and publication date) was created. A visual representation of information, or Galaxy View, was generated using the default text analysis algorithms. To generate a more coherent view of the database, the cluster number was limited to 20 clusters, and both title and abstract words were selected to create the clusters.

The Galaxy View is a proximity map, such that closely related records and clusters are placed near each other, while thematically distinct clusters are located far apart. The record clustering is determined by the numeric vector calculated for each record, based on word occurrence, distribution, and associations located in a selected component (our analysis parameter was both title and abstract words).

In the Galaxy View, each dot represents a record and each record represents a publication retrieved from MEDLINE. Within a cluster, each record can be identified and selected to view, in the information panel, a detailed information about the cluster label and the record. The cluster label is comprised by top three discriminating major terms. Major terms are the words or phrases located in the selected component that are most

Database:		
PubMed		
User query:		

("Temporomandibular Joint"[MeSH] OR "Myofascial Pain Syndromes" [MeSH] OR "Craniomandibular Disorders"[MeSH] OR "Occlusal Adjustment"[MeSH] OR temporomandibular joint[Text Word] OR temporomandibular joint's[Text Word] OR temporomandibular joints[Text Word] OR TMJ[Text Word] OR craniomandibular disorder[Text Word] OR craniomandibular disorders[Text Word] OR temporomandibular joint disorder[Text Word] OR temporomandibular joint disorders[Text Word] OR temporomandibular joint disease[Text Word] OR temporomandibular joint diseases[Text Word] OR tmj disease[Text Word] OR tmj diseases[Text word] OR temporomandibular disorder[Text Word] OR temporomandibular disorders[Text Word] OR tmj disorder [Text Word] OR tmj disordered[Text Word] OR tmj disorders[Text Word] OR myofascial pain syndrome[Text Word] OR myofascial pain syndromes[Text Word] OR myofascial trigger point[Text Word] OR myofascial trigger points[Text Word] OR occlusal adjustment[Text Word] OR occlusal adjustments[Text Word] OR occlusal equilibration [Text Word] OR occlusal equilibrations [Text Word] OR costen's syndrome[Text Word]) NOT ("animals"[MeSH:noexp] NOT humans[MESH])

Fig. 12.1 Search Strategy to access PubMed/MEDLINE database (from 1998 to 2008)

relevant to discriminating one record from another and they are the principal parameters used in clustering the records. Nearby clusters often share major terms, indicating that they have some themes in common. Detailed view of the selected clusters or records (e.g., publication type, author, title, abstract) can also be seen.

In the next phase, the clusters were queried to identify the major term, and determine the identity and number of clinical trials and systematic reviews. The search strategies used to identify the clinical trials and systematic reviews were based on the work of Haynes RB et al. [17] and Montori VM et al. [23]. The number of identified records and clusters was determined and tabulated using Excel for windows (Microsoft, USA) spreadsheets. A final analysis was done in a descriptive fashion.

12.3 Results: TMJD Literature

Our search strategy identified 6,196 publications in MEDLINE on TMJD from 1998 to 2008. Of these

5,138 could be imported into OmniViz™. The number of publications that are imported into OmniViz™ is lower than the number retrieved in the MEDLINE search, because OmniViz™, by default, during data importation, is set to ignore records that have titles but no abstract. Thus, the OmniViz™ TMJD database eliminated 1,058 publications.

Distributions of the publications, clinical trials, and systematic reviews per year are shown in Table 12.1. From 1998 to 2008, the 5,138 publications were distributed as follows. There were: 460 clinical trials and 100 systematic reviews. On an average, by year, there were 467 ± 65 publications, 42 ± 9 clinical trials, and 9 ± 4 systematic reviews (mean $\pm$ SD). Clinical trials and systematic reviews represent, respectively, 9 and 2% of the TMJD literature. During the most recent 5 years, 50% of the publications and clinical trials, and 61% of the systematic reviews were published. These figures indicate an increasing interest in TMJD, and also emphasize the lack of high quality studies (systematic reviews and clinical trials) in the TMJD literature.

Table 12.1 TMJD publications, clinical trials, and systematic reviews from 1998 to 2008

Year	Publications ($n > 5138$)	Clinical trials ($n > 460$)	Proportion clinical trials/ publications (%)	Systematic reviews ($n > 100$)	Proportion systematic reviews/ publications (%)
1998	401 (7.8%)	31 (6.7%)	7.7	4 (4.0%)	1.0
1999	413 (8.0%)	30 (6.5%)	7.3	7 (6.9%)	1.7
2000	419 (8.2%)	41 (8.9%)	9.8	4 (4.0%)	1.0
2001	440 (8.6%)	32 (7.0%)	7.3	11 (10.9%)	2.5
2002	427 (8.3%)	46 (10.0%)	10.8	4 (4.0%)	0.9
2003	470 (9.1%)	50 (10.9%)	10.6	8 (7.9%)	1.7
2004	465 (9.1%)	40 (8.7%)	8.6	11 (10.9%)	2.4
2005	470 (9.1%)	44 (9.6%)	9.4	8 (7.9%)	1.7
2006	456 (8.9%)	37 (8.0%)	8.1	12 (11.9%)	2.6
2007	603 (11.7%)	55 (12.0%)	9.1	17 (16.8%)	2.8
2008	574 (11.2%)	54 (11.7%)	9.4	14 (13.9%)	2.4
Mean	467	42	8.9	9	1.9
SD	65	9	1.2	4	0.7
Minimum	401	30	7.3	4	0.9
Maximum	603	55	10.8	17	2.8

12.4 Results: Using OmniViz™ Galaxy Views

Figures 12.2–12.4 show Galaxy views of TMJD literature from 1998 to 2008 and they provide the visual assessment of the data in Table 12.2.

In the Galaxy views, each blue dot represents a publication, each black dot represents a selected publication, and the publications were organized into 20

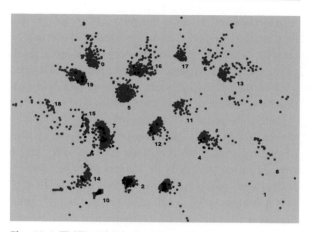

Fig. 12.4 TMJD published systematic reviews (*n*=100). This figure overlays published systematic reviews (black dots) on published articles (blue dots) displayed in Figure 12.2. Each red dot represents 1 systematic review. The presence of black dots in clusters [2–4, 7, 10, 12, 14–16 and 19] and the absence of black dots in clusters [0, 1, 5, 6, 8, 9, 11, 13, 17 and 18] indicates the need for and the presence of clinical trials among published articles, respectively. In comparing Figure 12.4 with Figure 12.3, one also notes clusters where there are clinical trials and no systematic reviews (clusters 0, 5, 11, 13 and 17), and clusters where there are no clinical trails or systematic reviews (clusters 1, 6, 8, 9 and 18)

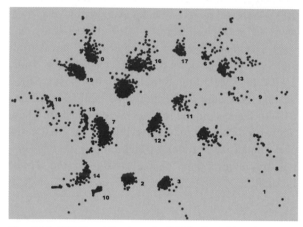

Fig. 12.2 TMJD publications (*n*=5138). Each blue dot represents 1 published article (record) and each number represents 1 cluster. The clusters were numbered from 0 to 19, and both title and abstract words were selected to create the clusters. Closely related records/clusters are placed near each other, while thematically distinct record/clusters are located far apart

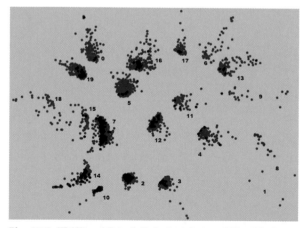

Fig. 12.3 TMJD published clinical trials (*n* = 460). This figure overlays published clinical trials (black dots) on published articles (blue dots) displayed in Figure 12.2. Each black dot represents 1 clinical trial. The presence of black dots in clusters [0, 2–5, 7, 10–17 and 19] and the absence of black dots in clusters [1, 6, 8, 9 and 18] indicates the need for and the presence of clinical trials among published articles, respectively

thematic clusters, numbered from 0 to 19. Closely related publications and clusters are placed near each other while thematically distinct clusters are located farther apart. For example, clusters seven and 15 are closely related, indicating that they share the top three discriminating words, referred to as major terms. This can be identified in Table 12.2; in cluster seven, the major terms are surgery, MRI, and internal derangement, and in cluster 15, the major terms are image, MRI, and surgery. Nevertheless, the sequence of the major terms also gives a hint about the cluster topic; thus, cluster seven is likely to have more surgical therapies publications than cluster 15. Clusters one, eight, and nine have a small number of publications and they are located farther apart, indicating almost no cohesion. They address topics more related to denture, prosthesis, and implant. They are the outlier clusters in the Galaxy view.

Galaxy views of clinical trials and systematic reviews publications are shown in Figs. 12.3 and 12.4, respectively. The largest number of clinical trials and systematic reviews are located in cluster two, 154 (33.5%) and 28 (28%), respectively. This cluster addressed topics related to TMJD, occlusion, and

Table 12.2 Clusters IDs and labels of the TMJD literature. Distribution of publications, clinical trials, and systematic reviews

Cluster ID	Cluster Label (Major terms)	Publications (n=5,138)	Clinical trials (n=460)	Proportion clinical trials/publications (%)	Systematic reviews (n=100)	Proportion systematic reviews/publications (%)
0	Disk, position, internal derangement	181 (3.5%)	3 (0.7%)	1.7	0 (0.0%)	0.0
1	Occlusion, denture, complete dentures	3 (0.1%)	0 (0.0%)	0.0	0 (0.0%)	0.0
2	Temporomandibular disorder, occlusion, headache	1000 (19.5%)	154 (33.5%)	15.4	28 (28.0%)	2.8
3	Temporomandibular disorder, occlusion, bruxism	349 (6.8%)	17 (3.7%)	4.9	18(18.0%)	5.2
4	Occlusion, contact, prothesis	117 (2.3%)	5 (1.1%)	4.3	6 (6.0)	5.1
5	Surgery, ankylosis, condylar	315 (6.1%)	7 (1.5%)	2.2	0 (0.0%)	0.0
6	Condylar, position, kinematic	54 (1.1%)	0 (0.0%)	0.0	0 (0.0%)	0.0
7	Surgery, MRI, internal derangement	872 (17.0%)	79 (17.2%)	9.1	14 (14.0%)	1.6
8	Occlusion, prosthesis, denture	21 (0.4%)	0 (0.0%)	0.0	0 (0.0%)	0.0
9	Stress, load, implant	20 (0.4%)	0 (0.0%)	0.0	0 (0.0%)	0.0
10	Myofascial pain, trigger points, headache	393 (7.6%)	90 (19.6%)	22.9	15 (15.0%)	3.8
11	Activity, electromyographic, position	67 (1.3%)	5 (1.1%)	7.5	0 (0.0%)	0.0
12	Condylar, occlusion, fracture	424 (8.3%)	27 (5.9%)	6.4	4 (4.0%)	0.9
13	Position, condylar, occlusion	138 (2.7%)	5 (1.1%)	3.6	0 (0.0%)	0.0
14	Activity, myofascial trigger points, Temporomandibular disorder	120 (2.3%)	29 (6.3%)	24.2	3 (3.0%)	2.5
15	Image, MRI, surgery	72 (1.4%)	4 (0.9%)	5.6	3 (3.0%)	4.2
16	Condylar, position, disk	216 (4.2%)	12 (2.6%)	5.6	4 (4.0%)	1.9
17	Surgery, fracture, condylar	75 (1.5%)	3 (0.7%)	4.0	0 (0.0%)	0.0
18	Cell, cartilage, gene	42 (0.8%)	0 (0.0%)	0.0	0 (0.0%)	0.0
19	Disk, internal derangement, surgery	659 (12.8%)	20 (4.3%)	3.0	5 (5.0%)	0.8
Mean		257	23	6.0	5	1.4
SD		288	40	7.1	8	1.9
Minimum		3	0	0.0	0	0.0
Maximum		1,000	154	24.2	28	5.2

headache. Nevertheless, publications which address myofascial trigger points (cluster 14) presented the best of clinical trial/publication proportion, 24.2%, and publications which examined TMJD, occlusion, and bruxism (cluster three) presented the best systematic review/publication proportion, 5.2%. Interestingly, clusters with the highest number of publications do not have the highest number of clinical trials or systematic reviews (e.g., cluster 19), and clusters with the highest number of clinical trials do not have the highest number of systematic reviews (e.g., cluster 14). Therefore, there appears to be an imbalance in the distribution of publications, clinical trials, and systematic reviews, suggesting possible knowledge gaps in the TMJD literature.

Moreover, clusters 1, 6, 8, 9, and 18 have no clinical trial or systematic review, and clusters 0, 5, 11, 13, and 17 have no systematic reviews. These clusters could be used as potential sources of new systematic reviews and/or clinical trials, but looking more closely in their major terms, one can identify the following: Clusters 1, 8, and 9 are the outliers, and clusters 6, 13, and 18 examined more topics related to laboratorial studies and basic science, leaving clusters 0, 5, 11, and 17 as potential sources of clinical trials and systematic reviews. Their publications addressed the following topics: TMJ internal derangement, TMJ ankylosis surgical treatment, TMJ electromyography, and surgical treatment of condylar fractures, respectively.

12.5 Discussion: Understanding Our TMJD Literature Analysis

The purpose of this analysis was threefold. The first was to generate a distribution and visual map of a TMJD literature using OmniViz™. The second was to categorize and locate high quality studies (clinical trials and systematic reviews). The third was to suggest possible topics for new systematic reviews and randomized clinical trials. The results indicated that over the last 11 years, there appeared to be a significant body of literature focusing on TMJD, only a small percentage of this literature comprises clinical trials and systematic reviews, and there are four potential topics for new high-quality studies.

The implied results are, perhaps, more interesting than the actual results. First, there were on an average 467 publications, 42 clinical trials, and nine systematic

reviews published per year addressing TMJD. If all of these publications are of high clinical applicability, these results suggest that one would need to read, digest, and implement into clinical practice between one and nine articles per week, 52 weeks per year, to keep current.

Second, all categories of clinical information generally increased over the 11-year period. For example, 61% of the systematic reviews were published in the most recent 5 years. Given this trend, one can expect the volume of literature to increase continually in the near future.

Third, the current percentage of clinical trials and systematic reviews, in comparison to the body of TMJD literature, is suboptimal, 9 and 2%, respectively. Moreover, the Galaxy view was comprised by 20 clusters, of which one individual cluster, in which topics are TMJD, occlusion, and headache, has the largest number of clinical trials and systematic reviews of 33.5 and 28%, respectively, five clusters had no clinical trial or systematic review, and five clusters no systematic review. This suggests an unbalanced body of TMJD high quality literature and leads one to an interesting dilemma: How can one best care for TMJD patients if there are few high quality studies upon which to base this care and they mainly examined an individual topic?

Forth, the evolution of an increasingly unbalanced body of literature suggests the need for additional high quality studies. This is congruent with previous systematic reviews [10, 11, 22, 25, 29]. However, our analysis suggests the following as potential topics: TMJ internal derangement, TMJ ankylosis surgical treatment, TMJ electromyography, and surgical treatment of condylar fractures.

Our analysis used OmniViz™ to integrate text, numeric, and categorical information and visually represent TMJD literature. With the Galaxy views, we were able to promptly identify knowledge gaps in the TMJD literature based on the distribution of clinical trials and systematic reviews in the 20 thematic clusters. Although, this is one alternative approach to understand TMJD literature, the scientific and quantitative study of publications or bibliometrics is not a new discipline, [18, 21, 35]. The subject has developed rapidly since the 1960s, largely because of the theoretical work of Derek de Solla Price at Yale [26] and the practical work of Eugene Garfield [13, 14]. In many ways, bibliometrics is to scientific papers as epidemiology is to patients, because, publication counts are a conventional metric of scientific output. Bibliometrics analysis has also been linked to funding and the financial bottom line of research [5].

Bibliometrics has many creative possibilities and can help in mapping the intellectual growth of a discipline and paving the way to a more sophisticated approach to evidence-based practice [5, 21]. In the traditional model of online evidence services, clinicians have access to a number of online information sources, such as journals, databases, and Medline, each with its own idiosyncrasies and search interfaces [4]. This means that users need to know which resources are most suitable for their current question and how the search query must be formulated for a given resource. Software tools, such as OmniViz™, address many of the limitations of these models by providing a mechanism to search a specific database, by translating query languages of each resource into a respective user queries, and to visually represent this information.

It should be noted that this study had four limitations and is only an approximation of reality. Some methods may have resulted in underestimations or overestimations of the reported TMJD literature. First, only MEDLINE was examined. Had the analysis included other databases (such as EMBASE) the number of citations would have increased. Second, certain relevant studies may have been omitted, whereas other irrelevant articles may have been included. As an attempt to address this limitation, we used EviDents search engine and current search strategies [17, 23] used by PubMed to identify clinical trials and systematic reviews. Third, the key words used in the OmniViz™ data clustering were limited to title and abstract vocabulary. This selection was meant to be inclusive, but it may have excluded some relevant articles. Finally, the cited publications were not critically appraised and this may also overestimate the actual clinically useful literature. This is because the analysis made no attempt to evaluate the methodological quality of the publications. We address this issue in our previous work [1].

Our results suggest the importance of computer-based clinical knowledge systems as an alternative tool to approach a controversial topic such as TMJD. Thus, the next steps are to sample, critically appraise, stratify, and electronically catalog the identified literature to provide an accessible and ongoing electronic database. Such a database could be useful for multiple audiences. These audiences include academics concerned about the evidence base for curricular decisions; patients and clinicians making decisions about clinical care; researchers interested in identifying gaps in the available knowledge base; corporate entities interested in developing new products; policy makers who fund clinical research; healthcare purchasers who make decisions about care compensation; and finally for professional societies that seek to provide guidance for their membership.

12.6 Clinical Implications

Much has been written about the TMJD, but where do we stand today as a result of all this discussion? One would hope that all the patients were receiving rational therapy based on a combination of knowledge about their TMJD specific problem, and treatment outcome data from high quality (clinical trials and systematic reviews) studies. However, our analysis of the literature on TMJD reveals that neither of these objectives has been totally accomplished at this time, or that this is not what is occurring in most TMJD topics.

The above statements should not be interpreted as entirely negative, because in fact, there has been significant progress, both in understanding TMJD and in rationally treating patients with these conditions. The increasing volume of clinical literature suggests that clinicians are providing a special attention to TMJD patients with associated problems, such as headache. The main problem lies in the unbalanced distribution of publications, clinical trials, and systematic reviews, suggesting possible knowledge gaps in the TMJD literature. This imbalance suggests that the efficacy of care is not being well documented. To stay current and make informed clinical decisions when faced with an onslaught of information, health care professionals need evidence-based knowledge-base systems that can provide support to their decision making process and optimize their clinical outcomes.

Most high quality publications end with the author urging the scientists to continue searching for more answers to the main topical issue so that better treatments can be provided (eg. [10, 11, 22, 25, 29]). However, to extrapolate this sentiment to the care of individual TMJD patients would be difficult. All patients vary with regard to their pathology and clinical characteristics, leading the clinician to adopt a multidisciplinary symptom-oriented approach to care [19, 20, 30, 34]. Our analysis suggested some TMJD topics (such as TMJ internal derangement, TMJ ankylosis surgical treatment, TMJ electromyography, and surgical treatment of condylar fractures) for which the aforementioned concerns demands more attention from researchers, if one is to provide quality patient care.

Moreover, the idea of using existing high quality studies is a logical and intuitively appealing concept; our experience suggests that it is not a foregone conclusion [1]. For example, systematic reviews in the form of overviews or meta-analysis are considered the most reliable method for summarizing large volumes of research evidence and they are recognized as the highest level of research evidence [2, 24, 27, 28, 31]. However, if researchers did not master the method of performing systematic reviews, these reviews, especially those that are meta-analyses, could be misused easily and could produce inaccurate, biased, or misleading outcomes.

Our previous work identified systematic reviews comparing surgical and nonsurgical TMJD treatment and evaluated their methodological quality and the evidence grade within the systematic reviews [1]. The search strategy identified 211 reports; of which two were systematic. In these systematic reviews, between 9 and 15% of the trials were graded as high quality, and 2 and 8% of the total number of patients were involved in these studies. The results indicated that in spite of the widespread impact of TMJD, and the multitude of potential interventions, clinicians have expended sparse attention to systematically implementing and evaluating clinical trial methodology that would improve validity and reliability of outcome measures.

The most troubling aspect of these findings involves the ethics of trials that do not meet international standards of conduct, and the care of patients that is not based on high levels of evidence. The potential implication of this failing is clearest to understand in terms of the U.S. Supreme Court ruling in Daubert v. Merrell Dow. In this case, the Supreme Court applied the Federal Rules of Evidence for causality of harm, based on the highest level of evidence. This ruling supplanted the common-law test of Frye v. United States, which based rulings on local practice customs [1]. Thus one might imagine that legal suits could arise from the application of trial methodology or clinical practice that does not meet international standards.

12.7 Conclusions

Within the limitations of this analysis, there is an imbalance in the distribution of publications, clinical trials, and systematic reviews. This raises two concerns. First, there are few high quality studies to base clinical care on, and second, there is a clear need for considerably more attempts to identify knowledge gaps in the TMJD literature. Our analysis suggests the following as potential topics for new high quality studies: TMJ internal derangement, TMJ ankylosis surgical treatment, TMJ electromyography, and surgical treatment of condylar fractures.

References

1. Bessa-Nogueira RV, Vasconcelos BC, Niederman R (2008) The methodological quality of systematic reviews comparing temporomandibular joint disorder surgical and nonsurgical treatment. BMC Oral Health 8:27
2. Carr AB (2002) Systematic reviews of the literature: the overview and meta-analysis. Dent Clin North Am 46:79–86
3. Cavalcanti do Egito Vasconcelos B, Bessa-Nogueira RV, Rocha NS (2006) Temporomandibular joint arthrocentesis: evaluation of results and review of the literature. Braz J Otorhinolaryngol 72:634–638
4. Coiera E, Walther M, Nguyen K et al (2005) Architecture for knowledge-based and federated search of online clinical evidence. J Med Internet Res 7:e52
5. Deshazo JP, Lavallie DL, Wolf FM (2009) Publication trends in the medical informatics literature: 20 years of "Medical Informatics" in MeSH. BMC Med Inform Decis Mak 9:7
6. Dimitroulis G (1998) Temporomandibular disorders: a clinical update. BMJ 317:190–194
7. Dolwick MF (2007) Temporomandibular joint surgery for internal derangement. Dent Clin North Am 51:195–208, vii–viii
8. Dworkin SF, LeResche L (1992) Research diagnostic criteria for temporomandibular disorders: review, criteria, examinations and specifications, critique. J Craniomandib Disord 6:301–355
9. Dworkin SF, Huggins KH, LeResche L et al (1990) Epidemiology of signs and symptoms in temporomandibular disorders: clinical signs in cases and controls. J Am Dent Assoc 120:273–281
10. Ernst E, White AR (1999) Acupuncture as a treatment for temporomandibular joint dysfunction: a systematic review of randomized trials. Arch Otolaryngol Head Neck Surg 125:269–272
11. Forssell H, Kalso E, Koskela P et al (1999) Occlusal treatments in temporomandibular disorders: a qualitative systematic review of randomized controlled trials. Pain 83:549–560

12. Fricton J (2006) Current evidence providing clarity in management of temporomandibular disorders: summary of a systematic review of randomized clinical trials for intra-oral appliances and occlusal therapies. J Evid Based Dent Pract 6:48–52

13. Garfield E (1964) "Science citation index"–a new dimension in indexing. Science 144:649–654

14. Garfield E (1972) Citation analysis as a tool in journal evaluation. Science 178:471–479

15. Greene CS (1995) Etiology of temporomandibular disorders. Semin Orthod 1:222–228

16. Greene CS (2001) The etiology of temporomandibular disorders: implications for treatment. J Orofac Pain 15:93–105; discussion 106–116

17. Haynes RB, McKibbon KA, Wilczynski NL et al (2005) Optimal search strategies for retrieving scientifically strong studies of treatment from medline: analytical survey. BMJ 330:1179

18. Lewison G, Devey ME (1999) Bibliometric methods for the evaluation of arthritis research. Rheumatology (Oxford) 38:13–20

19. Madland G, Feinmann C (2001) Chronic facial pain: a multidisciplinary problem. J Neurol Neurosurg Psychiatry 71:716–719

20. Makofsky HW, August BF, Ellis JJ (1989) A multidisciplinary approach to the evaluation and treatment of temporomandibular joint and cervical spine dysfunction. Cranio 7:205–213

21. Mavropoulos A, Kiliaridis S (2003) Orthodontic literature: an overview of the last 2 decades. Am J Orthod Dentofacial Orthop 124:30–40

22. McNeely ML, Armijo Olivo S, Magee DJ (2006) A systematic review of the effectiveness of physical therapy interventions for temporomandibular disorders. Phys Ther 86:710–725

23. Montori VM, Wilczynski NL, Morgan D et al (2005) Optimal search strategies for retrieving systematic reviews from medline: analytical survey. BMJ 330:68

24. Mulrow CD (1994) Rationale for systematic reviews. BMJ 309:597–599

25. Popowich K, Nebbe B, Major PW (2003) Effect of Herbst treatment on temporomandibular joint morphology: a systematic literature review. Am J Orthod Dentofacial Orthop 123:388–394

26. Price DJ (1965) Networks of scientific papers. Science 149:510–515

27. Sackett DL (1993) Rules of evidence and clinical recommendations for the management of patients. Can J Cardiol 9:487–489

28. Sackett DL, Straus SE, Richardson WS et al (2000) Evidence-based medicine: how to practice and teach EBM. Churchill Livingstone, Edinburgh

29. Shi Z, Guo C, Awad M (2003) Hyaluronate for temporomandibular joint disorders. Cochrane Database Syst Rev (1):CD002970

30. Stohler CS, Zarb GA (1999) On the management of temporomandibular disorders: a plea for a low-tech, high-prudence therapeutic approach. J Orofac Pain 13:255–261

31. Sutherland SE, Matthews DC (2004) Conducting systematic reviews and creating clinical practice guidelines in dentistry: lessons learned. J Am Dent Assoc 135:747–753

32. Tanaka E, Detamore MS, Mercuri LG (2008) Degenerative disorders of the temporomandibular joint: etiology, diagnosis, and treatment. J Dent Res 87:296–307

33. Turp JC, Motschall E, Schindler HJ et al (2007) In patients with temporomandibular disorders, do particular interventions influence oral health-related quality of life? A qualitative systematic review of the literature. Clin Oral Implants Res 18(Suppl 3):127–137

34. Turp JC, Jokstad A, Motschall E et al (2007) Is there a superiority of multimodal as opposed to simple therapy in patients with temporomandibular disorders? A qualitative systematic review of the literature. Clin Oral Implants Res 18(Suppl 3):138–150

35. Yang S, Needleman H, Niederman R (2001) A bibliometric analysis of the pediatric dental literature in MEDLINE. Pediatr Dent 23:415–418

The Efficacy of Horizontal and Vertical Bone Augmentation Procedures for Dental Implants: A Cochrane Systematic Review[1]

13

Marco Esposito, Maria Gabriella Grusovin, Pietro Felice, Georgios Karatzopoulos, Helen V. Worthington, and Paul Coulthard

Core Message

> Some patients may have insufficient bone to place dental implants, but there are many surgical techniques to increase the bone volume making implant treatment possible. Short implants appear to be more effective and cause fewer complications than conventional implants placed in resorbed lower jaws augmented with autogenous bone or bone substitutes (cow bone blocks). Bone can be regenerated in a horizontal and vertical direction using various techniques, but it is unclear which techniques are preferable. Complications especially for augmenting bone vertically are frequent. Some bone substitutes may cause less complications and pain than autogenous bone. Osteodistraction osteogenesis allows for more vertical bone augmentation than other techniques, which, on the other hand, can allow for horizontal augmentation at the same time.

> This review is based on a Cochrane systematic review entitled "Interventions for replacing missing teeth: horizontal and vertical bone augmentation techniques for dental implant treatment" published in The Cochrane Library (see www.cochrane.org for information). Cochrane systematic reviews are regularly updated to include new research and in response to comments and criticisms from readers. If you wish to comment on this review, please send your comments to the Cochrane website or to Marco Esposito. The Cochrane Library should be consulted for the most recent version of the review. The results of a Cochrane Review can be interpreted differently, depending on people's perspectives and circumstances. Please consider the conclusions presented carefully. They are the opinions of the review authors, and are not necessarily shared by the Cochrane Collaboration.

M. Esposito (✉)
G. Karatzopoulos
Oral and Maxillofacial Surgery,
School of Dentistry, The University of Manchester,
Higher Cambridge Street, Manchester,
M15 6FH Manchester, UK
e-mail: espositomarco@hotmail.com

M.G. Grusovin
The University of Manchester, Manchester,
UK and private practice, Gorizia, Italy

P. Felice
Department of Oral and Dental Sciences,
University of Bologna, Bologna, Italy

H.V. Worthington
P. Coulthard
Cochrane Oral Health Group, School of Dentistry,
The University of Manchester, Manchester, UK

[1]This paper is based on a Cochrane Review published in The Cochrane Library 2009, Issue 4 (see www.thecochranelibrary.com for information). Cochrane Reviews are regularly updated as new evidence emerges and in response to feedback, and The Cochrane Library should be consulted for the most recent version of the review.
Conflict-of-interest statement: Pietro Felice and Marco Esposito are among the authors of some of the included trials; however, they were not involved in the quality assessment of these trials.

13.1 Background

Missing teeth and supporting oral tissues have traditionally been replaced with dentures or bridges permitting restoration of chewing function, speech and aesthetics. Dental implants offer an alternative. These implants are inserted into the jawbones to support a dental prostheses and are retained because of the intimacy of bone growth onto their surface. This direct structural and functional connection between living bone and implant surface, termed osseointegration, was first described by Brånemark [5] and has undoubtedly been one of the most significant scientific breakthroughs in dentistry over the past 40 years.

Teeth may have been lost through dental disease or trauma or may be congenitally absent. In addition, teeth may be lost as part of a surgical procedure to resect part of a jaw because of pathology such as cancer. Sometimes, there is a lack of supporting bone in addition to the absent teeth due to atrophy, trauma, failure to develop or surgical resection. Dental implants can only be placed if there is sufficient bone to adequately stabilise them, and bone augmentation permits implant treatment that would otherwise not be an option for some of these patients. Bone augmentation procedures may be carried out some time prior to implant placement (two-stage procedure), or at the same time as implant placement (one-stage procedure), using various materials and techniques. When carried out prior to placement, this necessitates an additional surgical episode and then the area is left to heal for a period of time before the implants are placed.

There are different indications, numerous alternative techniques and various "biologically active" agents and biomaterials currently used to augment bone. Some materials used to augment the bone volume may be described as follows:

Autogenous bone grafts: these are bone grafts taken from an adjacent or remote site in the same patient and used to build up the deficient area and are considered to be the material of choice, i.e. the "gold standard". They are biologically compatible as they are from the same patient and provide a scaffold into which new bone may grow. Sites from within the mouth may be used for relatively small graft requirements or sites such as the iliac crest for larger bone volumes. All of these require surgery at a second site, and therefore, the morbidity must be considered. Of the many possible sites, each has its own merits and disadvantages. Sometimes, it may be possible to recycle bone taken from the site of implant placement when preparing the hole also by using a special filter to collect bone particles that would otherwise be lost and use this to build up a deficient area.

Allografts: these are bone grafts harvested from cadavers and processed by methods such as freezing or demineralising and freezing. The grafts are then sterilised and supplied by specially licenced tissue banks in several convenient ways such as bone particles or large blocks. They are resorbable. There may be some concern regarding their absolute non-infectivity.

Xenografts: these are graft materials derived from animals such as cow or coral. Animal bone, usually bovine bone, is processed to completely remove the organic component.

Alloplastic graft materials: these synthetic bone substitutes include calcium phosphates and bioactive glasses. Alloplasts provide a physical framework for bone ingrowth. Some surgeons use these materials in combination with autogenous bone grafts. These materials resorb completely or to some degree or not at all with time.

Barrier membranes for GBR: This technique uses special barrier membranes to protect defects from the ingrowth of soft tissue cells so that bone progenitor cells may develop bone uninhibited. Ingrowth of soft tissue may disturb or totally prevent osteogenesis in a defect or wound. Examples of membrane are expanded polytetrafluoroethylene, porcine collagen and polyglactin. Membranes can be resorbable or non-resorbable.

Bone promoting proteins (BMPs) and platelet rich plasma (PRP): BMPs are a family of proteins naturally present in bone and responsible for activation of bone development [35]. BMPs may encourage bone formation. They may be incorporated into any of the above graft types. Growth factors and PRP are used to promote bone formation.

Some surgical techniques used to augment bone volume include:

Onlay grafting: the graft material is laid over the defective area to increase width or height or both of the alveolar jawbone. The host bed is usually perforated with a small bur to encourage the formation of a blood clot between the graft and recipient bed. The graft is immobilised with screws or plates or with dental implants [20].

Inlay grafting: A section of jawbone is surgically separated and graft material sandwiched between two sections. Le Fort I osteotomy and interpositional bone graft procedure [25] has been used for patients requiring implant treatment [21].

Ridge expansion: the alveolar ridge is split longitudinally and parted to widen it and allow placement of an implant or graft material or both in the void. The longitudinal split can be limited by placing transverse cuts in the bone.

Distraction osteogenesis: the principals of distraction osteogenesis, in which a gradual controlled displacement of a surgically prepared fracture is used to increase bone volume, are not new but have recently been introduced into implant surgery to increase alveolar bone volume. The gap created during the displacement of the bone segment fills with immature non-calcified bone that matures during a subsequent fixation period. The associated soft tissues are also expanded as the bone segment is transported.

Zygomatic implants: a long implant may be placed to the upper jaw passing through the sinus into the body of the zygomatic bone [4]. This surgical technique is an alternative to bone augmentation in those patients with insufficient bone for placement of the usual type of dental implant. This comparison is not included in this review as the zygoma implant technique is not a technique for bone augmentation, but is evaluated in another Cochrane review [13].

Each type of augmentation material may be used in combination with a variety of different surgical techniques, so many permutations of treatment are possible and the situation is rather complicated. In addition, new techniques and "active agents" are continuously introduced in the clinical practise. Particular treatment options have strong proponents with surgeons claiming that a particular material or technique offers improved implant success.

This review will focus exclusively on techniques aimed at augmenting the bone in a horizontal or vertical direction. Several reviews have been published on this topic, though their findings were not based on the most reliable clinical trials; therefore, the information presented has to be interpreted with a great deal of caution [12, 17, 28, 34]. The reader can find information on the procedures for augmenting the maxillary sinus, post-extractive sites, bone fenestrations at implants in the previous version of this review [11]. Information about bone augmentation at implants affected by peri-implantitis can be found in another Cochrane review [10].

13.2 Objectives

To test (a) whether and when horizontal and vertical bone augmentation procedures are necessary and (b) which are the most effective horizontal and vertical bone augmentation techniques.

Augmentation procedures were divided into two broad categories:

1. Horizontal bone augmentation procedures: any technique aimed at making the recipient bone wider or thicker in order to receive dental implants of adequate diameter (usually of a 3.5-mm diameter or wider).
2. Vertical bone augmentation procedures: any technique aimed at making the recipient bone higher in a vertical dimension in order to receive dental implants of adequate length (usually 9 mm or longer). In many instances, a combination of horizontal and vertical bone augmentation is needed and these procedures were included in the vertical augmentation group.

13.3 Materials and Methods

13.3.1 Criteria for Considering Studies for this Review

All RCTs evaluating patients with missing teeth who may require horizontal and/or vertical alveolar bone augmentation prior to or during dental implant placement procedures to allow the placement of osseointegrated dental implants. Any bone augmentation technique, active agent (such as bone morphogenetic proteins, PRP) or biomaterials used in relation with dental implants was considered. For trials to be considered in this review, implants have to be placed and the outcome of the implant therapy has to be reported at least at the endpoint of the abutment connection procedure. The following time points were considered: abutment connection, 1, 3 and 5 years after loading. Outcomes measures were:

- Prosthesis failure: planned prostheses that could not be placed due to implant failure(s) and loss of the prostheses secondary to implant failure(s).
- Implant failure: implant mobility and removal of stable implants dictated by progressive marginal

bone loss or infection (biological failures). Implant mobility could be assessed manually or with instruments such as Periotest (Siemens AG, Benshein, Germany) or resonance frequency (Osstell, Integration Diagnostics, Göteborg, Sweden).

- Augmentation procedure failure: failure of the augmentation procedure (i.e. of the bone graft or the GBR procedure, etc.) not affecting the success of the implant.
- Major complications at treated/augmented sites (e.g. infection, nerve injury, haemorrhage, etc.).
- Major complications at bone donor sites (e.g. nerve injury, gait disturbance, infection, etc.).
- Patient satisfaction including aesthetics.
- Patient preference including aesthetics (only in split-mouth trials).
- Bone gain vertically or horizontally or both expressed in mm or percentage, including bone level changes over time.
- Aesthetics evaluated by dentist.
- Duration of the treatment time starting from the first intervention to the functional loading of the implants.
- Treatment costs.

Trials evaluating only histological outcomes were not considered in this review.

13.3.2 Search Strategy for Identification of Studies

For the identification of studies included or considered for this review, detailed search strategies were developed for each database searched. For more details, see the original Cochrane review [9]. The following databases were searched:

- The Cochrane Oral Health Group's Trials Register (to 9 January 2009)
- The CENTRAL (The Cochrane Library 2008, Issue 4)
- MEDLINE (1966 to 21 January 2009)
- EMBASE (1980 to 12 January 2009)

The most recent electronic search was undertaken on 21 January 2009. Several dental journals were hand searched up to January 2009. There were no language restrictions. All the authors of the identified RCTs were contacted, the bibliographies of all identified RCTs and relevant review articles were checked, and personal contacts were used in an attempt to identify

unpublished or ongoing RCTs. In the first version of this review, more than 55 oral implant manufacturers and an Internet discussion group (implantology@ yahoogroups.com) were contacted; however, this was discontinued due to poor yield.

Study selection and data extraction.

The titles and abstracts (when available) of all reports identified through the electronic searches were scanned independently by two review authors. For studies appearing to meet the inclusion criteria, or for which there were insufficient data in the title and abstract to make a clear decision, the full report was obtained. The full reports obtained from all the electronic and other methods of searching were assessed independently by two review authors to establish whether the studies met the inclusion criteria or not. Disagreements were resolved by discussion. Where resolution was not possible, a third review author was consulted. All studies meeting the inclusion criteria then underwent validity assessment and data extraction. Studies rejected at this or subsequent stages were recorded in the table of excluded studies, and reasons for exclusion recorded.

Data were extracted by two review authors independently using specially designed data extraction forms. The data extraction forms were piloted on several papers and modified as required before use. Any disagreement was discussed and a third review author consulted where necessary. All authors were contacted for clarification or missing information. Data were excluded until further clarification was available if agreement could not be reached. For each trial, the following data were recorded: year of publication, country of origin and source of study funding; details of the participants including demographic characteristics; details on the type of intervention; details of the outcomes reported, including method of assessment and time intervals.

13.3.3 Quality Assessment

Three main quality criteria were examined as follows:

1. Allocation concealment, recorded as adequate, unclear and inadequate.

Allocation concealment was considered adequate if it was centralised (e.g. allocation by a central office unaware of subject characteristics); pharmacy-controlled randomisation; pre-numbered or coded identical containers which were administered serially to participants; on-site computer system combined with allocation kept in a locked unreadable computer file that can be accessed only after the characteristics of an enrolled patient have been entered; sequentially numbered, sealed, opaque envelopes; and other approaches similar to those listed above, along with the reassurance that the person who generated the allocation scheme did not administer it. Some schemes may be innovative and not fit any of the approaches above, but still provide adequate conceal-ment. Approaches to allocation concealment which were considered clearly inadequate included any procedure that was entirely transparent before allocation, such as an open list of random numbers. Ideally, the surgeon should have known the group allocation just after implants were inserted. Those articles or authors stating that allocation concealment procedures were implemented, but did not provide details on how this was accomplished, were coded as "unclear".

2. Treatment blind to outcome assessors, recorded as yes, no, unclear, and not possible.
3. Completeness of follow-up (is there a clear expla-nation for withdrawals and drop outs in each treat-ment group?) assessed as: Yes (in the case that clear explanations for drop outs were given, a further subjective evaluation of the risk of bias assessing the reasons for the drop out was made) and No.

After taking into account the additional information provided by the authors of the trials, studies were grouped into the following categories:

(a) Low risk of bias (plausible bias unlikely to seri-ously alter the results) if all criteria were met.
(b) High risk of bias (plausible bias that seriously weakens confidence in the results) if one or more criteria were not met.

Further quality assessment was carried out to assess sample size calculations, definition of exclusion/inclu-sion criteria and comparability of control and test groups at entry. The quality assessment criteria were pilot tested using several articles.

13.3.4 Data Synthesis

For dichotomous outcomes, the estimates of effect of an intervention were expressed as odds ratios (OR) together with 95% CIs. For continuous outcomes, mean differences and standard deviations (SDs) were used to summarise the data for each group together with 95% CIs. The statistical unit was the patient and not the aug-mentation procedure or the implant. A meta-analysis was done only if there were studies of similar compari-sons reporting the same outcome measures. Odds ratios were combined for dichotomous data, and mean differ-ences for continuous data, using random-effects models.

The significance of any discrepancies in the esti-mates of the treatment effects from the different trials was to be assessed by means of Cochran's test for het-erogeneity and the I^2 statistic, which describes the per-centage total variation across studies that is due to heterogeneity rather than chance. Clinical heterogene-ity was to be assessed by examining the types of partici-pants and interventions for all outcomes in each study.

13.4 Results

Of the 19 potentially eligible trials [1–3, 7, 8, 14–16, 18, 19, 22, 23, 26, 27, 29–31, 33, 36], four were excluded because they reported only histological outcomes without reporting any implant related outcomes, one because it was just a research protocol presenting only histological outcomes and one because it presented the data of the various group combined [1, 2, 19, 29, 31, 36].

Of the 13 included trials, eight were conducted in Italy and five in the Netherlands [3, 7, 8, 14–16, 18, 22, 23, 26, 27, 30, 33].

Nine trials had a parallel group study design and four had a split-mouth design [15, 18, 26, 27]. One study included one patient treated bilaterally, and only data from a randomly selected side were included in this review [3].

For six trials it was declared that support was received from industry directly involved in the product being tested also in the form of free material [14, 15, 22, 26, 27, 33]. One trial received support from the implant manufacturer; however, the trial was not designed to test the implants, but the augmentation techniques [23]. The authors of six trials declared that no support was received from commercial parties whose products were being tested in the trials [3, 7, 8, 16, 18, 30].

Eleven trials were conducted at university, hospital, or specialist dental clinics and two trials in private practices [14, 23].

13.4.1 Characteristics of the Interventions

The following interventions were tested:
Different techniques for horizontal bone augmentation.

13.4.1.1 Is Horizontal Augmentation Necessary? (No Trial)

13.4.1.2 Which is the most effective horizontal augmentation technique? (three trials)

- Two-stage sinus lift with autogenous blocks and particulate bone together with buccal onlays mono-cortico-cancellous bone grafts, to reconstruct the width of the maxilla, fixed with titanium screws harvested from the iliac crest with or without PRP left to heal for 3 months in a split-mouth trial [27]. Barriers were not used. PRP was made using the Platelet Concentration Collection System kit (PCCS kit, 3i Implant Innovations Inc. Palm Beach Gardens, FL, USA). Fifty-four millilitre of blood were mixed with 6 mL of anti-coagulant (citrate dextrose) and processed with the platelet concentration system. To promote the release of growth factors from the platelets, 10% calcium chloride solution and the patient's serum, as a source of autologous thrombin, were added before actual reconstruction of the defect with the bone graft. The resulting gel was mixed with the bone graft and some gel was applied at the closure of the wound at the side treated with PRP. Three implants were inserted into the healed graft of each side and were left to heal for additional 6 months. All the augmentation procedures were performed under general anaesthesia. Surgical templates were used to optimise implant insertion. All implants were turned titanium self-tapping (Nobel Biocare, Göteborg, Sweden) and were rehabilitated with two implant supported prostheses.
- Two-stage buccal onlays monocortico-cancellous bone grafts fixed with two titanium (diameter 1.5 mm, Martin Medizin Technik, Tuttlingen, Germany) or resorbable poly (D,L-lactide) acid (PDLLA, diameter 2.1 mm, Resorb X, Martin Medizin Technik) screws in a split-mouth trial, to reconstruct the width of the maxilla [26]. Grafts were covered with resorbable barriers (Bio-Gide,

Geistlich Pharmaceutical, Wolhusen, Switzerland). Grafts were harvested from the iliac crest and bilateral sinus lifts were performed at the same time with autogenous blocks and particulate bone. After 3 months, implants were inserted into the healed graft of each side and were left to heal for an additional 6 months. All the augmentation procedures were performed under general anaesthesia. Surgical templates were used to optimise implant insertion. All implants were turned titanium self-tapping (Nobel Biocare, Göteborg, Sweden) and were rehabilitated with implant supported overdentures.

- Three different techniques to horizontally augment local ridge maxillary defects (from first to first premolars) for allowing placement of single implants were tested (25): (1) bone graft from the chin, (2) bone graft from the chin with a resorbable barrier (Bio-Gide, Geistlich Pharma, Wolhusen, Switserland) and (3) 100% bovine anorganic bone (Bio-Oss, spongiosa granules of 0.25–1 mm, Geistlich Pharma) with a Bio-Gide resorbable barrier. The cortical bone of the recipient sites was perforated to create a bleeding bone surface and to open the cancellous bone. Bone blocks from the chin were fixed with a 1.5-mm diameter titanium screw (Martin Medizin Technik, Tuttlingen, Germany) and particulate bone from the chin was placed around the fixed bone grafts. Implants were placed 3 months after autogenous bone grafting and 6 months after augmenting sites with Bio-Oss. Single ITI-EstheticPlus implants (Institute Straumann AG, Waldenburg, Switserland) were placed using templates and left healing submerged for 6 months. On the day of uncovering, provisional single crowns were screwed on the implants and were replaced 1 month later by final porcelain crowns with a zirconium oxide core (Procera, Nobel Biocare, Göteborg, Sweden).

13.4.2 Different Techniques for Vertical Bone Augmentation

13.4.2.1 Is Vertical Augmentation Necessary? (Two Trials)

- One trial addressed the issue of which is the best treatment alternative to provide an overdenture to patients with a resorbed mandible, i.e. symphyseal height 6–12 mm measured on lateral radiographs [33]. Three procedures were tested: (1) installation of four short implants (8 or 11 mm) left to heal for 3 months; (2) mandibular augmentation with an autologous bone graft from the iliac crest and (3) transmandibular Bosker implants. We were only interested in the former two procedures. Mandibles were augmented under general anaesthesia using the interpositional technique. In brief, the mandible was sectioned in the interforaminal area, and a bone block taken from the anterior ilium was positioned between the two segments that were stabilised with osteosynthesis wires and left to heal for 3 months. The wires were then removed, and four 13–18 mm long implants were placed and left to heal for an additional 3 months. Patients were not allowed to wear their dentures for the entire healing period (about 6 months). The short implants used were Twin Plus IMZ implants (Friatec, Mannheim, Germany), whereas the augmented mandibles were treated with four specially designed IMZ apical screw implants. No explanation was given why two different types of implants were used. Patients were rehabilitated with overdentures supported by an egg-shaped triple bar with a Dolder-clip retention system. The bars did not have cantilever extensions.

- One trial compared the 7 mm short implants vs. 10 mm or longer implants placed in atrophic posterior mandibles augmented with a bone substitute block (Bio-Oss, Geistlch Pharma, Wolhusen, Switserland) placed according to an inlay technique (32). Posterior mandibles with 7–8 mm of bone height above the mandibular canal and a width of at least 5.5 mm as measured on CT scans were treated under local anaesthesia. In brief, after a paracrestal buccal incision, a horizontal osteotomy was made 2–4 mm above the mandibular canal. Two oblique cuts were made, the bone segment was raised sparing the lingual periosteum and a Bio-Oss block was modelled and positioned between the two segments that were stabilised with osteosynthesis miniplates, covered with a resorbable membrane (Bio-Gide, Geistlch Pharma) and left to heal for 5 months. Patients were not allowed to wear their removable prostheses for 1 month after the augmentation procedure. Two to three implants (NanoTite, parallel walled, with external connection, Biomet 3i, Palm Beach, FL, USA) were placed 0.6 mm supracrestally and left to heal for 4 months in both groups.

Provisional screw-retained acrylic restorations were delivered and replaced after 4 months by screw-retained metal-ceramic restorations.

13.4.2.2 Which is the Most Effective Vertical Augmentation Technique? (Eight Trials)

- Vertical GBR with non-resorbable titanium-reinforced ePTFE barriers (Gore-Tex, WL Gore and Associates, Inc., Flagstone, USA) supported by particulate autogenous bone harvested from the mandibular ramus and when the bone was not sufficient also from the chin (two patients) vs. vertical distraction osteogenesis [7]. Two different vertical GBR procedures were used: six patients were treated with a one-stage approach (implants were inserted protruding 2–7 mm from the bone level and the augmentation procedure was performed on the same occasion; the abutment connection was performed after 6–7 months), whereas five patients were treated with a two-stage approach (first the bone at site was augmented, and after healing of 6–7 months, the implants were placed and left submerged for an additional 3–5 months). The two-stage approach was used when the risk of insufficient primary implant stability of implants was subjectively expected. With the two-stage approach one or two titanium miniscrews were used as additional support for the titanium-reinforced barriers. All barriers were stabilised with titanium fixating pins (Frios, Friadent GmbH, Mannheim, Germany) or miniscrews (Gebrüder Martin GmbH & Co., Tuttlingen, Germany) or both. The distraction procedure was accomplished by using osteodistractors (Gebrüder Martin GmbH & Co.) fixed to the bone segments with 1.5 mm large titanium screws. The distraction devices were activated after 1 week, twice a day (0.5 mm every 12 h) until the desired amount of distraction was obtained (4–9 mm). The bone segments were then left to consolidate for 2–3 months, the osteodistractors were then removed and dental implants placed and left submerged for 3–6 months. The augmentation procedures were performed under local anaesthesia, local anaesthesia with intravenous sedation and general anaesthesia according to operator and patient preferences. Surgical templates were used to optimise implant insertion. Two implant systems were used: Brånemark Mark III implants (Nobel Biocare, Göteborg, Sweden) in 19 patients and ITI SLA implants (Institute Straumann AG, Waldenburg, Switzerland) in two patients. The choice of two different implant systems was dictated by the system used by the referring dentists. All patients were rehabilitated with screw-retained metal-ceramic fixed prostheses.

- Autogenous onlay bone grafts harvested from the mandibular ramus vs. vertical distraction osteogenesis to vertically augment deficient mandibles [8]. Patients were grafted with a two-stage approach: first bone blocks were fixed with 1.5 mm diameter miniscrews (Gebrüder Martin GmbH & Co., Tuttlingen, Germany). Empty spaces were filled with cancellous bone chips. In case of severe vertical resorption, grafts were assembled in a multi-layered fashion. No barriers were used. Bone grafts were harvested from the mandibular ramus of the same side of reconstruction in six patients, while in two patients, where larger defects were present, bone was harvested bilaterally. After 4–5 months, implants were placed and left submerged for an additional 3–4 months. The distraction procedure was accomplished by using osteodistractors (Gebrüder Martin GmbH & Co.) fixed to the bone segments with 1.5 mm large titanium screws. The distraction devices were activated after 1 week, twice a day (0.5 mm every 12 h) until the desired amount of distraction was obtained (2–7 mm). The bone segments were then left to consolidate for 2–3 months, the osteodistractors were then removed and dental implants placed and left submerged for 3–4 months. The augmentation procedures were performed under local anaesthesia, local anaesthesia with intravenous sedation and general anaesthesia according to operator and patient preferences. Surgical templates were used to optimise implant insertion. ITI SLA implants (Institute Straumann AG, Waldenburg, Switzerland) were used. All patients were rehabilitated with screw-retained metal-ceramic fixed prostheses.

- One-stage vertical GBR using particulate autogenous bone harvested from intraoral locations covered with non-resorbable titanium-reinforced ePTFE barriers (Gore-Tex, WL Gore and Associates, Inc., Flagstone, USA), stabilised with miniscrews, vs. osteosynthesis plates (Gebrüder Martin GmbH & Co., Tuttlingen, Germany), appropriately adapted

and fixed with miniscrews, supporting resorbable collagen barriers (Bio-Gide®, Geistlich Pharma AG, Wolhusen, Switzerland) [23]. The augmentation procedures were performed under local anaesthesia or local anaesthesia with intravenous sedation according to operator and patient preferences. XiVe®S CELLplus (Friadent GmbH, Mannheim, Germany) implants were used. All patients were rehabilitated with provisional resin fixed prostheses replaced then by metal-ceramic definitive prostheses. One implant from each patient was used for the statistical calculations.

- Autogenous inlay bone grafts harvested from the iliac crest vs. distraction osteogenesis to vertically augment deficient posterior mandibles [3]. Patients were grafted with a two-stage approach: first a monocortical bone block was interposed between the basal bone and an osteotomised segment raised coronally without flap elevation at the lingual side to preserve blood supply and fixed with titanium miniplates and miniscrews (KLS Martin, Tuttlingen, Germany). No barriers were used. After 3–4 months, miniplates were removed and implants were placed and left submerged for 3–4 months. The distraction procedure was accomplished by using osteodistractors of various brands (Track by KLS Martin, Al-Mar by Cizeta, LactoSorb by Wakterl Lorenz Surgical, the latter being a resorbable device) fixed to the bone segments with various titanium or resorbable screws. The distraction devices were activated after 1 week, twice a day (0.5–1 mm/day for 5–7 days) until the desired amount of distraction was obtained (7–15 mm). In two cases a prosthetic device was used to avoid lingual tipping. The bone segments were then left to consolidate for 3–4 months, the osteodistractors were removed and dental implants placed and left submerged for 3/4 months. All augmentation procedures were performed under general anaesthesia. Dental implants of several brands were used (A-Z implant, Biohorizons, Biomet 3i, Friadent, Nobel Biocare). All patients were rehabilitated with partial provisional prostheses for 14–16 months until definitive prostheses were delivered.

- Autogenous inlay bone grafts harvested from the iliac crest vs. blocks of anorganic bovine bone (Bio-Oss®, Geistlich Pharma AG, Wolhusen, Switzerland) for vertically augmenting deficient posterior mandibles [15]. Patients were grafted with a two-stage approach: first a monocortical bone block was interposed between the basal bone and an osteotomised segment raised coronally without flap elevation at the lingual side to preserve blood supply and fixed with titanium miniplates and miniscrews (KLS Martin, Tuttlingen, Germany) and covered with a resorbable barrier (Bio-Gide®, Geistlich Pharma AG). The contra-lateral side was treated with a similar technique, but using a Bio-Oss bone block instead. The removable prostheses were allowed for 1 month after the augmentation procedure. After 4 months, miniplates were removed and implants were placed and left submerged for 4 months. All augmentation procedures were performed under general anaesthesia and patients remained hospitalised for 3 days. Dental implants of three different brands were used (Nanotite Biomet 3i cylindrical implants with external connection, Ankylos and XiVe Dentsply-Friadent implants). All patients were rehabilitated with fixed partial provisional acrylic prostheses for 4 months until definitive metal-ceramic fixed prostheses were delivered.

- Two-stage vertical GBR using non-resorbable titanium-reinforced ePTFE barriers (Gore-Tex, WL Gore and Associates, Inc., Flagstone, USA), stabilised with miniscrews, comparing particulate autogenous bone harvested from the retromolar area with trephine drills and subsequently particulated with a bone mill vs. an allograft made of malleable allogenic bone matrix (Regenaform, Regeneration Technologies, Alachua, FL, USA) [18]. This allograft is a combination of assayed demineralized bone matrix (DFDBA) with cortico-cancellous bone chips uniformly dispersed in a termoplastic biological carrier which became malleable when warmed between 43 and 49°. The augmentation procedures were performed under local anaesthesia with sedative pre-medication half an hour prior to surgery. Two mini-implants were used as "poles" to support the barrier. They were placed to protrude for the required height. One pole was a stainless steel mini-screw (6–12 mm long; Ace Dental Implant System, Brockton, MA, USA), and the other was an immediate provisional implant (IPI, Steri-Oss, Nobel Biocare, Göteborg, Sweden). This micro-implant (2 mm in diameter and 10 mm in length) was removed at implant installation with a 4-mm diameter trephine bur for histological examination. Several drill holes were made on the cortical

bone to ensure bleeding. After 6 months of submerged healing, the barriers and the mini-implant were removed and Brånemark MK III (Nobel Biocare) implants with a TiUnite surface were placed. After 5 month of healing, implant stability was tested and abutments were placed.

- Ultrasound or placebo were applied using a sonic-accelerated fracture-healing system (SAFHS model 2000, Smith and Nephew, Memphis, TN, USA) by patients subjected to vertical osteodistraction osteogenesis in the anterior mandible when active osteodistraction was initiated after a latency period of about 5 days [30]. Ultrasound self-treatment involved a daily treatment of 20 min for about 50 days on the skin of the chin covering the osteodistraction gap using 1.5 MHz pressure wave in pulses of 200 µs. Between pulses there was an 800-µs pause (on:off period > 1:4). Patient compliance was monitored by a memory chip inside the ultrasound equipment. Six weeks post-distraction, the distraction devices were removed and two 12 mm long ITI Bonefit implants (Straumann AG, Waldenburg, Switserland) were inserted and left to heal for 3 months before being loaded with an overdenture.

- Inlays vs. onlays autogenous bone grafts harvested from the iliac crest to vertically augment deficient posterior mandibles [16]. Patients were grafted with a two-stage approach: a monocortical bone block was either interposed between the basal bone and the osteotomised segment raised coronally without flap elevation at the lingual side to preserve blood supply or placed as an onlay. Grafts were fixed with titanium miniplates or miniscrews (Gebrüder Martin GmbH & Co, Tuttlingen, Germany). The grafted areas were covered with resorbable barriers (Bio-Gide®, Geistlich Pharma AG). All augmentation procedures were performed under general anaesthesia. Patients were instructed not to wear removable prostheses for 1 month after the augmentation procedure. After 3–4 months miniplates/screws were removed and two dental implants were placed and left submerged for 4 months. Dental implants of several brands were used (Biomet 3i and XiVe Dentsply-Friadent implants for the inlay group and Astra Tech, Biolok and Alpha Bio implants for the onlay group). All patients were rehabilitated with screw-retained acrylic partial provisional prostheses for 4–5 months until definitive screw-retained prostheses were delivered.

13.4.3 Characteristics of Outcome Measures

- Prosthesis failure [3, 7, 8, 14–16, 18, 22, 23, 26, 27, 30, 33].
- Implant failure [3, 7, 8, 14–16, 18, 22, 23, 26, 27, 30, 33].
- Augmentation procedure failure [3, 7, 8, 14–16, 18, 22, 23, 26, 27, 30, 33].
- Major complications at augmented site [3, 7, 8, 14–16, 18, 22, 23, 26, 27, 30, 33].
- Major complications at bone donor site [3, 7, 8, 15, 16, 18, 22, 23, 26, 27, 33].
- Patient satisfaction including aesthetics [22, 33]. We could not use the data of one trial since they were not presented by study groups [22].
- Patient preference including aesthetics (only in split-mouth trials) [15].
- Bone gain vertically or horizontally or both expressed in mm or percentage including bone level changes over time: vertical bone gain was measured in mm by direct measurement in seven studies [3, 7, 8, 15, 16, 18, 23]. Peri-implant marginal bone level changes were assessed in five trials (7, 8, 15, 16, 22), but in three trials (16, 25, 33) data were presented in a way we could not use. One study included different types of implants followed at different follow-up time [16]. The resorption pattern of the mandible after implant insertion was evaluated in one study using the oblique lateral radiographic technique, but insufficient data were presented to enable us to evaluate bone height changes [33].
- Aesthetics assessed by dentist: one trial; however, we could not use the data since they were not presented by study groups [22].
- Duration of the treatment period starting from the first intervention to the functional loading of the implants: all trials.
- Treatment costs: no trials. However, this outcome measure was indirectly extrapolated by us for all trials.

13.4.4 Duration of Follow-Up

- Four-month post-loading [14].
- One-year post-loading [15, 16, 18, 22].
- One-year and half post-loading [3].
- Two-year post-loading [26, 27, 30, 33].
- Three-year post-loading [7, 8, 23].

13.4.5 Risk of Bias in Included Studies

The final quality scoring after having incorporated the additional information kindly provided by the authors of the trials is summarised in Table 13.1. For each

Table 13.1 Risk of bias assessment after having included additional explanations provided by the authors of the included trials

Study	Allocation concealment	Outcome assessor blind	Withdrawals	Risk of bias
Stellingsma et al. [33]	Unclear	No	Yes, reasons given	High
Chiapasco et al. [7]	Inadequate	No	None	High
Raghoebar et al. [27]	Unclear	Yes	None	High
Raghoebar et al. [26]	Unclear	No	None	High
Chiapasco et al. [8]	Adequate	Yes, when possible	None	Low
Meijndert et al. [22]	Unclear	Yes	Yes, reasons given	High
Merli et al. [23]	Adequate	Yes, when possible	None	Low
Bianchi et al. [3]	Adequate	Yes, when possible	None	Low
Felice et al. [15]	Inadequate	Yes, when possible	None	High
Fontana et al. [18]	Adequate	Yes	None	Low
Schortinghuis et al. [30]	Adequate	Yes	None	Low
Felice et al. [14]	Adequate	Yes	None	Low
Felice et al. [16]	Adequate	Yes	None	Low

trial, we assessed whether it was at low or high risk of bias. Seven studies were judged to be at low risk of bias and the remaining at high risk of bias [3, 14, 16, 18, 23, 25, 30].

13.4.6 Allocation Concealment

While assessing the information presented in the articles, allocation concealment was scored adequate for three trials (18, 26, 32), inadequate for one trial (29) and unclear for all other trials. All authors replied to our request for clarification [7, 14, 15, 23]. While evaluating authors' replies, one trial scored as being adequately concealed became not concealed 18; five trials were judged to be properly concealed (24, 28, 30, 31, 33), whereas four trials remained unclear 21, 23, 25, 34 [3, 6–8, 14–16, 18, 23, 26, 27, 30].

13.4.7 Blinding

While assessing the information presented in the articles for the outcome measures of interest in the present review that were possible to be masked, blinding of the outcome assessor was scored as unclear for all trials with five exceptions [15, 22, 23, 27, 30]. Three trials were scored as blinded (21, 25, 31) and two as blinded when possible (26, 29) [15, 22, 23, 27, 30]. All authors replied to our request for clarification. When evaluating authors' replies, the outcome assessors of two trials were considered blinded (30, 33), of three trials blinded when possible (24, 28, 32) since complete blinding was not possible, and those of three trials as not blinded (18, 23, 34) [3, 7, 8, 14, 16, 18, 26, 32].

13.4.8 Completeness of Follow-Up

When assessing the information presented in the articles, information on drop outs was clearly presented in all trials, with one exception [7]. The authors confirmed that there were no withdrawals [7].

13.4.8.1 Main Inclusion Criteria

- Severely resorbed maxillae (classes V–VI according to Cawood with maxillary sinuses having

<5 mm in height of residual alveolar bone with reduced stability and retention of upper dentures) [6, 26, 27].
- Severely resorbed mandibles, i.e. symphyseal height 6–12 mm as measured on standardised lateral radiographs of patients who have been edentulous for at least 2 years and experienced severe functional problems with their lower dentures [32].
- Residual bone height over the mandibular canal of 5–9 mm [3].
- Residual bone height over the mandibular canal of 5–7 mm and bone width of at least 5 mm [15].
- Residual bone height over the mandibular canal of 7–8 mm and bone width of at least 5.5 mm [14].
- Residual bone height over the mandibular canal of at least 4.5–11 mm and bone width of at least 5 mm [16].
- Patients with bilateral posterior mandibular partial edentulism (Applegate-Kennedy Class I) having a defect of more than 3 mm considering the deepest portion of the edentulous ridge in relation to the bone adjacent the last tooth [18].
- Edentulous ridges requiring vertical regeneration [7, 8, 23].
- Horizontal bone deficiency in a maxillary site (incisor, cuspid or first bicuspid) requiring a single implant [22].

13.4.8.2 Main Exclusion Criteria

- Smoking more than 20 cigarettes per day [23].
- Smoking more than 15 cigarettes per day [3, 7, 8, 15].
- Smoking more than ten cigarettes per day [18].
- Smokers [22].
- Intravenous bisphosphonate [14–16].
- Severe knife-edge ridges [3, 7, 8].
- History of reconstructive, pre-prosthetic surgery or previous oral implantology [15, 16, 22, 26, 27].
- Edentulous period less than 3 months [14, 18].
- Edentulous period less than 1 year [26, 27].
- Mucosal disease, such as lichen planus, in the areas to be treated [3, 7, 8, 15, 16].

13.4.9 Sample Size

A priori calculation for the sample size was undertaken in three trials [14, 15, 23]. The calculation of one trial was based on the complications that occurred in

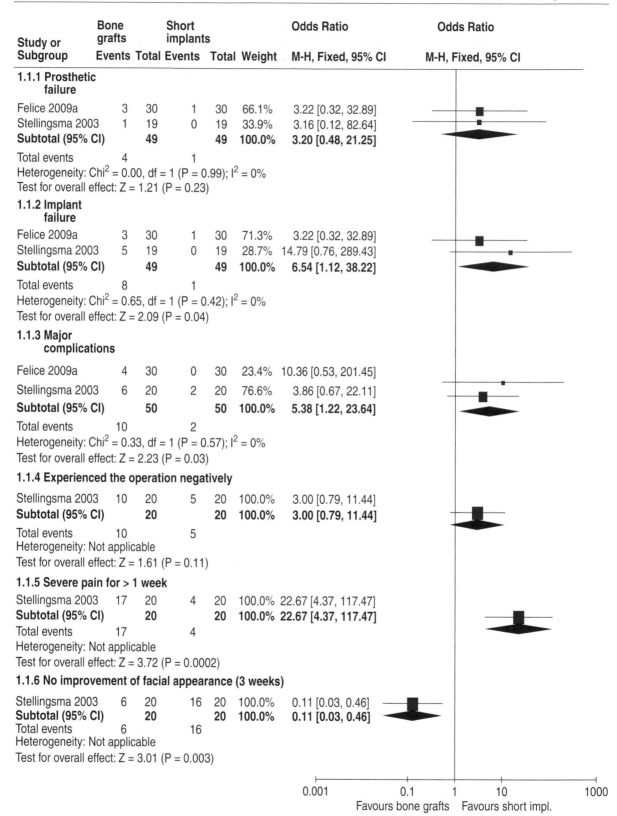

Fig. 13.1 Forest plots illustrating the meta-analysis of two trials comparing short implants vs. augmentation of the mandible. Shot implants had statistically less implant failures and complications than longer implants placed in augmented mandibles

occurred. Two augmentation procedures were considered a complete failure because the planned augmentation was not obtained and 7 mm short implants had to be used instead of the planned 10 mm or longer implants. These graft failures were associated with the fracture of the Bio-Oss blocks at the augmentation procedure. In the augmented group three patients lost one implant each vs. one patient in the short implant group and the related prostheses could not be placed when planned; however, all failed implants were successfully replaced and loaded. No statistically significant differences between groups were observed. With respect to cost and treatment time, short implants were loaded about 4 months after initiation of the treatment, whereas longer implants placed in augmented bone about 9 months after treatment start. The cost of one additional surgical intervention and of the Bio-Oss block for patients treated with the augmentation procedure should also be considered. The trial was judged to be at low risk of bias.

The meta-analysis of these two trials for the outcome measures (prostheses failures, implant failures and complications) resulted in statistically significant more implant failures OR > 6.54 (95% CI 1.12–38.22) and complications OR > 5.38 (95% CI 1.22–23.64) in the vertically augmented group (Fig. 13.1) [14, 33].

13.4.11.2 Which is the Most Effective Augmentation Technique? (8 Trials with 118 Patients)

- One trial compared distraction osteogenesis in 11 patients vs. GBR with non-resorbable barriers and particulate autogenous bone grafts taken from the mandibular ramus (if not sufficient also from the chin) in ten patients for vertically augmenting edentulous ridges for 3 years after loading [7]. No patient dropped out. Two complications occurred in two patients of the osteodistraction group: the bone fragment inclined lingually during the distraction phase probably due to the traction on the osteotomized segment by muscle forces of the floor of the mouth. The complications were successfully treated by applying an orthodontic traction until the bone segment consolidated in the desired position. Five complications occurred in four patients of the GBR group: three barrier exposures occurred, one of

which was associated with an infection, and two transient paraesthesiae of the chin area lasting 1 and 4 weeks. Both paraesthesiae were associated with the only two procedures for harvesting bone from the chin. All procedures for harvesting bone from the ramus were complication free. There was no statistically significant difference for complications between the two procedures. No implants or prostheses failed over the 3-year follow-up period. The mean bone gain after the augmentation procedure was reported for both groups, but without explaining how it was recorded or which were the reference points. Also data on peri-implant bone loss were unclear and could not be used. With respect to cost and treatment time, in the GBR group the cost of the barriers and the fixing pins should be considered vs. the cost of the intraoral distractor and related orthodontic therapy when needed. In the osteodistraction group, the time of exposing the implants ranged between 6 and a half months (mandibles) to 9 and a half months (maxillae) and patients were not allowed to use prostheses for about 3 and a half months. In the GBR group, the time of exposing the implants ranged between 6 and 7 months, when implants were placed simultaneously with the GBR procedure, and to 9–12 months, when implants were placed after the ridge had been vertically augmented. Patients were left without removable prostheses for 6–7 months. The trial was judged to be at high risk of bias.

- One trial compared distraction osteogenesis in nine patients vs. autogenous onlay bone grafts taken from the mandibular ramus in eight patients for vertically augmenting mandibular edentulous ridges for 3 years after loading [8]. No patient dropped out. Three complications occurred in three patients of the osteodistraction group: the bone fragment inclined lingually during the distraction phase probably due to the traction on the osteotomized segment by muscle forces of the floor of the mouth. The complications were successfully treated by applying an orthodontic traction until the bone segment consolidated in the desired position. In the third patient, distraction was interrupted before completion because of the impossibility to move further the distracted segment. This was probably caused by an incorrect design of the vertical osteotomic lines. Shorter implants (6 mm instead of the planned 8 mm) could be placed anyway. Four complications occurred in four patients of the bone graft group: three paraesthesiae of the alveolar inferior nerve, two transient but one permanent. In the last patient the graft became exposed and was partially lost. The treatment could be completed anyway using short implants. There was no statistically significant difference for complications between the two groups. No implants or prostheses failed over the 3-year follow-up period. The mean bone gain after the augmentation procedure was 5.3 + 1.58 mm for the osteodistracted sites and 5.0 + 1.07 mm for the grafted sites. No statistically significant differences were observed regarding marginal peri-implant bone loss between groups at 1 and 3 years. Three years after loading, implants in osteodistracted sites lost on average 0.9 mm of peri-implant bone vs. 1.3 mm in grafted sites. With respect to cost and treatment time, in the bone graft group only the cost of the fixing pins should be considered vs. the cost of the intraoral distractor and related orthodontic therapy when needed, making bone grafting cheaper. In the bone graft group, the time occurring for exposing the implants ranged between 8/9 months. Patients were left without removable prostheses for at least 2 months. In the osteodistraction group the time to expose implants was 7/8 months and patients were not allowed to use prostheses for about 3 months. The trial was judged to be at low risk of bias.

- One trial compared one-stage particulate autogenous bone grafts from intraoral locations in 11 patients treated with non-resorbable titanium-reinforced barriers vs. 11 patients treated with resorbable barriers supported by osteosynthesis plates (26). One implant per patient was used for the statistical calculations. No patient dropped out. Four complications occurred in the resorbable group: two abscesses that determined the failure of the grafting procedures, and two minor complications not affecting the outcome of the therapy (barrier exposure without sign of infection, and a swelling suggesting an early infection successfully treated with antibiotics). Five complications occurred in the non-resorbable group: one infection that determined the failure of the graft and three fistulas in three patients. The last complication was lymph nodes swelling 1 month after intervention suggesting an infection that was treated with systemic antibiotics. No study implant failed and all planned prostheses could be delivered. Both treatments resulted in statistically significant vertical bone gain (2.2 mm for the resorbable group and 2.5 mm for the non-resorbable group); however, no statistically significant differences were found among the two procedures (Fig. 13.2). Three years after loading, both groups lost peri-implant bone in a statistically significant way (about 0.5 mm) and there was no difference in bone loss between groups (Fig. 13.2). With respect to cost and treatment time, for the resorbable group the cost of one or two barriers, the osteosynthesis plates and related fixating pins should be considered vs. the cost of a titanium-reinforced barrier and related pins in the non-resorbable group, which could be slightly cheaper. The healing time for both groups was about four

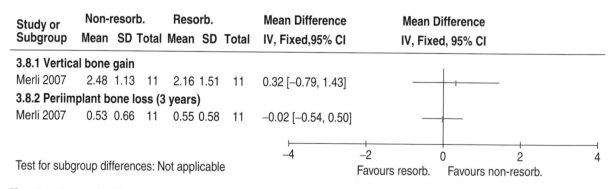

Fig. 13.2 Forest plot illustrating clinical vertical bone gain at abutment connection and radiographic peri-implant bone levels 3 years after loading of two regenerative techniques for vertical augmentation with autogenous bone using non-resorbable titanium-reinforced barrier or resorbable barriers supported by osteosynthesis plates. Both procedures determined a statistically significant gain of bone with no statistical differences among the two techniques. Only about 0.5 mm of peri-implant bone was lost 3 years after loading

and a half months, slightly less than originally planned (5 months), due to premature removal of some infected barriers. The trial was judged to be at low risk of bias.

- One trial compared distraction osteogenesis in five patients vs. autogenous inlay bone grafts taken from the iliac crest in six patients for vertically augmenting mandibular edentulous ridges of 5–9 mm height above the mandibular canal for at least 1 year and half after loading [3]. No patient dropped out. Three complications occurred in the distraction group and one in the inlay group. In the distraction group two patients developed progressive lingual inclination of the distraction segments possibly due to traction by the muscles of the floor of the mouth. Orthodontic traction was applied to avoid consolidation of the distracted segments in an unfavourable position. One patient developed a minor infection at implant insertion time resolved with local debridement. There were no statistically significant differences for complications between groups. In the inlay group recovery of the donor sites was uneventful in all cases with no complications. One patient developed a post-augmentation dehiscence of the distal fixation screw, infection and partial resorption of the cranial segment. This was resolved with local debridement. Those complications did not jeopardise the success of the augmentation procedures. No study implant failed and all planned prostheses could be delivered. Both treatments resulted in vertical bone gain (8.4 mm for the distraction group and 5.1 mm for the inlay group), with osteodistraction gaining statistically more bone (Fig. 13.3). With respect to costs, for the distraction group the cost of the distractor device should be considered vs. the cost of the osteosynthesis plates in the inlay group, which could be slightly cheaper. The time needed to

achieve the desired outcome was similar. The trial was judged to be at low risk of bias.

- One split-mouth trial compared autogenous bone blocks taken from the iliac crest vs. anorganic bovine bone blocks used as inlays in ten patients for vertically augmenting posterior mandibular edentulous ridges of 5–7 mm height above the mandibular canal for 1 year after loading [15]. No patient dropped out. Three complications occurred in three patients: two infections at the sites grafted with autogenous bone, one determining the complete failure of the graft and the other a partial loss of the graft vs. a minor soft tissue dehiscence at a Bio-Oss treated site. Because of the complete failure of one autogenous bone graft, the two planned implants and their prostheses could not be placed. One implant failed in the Bio-Oss group 11 weeks after loading. It was successfully replaced and a new prostheses was made. There were no statistically significant failures for prostheses and implant failures as well as complications. Both treatments resulted in vertical bone gain (6.2 mm for the bone substitute group and 5.1 mm for the autogenous bone group), and the difference of 1.1 mm was not statistically significant. One-year after loading, both groups lost statistically significant peri-implant marginal bone (0.82 mm the autogenous bone group and 0.59 mm the Bio-Oss group), but the 0.21 mm of difference between the two groups was not statistically significant. When asked for their preference 1 month after delivery of the definitive prostheses, eight out of ten patients preferred the bone substitute vs. two patients who had no preference since both interventions were fine for them. This difference was statistically significant (OR > 0.03, 95% CI 0.00–0.64, $p > 0.02$). With respect to costs, the cost of the bone substitutes should be considered vs. the

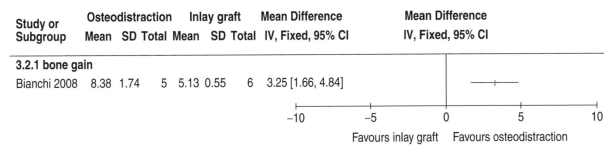

Fig. 13.3 Forest plot comparing osteodistraction with inlay bone grafts for vertically augmenting posterior mandibles. Statistically significant more vertical bone gain was obtained with osteodistraction

need of an additional operation to retrieve autogenous bone for the iliac crest which has to be conducted in general anaesthesia. The time needed to achieve the desired outcome was similar. The trial was judged to be at high risk of bias.

- One split-mouth trial evaluated vertical GBR with titanium-reinforced barriers supported by two "poles" comparing particulate autogenous bone harvested from the retromolar area with a thermoplastic allogenic bone substitute (Regenaform) in five patients for vertically augmenting posterior mandibular edentulous ridges up to 1 year after loading [18]. No patient dropped out. Two complications occurred in one patient, one at each of treated site. The side treated with autogenous bone showed an infection without barrier exposure 2 months after augmentation. The barrier and the small tissue portion affected by the infection were removed. On the contra-lateral side a buccal bone dehiscence developed around one of the implants. It was treated with autogenous bone and a resorbable barrier. Those complications did not jeopardise the success of the augmentation procedures. No study implant failed and all planned prostheses could be delivered. Both treatments resulted in vertical bone gain (4.7 mm for the bone substitute group and 4.1 mm for the autogenous bone group), and the difference of 0.6 mm was statistically significant (Fig. 13.4). With respect to costs, the cost of the bone substitutes should be considered vs. the need of an additional flap operation to retrieve autogenous bone. The time needed to achieve the desired

outcome was similar. The trial was judged to be at low risk of bias.

- One trial evaluated the effect of ultrasounds on vertical distraction osteogenesis in anterior atrophic mandibles [30]. Five patients were treated with ultrasounds and four patients with a placebo. The ultrasounds or placebo were delivered at the start of the active osteodistraction phase for about 45 days. No patient dropped out. No complication occurred, no implant failed and all planned prostheses could be delivered and followed for 2 years after loading. The distraction distance obtained was 4.6 mm for the ultrasound group and 5.8 mm for the placebo group. The difference of 1.2 mm was not statistically significant, but clearly in favour of the placebo group. With respect to costs, the cost of the ultrasound equipment should be considered. The time needed to achieve the desired outcome was similar, though patients had to spend about 20 min/day for about 45 days to deliver the treatment. The trial was judged to be at low risk of bias.

- One trial evaluated inlays (in ten patients) vs. onlays (in 13 patients) of autogenous bone grafts harvested from the iliac crest to vertically augment deficient posterior mandibles of 4.5–10 mm height above the mandibular canal for 1 year after loading [16]. The number of patients in each group was unbalanced because toss of a coin was used to randomise patients. No patient dropped out. Four complications occurred in four patients of the inlay group (three dehiscence/infection with partial exposure of the miniplates, one determining the failure of the

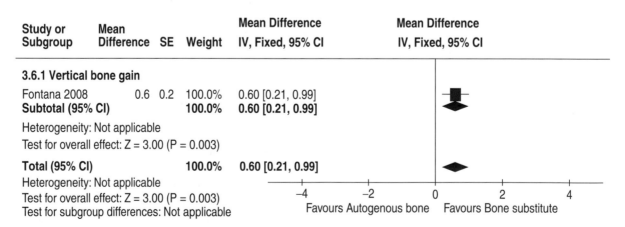

Fig. 13.4 Forest plot comparing autogenous bone with a bone substitute for vertically augmenting posterior mandibles. Statistically significant more vertical bone gain was obtained using a bone substitute

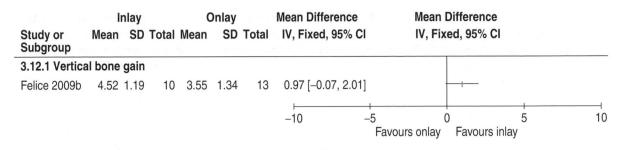

| Study or Subgroup | Inlay | | | Onlay | | | Mean Difference IV, Fixed, 95% CI | Mean Difference IV, Fixed, 95% CI |
	Mean	SD	Total	Mean	SD	Total		
3.12.1 Vertical bone gain								
Felice 2009b	4.52	1.19	10	3.55	1.34	13	0.97 [–0.07, 2.01]	

Fig. 13.5 Forest plot comparing inlay vs. only blocks of autogenous bone for vertically augmenting posterior mandibles. No statistically significant difference was observed ($p > 0.07$) but trends (borderline significance) clearly favoured the inlay blocks

augmentation procedure and one peri-implantitis) vs. six complications in five patients from the onlay group (three dehiscence/infection with partial exposure of the miniplates, one determining the failure of the augmentation procedure, two altered chin/lip sensation, one lasting for 6 months and one permanent and one peri-implantitis in the same patient who had paraesthesia for 6 months). No implant failed. Both treatments resulted in vertical bone gain (3.5 mm for the onlay group and 4.5 mm for the inlay group), and the difference between the two procedures of 1 mm was not statistically significant (Fig. 13.5), but was very close to significance ($p > 0.07$). There were no differences in costs and treatment time. The trial was judged to be at low risk of bias.

13.5 Discussion

This review was originally conceived as having a broad focus and was aimed to include any RCT dealing with any aspect of bone augmentation in relation to dental implant rehabilitation. In the present update we decided to split the original review in three more focused reviews: the present one dealing with horizontal and vertical bone augmentation procedures, one dealing with procedures to augment the maxillary sinus, and a third one dealing with minor augmentation procedure at extraction sockets, immediate implants and implants with bone fenestration. We are fully aware that there are limitations in this classification, as in many classifications, since the exact borders among the different categories may not always be clearly identified. Trials reporting only histological outcomes or which did not

report any implant related outcome were not considered of interest since they would not be able to provide reliable clinical information for the prognosis of dental implant rehabilitation.

Only in three trials was a sample size calculation undertaken 26, 29, 32; however, the planned sample sizes could be achieved only in one trial 29 [14, 15, 23]. Sample sizes of all studies were relatively small. It is, therefore, likely that many of these studies were underpowered to demonstrate any significant difference in outcome measures between groups. Nevertheless, some of the included trials did provide limited but indeed useful clinical information and indications that should be carefully evaluated by clinicians when deciding whether to perform an augmentation procedure or not, or which augmentation procedure to select. We have spent a great deal of time contacting RCTs' authors, who have kindly provided useful unpublished information on their trials. We feel that these contacts have made the present review more complete and useful for the readers. It is also worth observing that all authors of the included trials replied to our requests of clarifications. It is unusual to have such a high response rate. This might be partly explained by the serious research interests of the investigators conducting RCTs in the area, and may be indicative of a growing consciousness that high quality systematic reviews can be of great benefit to the entire society. We also noticed a considerable increase in the number of RCTs published over the last years. This should be viewed positively since it may indicate that in the near future some currently unanswered clinical questions might finally get an evidence-based answer, going over the traditional "opinion-biassed" approach to clinical decision-making. The priority now is to concentrate research efforts on a few important clinical questions, increasing the sample size, and decreasing the number of treatment variables in the trials. This might be obtained through collaborative efforts among various research groups.

We tried to evaluate first, whether a certain augmentation procedure is necessary, and second, which could be the most effective augmentation techniques. This distinction is relevant since it is possible that many complicated, painful and even potentially dangerous procedures that are widely performed today have no evidence-based justification and do not improve the prognosis or the patients' quality of life.

No trial evaluated whether and when horizontal bone augmentation is necessary, but two trials evaluated whether vertical bone augmentation procedures are needed or whether shorter implants could be used instead [14, 33]. One trial (17) investigated whether it was better to use iliac crest bone for inlay augmentation procedures to allow the placement of 13–18 mm long implants rather than placing 8–11 mm short implants without augmentation to treat atrophic anterior mandibles with a residual bone height of 6–12 mm [33]. The other trial (32) compared an inlay augmentation technique with Bio-Oss blocks to allow the placement of at least 10 mm long implants, with 7 mm long implants for treating posterior mandibles with a residual bone height above the mandibular canal of 7–8 mm [14]. The meta-analysis of these two trials showed that vertical augmentation was associated with statistically significantly more implant failures and complications than short implants. Caution should be exercised when extrapolating these results since in one trial (17) 11 mm implants were used that are not considered to be short, and the other trial (32) had only a follow-up of 4 months after loading [14, 33]. Nevertheless, when considering resorbed mandibles, inlay augmentation techniques to allow the placement of longer implants may not be the optimal treatment choice. It is, therefore, useful to underline that when evaluating the only two properly designed trials to test whether augmentation procedures are needed, the augmentation procedures resulted in more serious complications (including a life threatening sublingual oedema), major discomfort and pain, significantly more costs for society, longer treatment time and clinically poorer outcomes [14, 33]. These examples should clearly illustrate that a more critical approach should be taken when evaluating the need for vertical bone augmentation procedures for dental implants.

When evaluating which are the most effective augmentation techniques for horizontal ridge augmentation for single implants, only one trial was designed in a way to provide clinical useful information [22]. This trial, which had the largest sample size included in this review, compared three different two-stage techniques to horizontally augment bone to allow placement of single implants [22]. Thirty-one patients were included in each group and aesthetic outcomes were assessed both by the patients and a blinded experienced evaluator. Unfortunately, most of the data were presented aggregated and not by study group, meaning that it was not possible to use them to compare advantages or disadvantages of the individual techniques. For 62 patients, a block of bone was retrieved from the chin, whereas in 31 patients the defects were reconstructed with 100% bone substitute (Bio-Oss) and a resorbable barrier. Despite these relatively high numbers, the authors confirmed to us that not a single complication occurred. These are remarkable results not confirmed by other trials included in the present review. Only two implants failed early in the bone substitute group, although they were successfully replaced. The healing period used for the bone substitute group was 3 months longer, but on the other hand, no autogenous bone was needed to complete the procedure. At present, it is still difficult to recommend which should be the procedure to be used and additional information is needed to confirm these results. The other two trials evaluating aspects for horizontal bone augmentation had too small sample sizes to provide any reliable evidence [26, 27]. In fact, only five patients treated with a split-mouth design were recruited to evaluate the clinical efficacy, if any, of PRP [27]. When comparing titanium vs. resorbable screws for holding buccal onlay autogenous grafts, despite no significant differences being observed, although the sample size of eight patients was too small to be able to detect any difference, the observation that two resorbable screws broke at insertion and that a considerable amount of remnants of the resorbable screws were still visible after 9 months and were surrounded by fibrotic tissue rich in giant cells may suggest that titanium screws are still the best choice [26].

When evaluating which are the most effective augmentation techniques for vertical ridge augmentation, eight trials were included [3, 7, 8, 15, 16, 18, 23, 30]. Osteodistraction osteogenesis, various GBR techniques, autogenous onlay block grafting and inlay grafting with both autogenous bone and bone substitutes can be successful for augmenting bone vertically; however, there is insufficient evidence to suggest if one technique is preferable. The osteodistraction technique may not be used in all circumstances (for instance in the presence of thin knife-edge bone) as it is more expensive than GBR and bone grafting, but may reduce treatment time and allow for more vertical ridge augmentation, if needed. On the other hand, GBR and onlay bone grafting techniques also allow for simultaneous bone widening, if needed. All the vertical augmentation techniques evaluated were associated with high complication rates ranging from 60 (28) to 20% (29) with only one study on osteodistraction osteogenesis that reported no complications (31) [3, 15, 30]. However, in few cases (10% in (29) and 15% (26)) the vertical augmentation resulted in the failure of augmentation procedure. It is, therefore, recommended that both clinicians and patients carefully evaluate the pros and cons in relation to the desired outcome before deciding whether to use vertical ridge augmentation techniques. Results from some of these trials (24, 26) also suggested that the vertically augmented bone can be successfully maintained up to 3 years after loading with just a minimal bone loss in the range of 0.5–1 mm [8, 23].

One study evaluated the efficacy of ultrasounds to stimulate osteogenesis at vertically distracted mandibular bone [30]. Ultrasounds are used to stimulate healing in bone fractures, especially in delayed healing and non-union fractures. The results of this pilot study suggested that ultrasounds had no positive effects on bone healing. When looking at the data it can be observed that ultrasound treated sites were distracted for 4.6 mm and placebo sites for 5.8 mm. The difference among the two procedures in amount of distracted bone (1.2 mm) was not statistically significant, but it was clearly in favour of the placebo group. Ultrasounds were applied when the active osteodistraction phase was initiated. A possible interpretation of the results is that ultrasounds were effective in stimulating bone healing, and this could explain why the placebo group gained more bone. It is possible that ultrasounds were delivered at the wrong time (the active osteodistraction phase) and stimulated bone healing, reducing the osteodistraction potential. The results of this study remain difficult to interpret, but it is possible that ultrasounds should be delivered when the active osteodistraction phase is completed.

Autogenous bone is often considered the "gold standard" material for bone augmentation. Three trials compared autogenous bone with bone substitutes and curiously the indications that these trials gave were not consistently in favour of autogenous bone [15, 18, 22]. When augmenting bone horizontally to allow the placement of single implants, a bone substitute (Bio-Oss) could be successfully used [22]. Implants placed in bone augmented with Bio-Oss showed trends to increased failure rates, though all failed implants could be successfully replaced without the need of additional augmentation. Another disadvantage with Bio-Oss was that the healing time was increased by 3 months, and on the other hand, no autogenous bone had to be collected from the chin, meaning also a less invasive operation, and therefore, additional information are needed to establish which could be the most cost-effective procedure. A split-mouth pilot study evaluated whether anorganic bovine bone blocks (Bio-Oss) could replace autogenous bone harvested from the iliac crest for vertical augmenting atrophic posterior mandibles with an inlay technique (29). Though no statistical differences for clinical outcomes could be found, eight out of ten patients preferred the augmentation procedure with the bone substitute and this was statistically significant. In addition, general anaesthesia is not needed when using blocks of bone substitute block to augment atrophic. Finally, another split-mouth pilot study, including only five patients, compared a malleable bone substitute (Regenaform) with particulate autogenous bone for vertical GBR at posterior mandibles [18]. Significantly more bone (0.6 mm) was vertically augmented at the sides treated with the bone substitute. While a 0.6-mm of additional vertical bone gain may not have a significant clinical impact, it is also true that the bone substitute behaved similarly, if not better, than autogenous bone.

With respect to generalisation of the results of the present review to general practise, many of the augmentation procedures evaluated were rather complex, were performed by experienced and skilful clinicians, patients were undergoing strict post-operative control regimens, complications were common, and in few instances, serious. Caution is, therefore, recommended while deciding to use any augmentation procedure. The first clinical question that clinicians should ask themselves is which could be the added benefits for the patient by applying such procedures. Then the expected benefits need to be carefully weighed against the risk of complications of the chosen procedure.

13.6 Conclusions

These conclusions are based on few trials with small or very small sample sizes, relatively short follow-ups and being sometimes judged to be at high risk of bias; therefore they should be viewed with great caution.

- Two trials investigated whether vertical augmentation procedures are necessary to allow placement of longer implants when compared to simple placement of short implants.

Vertical augmentation of resorbed mandibles with inlay techniques resulted in statistically significantly more implant failures, complications, pain, days of hospitalisation, costs, and longer treatment time than using short implants; therefore the current available scientific evidence does not justify these procedures for placing longer implants in resorbed mandibles. However, the long-term prognosis of shorter implants is yet unknown.

- Three trials investigated which are the most effective techniques for horizontal bone augmentation.
- Various augmentation techniques are able to regenerate bone in a horizontal direction; however, there is insufficient evidence to indicate which technique could be preferable. It appears that a bone substitute (Bio-Oss) can be used with a slightly higher risk (not statistically significant) of having an implant failure.
- There is insufficient evidence supporting or confuting the efficacy of various active agents such as PRP in conjunction with implant treatment.
- Titanium screws might be preferable to resorbable poly (D,L-lactide) acid screws to fix onlay bone blocks.
- Eight trials investigated which are the most effective techniques for vertical bone augmentation.
- Various augmentation techniques are able to augment bone in a vertical direction; however, there is insufficient evidence to indicate which could be the preferable technique.
- Bone substitutes, such as Bio-Oss blocks, may be a valid, cheaper alternative to autogenous bone particularly when harvested from extra-oral locations since they are associated to less post-operative morbidity.
- Osteodistraction allows for more vertical augmentation, but is of little use in the presence of thin ridges.

- Complications were common, and in some cases, determined the failure of the augmentation procedure.
- Clinicians and patients should carefully evaluate the benefits and risks in relation to the desired outcome when deciding whether to use vertical ridge augmentation techniques.

In order to understand when bone augmentation procedures are needed and which are the most effective techniques, larger and well-designed trials are needed. Such trials should be reported according to the Consolidated Standards of Reporting Trials (CONSORT) guidelines [24] (http://www.consort-statement.org/). It is difficult to provide clear indications with respect to which augmentation procedures should be tested first; however, once established in which clinical situations augmentation procedures are actually needed, priority could be given to those interventions which look simpler, less invasive, involve less risk of complications and reach their goals within the shortest timeframe. Indications for using various bone substitutes should be explored in more detail and it should be evaluated which donor sites could provide the sufficient amount of bone with less risk of complications and patient discomfort. Patient-centred outcomes should also be considered when designing such trials.

Acknowledgements We wish to thank Sylvia Bickley (Cochrane Oral Health Group) and Anna Littlewood for their assistance with literature searching; Luisa Fernandez Mauleffinch and Philip Riley (Cochrane Oral Health Group) for their help with the preparation of this review; Stella Kwan who co-authored a previous version of this review; Matteo Chiapasco, Filippo Fontana, Giuseppe Lizio, Gerry Raghoebar, Jurjen Schortinghuis and Kees Stellingsma for providing us with additional information on their trials. We would also like to thank the following referees: Stephen Chen, Matteo Chiapasco, Christer Dahlin, Mats Hallman, Jayne Harrison, Jan Hirsch, Ian Needleman, Gerry Raghoebar and Bill Shaw.

References

1. Antoun H, Sitbon JM, Martinez H, Missika P (2001) A prospective randomized study comparing two techniques of bone augmentation: onlay graft alone or associated with a membrane. Clin Oral Implants Res 12:632–639
2. Bettega G, Brun JP, Cracowski JL, Vérain A, Raphael B (2005) Use of autologous platelet concentrates during pre-implantation maxillary reconstruction. Revue de Stomatologie et de Chirurgie Maxillofaciale 106:189–191
3. Bianchi A, Felice P, Lizio G, Marchetti C (2008) Alveolar distraction osteogenesis versus inlay bone grafting in

posterior mandibular atrophy: a prospective study. Oral Surg Oral Med Oral Pathol Oral Radiol Endod 105:282–292

4. Brånemark PI, Gröndahl K, Öhrnell LO, Nilsson P, Petruson B, Svensson B et al (2004) Zygoma fixture in the management of advanced atrophy of the maxilla: technique and long-term results. Scand J Plast Reconstr Surg 38:70–85

5. Brånemark P-I, Hansson BO, Adell R, Breine U, Lindström J, Hallén O et al (1977) Osseointegrated implants in the treatment of the edentulous jaw. Experience from a 10-year period. Almqvist & Wiksell International, Stockholm

6. Cawood JI, Howell RA (1991) Reconstructive preprosthetic surgery. I. Anatomical considerations. Int J Oral Maxillofac Surg 20:75–82

7. Chiapasco M, Romeo E, Casentini P, Rimondini L (2004) Alveolar distraction osteogenesis vs. vertical guided bone regeneration for the correction of vertically deficient edentulous ridges: a 1-3-year prospective study on humans. Clin Oral Implants Res 15:82–95

8. Chiapasco M, Zaniboni M, Rimondini L (2007) Autogenous onlay bone grafts vs. alveolar distraction osteogenesis for the correction of vertically deficient edentulous ridges: a 2-4-year prospective study on humans. Clin Oral Implants Res 18:432–440

9. Esposito M, Grusovin MG, Felice P, Karatzopoulos G, Worthington HV, Coulthard P (2009) Interventions for replacing missing teeth: horizontal and vertical bone augmentation techniques for dental implant treatment. Cochrane Database of Systematic Reviews

10. Esposito M, Grusovin MG, Kakisis I, Coulthard P, Worthington HV (2008) Interventions for replacing missing teeth: treatment of perimplantitis. Cochrane Database of Systematic Reviews. Wiley, Chichester, UK

11. Esposito M, Grusovin MG, Kwan S, Worthington HV, Coulthard P (2008) Interventions for replacing missing teeth: bone augmentation techniques for dental implant treatment. Cochrane Database of Systematic Reviews. Wiley, Chichester, UK

12. Esposito M, Hirsch J-M, Lekholm U, Thomsen P (1998) Biological factors contributing to failures of osseointegrated oral implants. (I) Success criteria and epidemiology. Eur J Oral Sci 106:527–551

13. Esposito M, Worthington HV, Coulthard P (2005) Interventions for replacing missing teeth: dental implants in zygomatic bone for the rehabilitation of the severely deficient edentulous maxilla. Cochrane Database of Systematic Reviews. Wiley, Chichester, UK

14. Felice P, Cannizzaro G, Checchi V, Pellegrino G, Censi P, Esposito M (2009) Vertical bone augmentation versus 7 mm long dental implants in posterior atrophic mandibles. A randomized controlled clinical trial. Eur J Oral Implantol 2:7–20

15. Felice P, Marchetti C, Piattelli A, Pellegrino G, Checchi V, Worthington H et al (2008) Vertical ridge augmentation of the atrophic posterior mandible with interpositional block grafts: bone from the iliac crest versus bovine anorganic bone. Results up to delivery of the final prostheses from a split-mouth, randomised controlled clinical trial. Eur J Oral Implantol 1:183–187

16. Felice P, Pistilli R, Lizio G, Pellegrino G, Nisii A, Marchetti C (2009) Inlay versus onlay iliac bone grafting in atrophic posterior mandible: a prospective controlled clinical trial for

the comparison of two techniques. Clin Implant Dentistry Relat Res 11:e69–e82

17. Fiorellini JP, Nevins ML (2003) Localized ridge augmentation/ preservation. A systematic review. Ann Periodontol 8:321–327

18. Fontana F, Santoro F, Maiorana C, Iezzi G, Piattelli A, Simion M (2008) Clinical and histologic evaluation of allogenic bone matrix versus autogenous bone chips associated with titanium-reinforced e-PTFE membrane for vertical ridge augmentation: a prospective pilot study. Int J Oral Maxillofac Implants 23:1003–1012

19. Friedmann A, Strietzel FP, Maretzki B, Pitaru S, Bernimoulin JP (2002) Histological assessment of augmented jaw bone utilizing a new collagen barrier membrane compared to a standard barrier membrane to protect a granular bone substitute material. Clin Oral Implants Res 13:587–594

20. Kahnberg K-E, Nyström E, Bartholdsson L (1989) Combined use of bone grafts and Brånemark fixtures in the treatment of severely resorbed maxillae. Int J Oral Maxillofac Implants 4:297–304

21. Keller EE (1992) The maxillary interpositional composite graft. In: Worthington P, Brånemark P-I (eds) Advanced osseointegration surgery: applications in the maxillofacial region. Quintessence, Chicago, pp 162–174

22. Meijndert L, Meijer HJ, Stellingsma K, Stegenga B, Raghoebar GM (2007) Evaluation of aesthetics of implant-supported single-tooth replacements using different bone augmentation procedures: a prospective randomized clinical study. Clin Oral Implants Res 18:715–719

23. Merli M, Migani M, Esposito M (2007) Vertical ridge augmentation with autogenous bone grafts: resorbable barriers supported by ostheosynthesis plates versus titanium-reinforced barriers. A preliminary report of a blinded, randomized controlled clinical trial. Int J Oral Maxillofac Implants 22:373–382

24. Moher D, Schulz KF, Altman DG (2001) The CONSORT statement: revised recommendations for improving the quality of reports of parallel-group randomised trials. Lancet 357:1191–1194

25. Obwegeser HL (1969) Surgical correction of small or retro-displaced maxillae. The "dish-face" deformity. Plast Reconstr Surg 43:351–365

26. Raghoebar GM, Liem RS, Bos RR, van der Wal JE, Vissink A (2006) Resorbable screws for fixation of autologous bone grafts. Clin Oral Implants Res 17:288–293

27. Raghoebar GM, Schortinghuis J, Liem RS, Ruben JL, van der Wal JE, Vissink A (2005) Does platelet-rich plasma promote remodeling of autologous bone grafts used for augmentation of the maxillary sinus floor? Clin Oral Implants Res 16:349–356

28. Rocchietta I, Fontana F, Simion M (2008) Clinical outcomes of vertical bone augmentation to enable dental implant placement: a systematic review. J Clin Periodontol 35:203–215

29. Roccuzzo M, Ramieri G, Bunino M, Berrone S (2007) Autogenous bone graft alone or associated with titanium mesh for vertical alveolar ridge augmentation: a controlled clinical trial. Clin Oral Implants Res 18:286–294

30. Schortinghuis J, Bronckers AL, Gravendeel J, Stegenga B, Raghoebar GM (2008) The effect of ultrasound on osteogenesis in the vertically distracted edentulous mandible: a double-blind trial. Int J Oral Maxillofac Surg 37:1014–1021

31. Schortinghuis J, Bronckers ALJJ, Steganga B, Raghoebar GM, de Bont LGM (2005) Ultrasound to stimulate early

bone formation in a distraction gap: a double blind randomised clinical pilot trial in the edentulous mandible. Arch Oral Biol 50:411–420

32. Steinemann SG (1998) Titanium – the material of choice? Periodontology 2000(17):7–21

33. Stellingsma K, Bouma J, Stegenga B, Meijer HJ, Raghoebar GM (2003) Satisfaction and psychosocial aspects of patients with an extremely resorbed mandible treated with implant-retained overdentures. A prospective, comparative study. Clin Oral Implants Res 14:166–172

34. Tolman DE (1995) Reconstructive procedures with endosseous implants in grafted bone: a review of the literature. Int J Oral Maxillofac Implants 10:275–294

35. Valentin-Opran A, Wozney J, Csimma C, Lilly L, Riedel GE (2002) Clinical evaluation of recombinant human bone morphogenetic protein-2. Clin Orthop Relat Res 395: 110–120

36. Van der Zee E, Oosterveld P, Van Waas MA (2004) Effect of GBR and fixture installation on gingiva and bone levels at adjacent teeth. Clin Oral Implants Res 15:62–65

Conclusion: Toward Optimization of the Evidence-Based Paradigm in Medicine and Dentistry

Evidence-Based Medicine: What does it Mean and Where Are We Going?

14

Sergio Frustaci, Gian Maria Miolo, Angela Buonadonna, Diana Crivellari, and Simona Scalone

Core Message

> Although most health professionals are familiar with the term evidence-based medicine (EBM) and have some idea of what it means, it is surprisingly rare to see it actually being used. Despite its ancient origins, EBM remains a relatively young discipline whose positive impacts are just beginning to be validated, and it will continue to evolve.

14.1 Introduction

The term evidence-based medicine (EBM) first appeared in a 1992 JAMA article [28], which explicitly stated that all clinical actions in the fields of diagnosis, prognosis, and therapeutic decision making should be based on sound quantitative evidence deriving from high-quality epidemiological and clinical research.

S. Frustaci (✉)
G.M. Miolo
A. Buonadonna
Division of Medical Oncology B, Centro di Riferimento Oncologico, Istituto Nazionale Tumori,
Via F. Gallini, 2, Aviano, Italy
e-mail: sfrustaci@cro.it

D. Crivellari
S. Scalone
Division of Medical Oncology C, Centro di Riferimento Oncologico, Istituto Nazionale Tumori, Via F. Gallini, 2, Aviano, Italy

EBM, commonly defined as "the conscientious, explicit, and judicious use of the current best evidence in making decisions about the care of individual patients," requires the integration of "clinical expertise with the best available external clinical evidence from systematic research" [73].

EBM proponents attempt to objectify medical practice through the use of the best available, most-rigorously tested screening, diagnostic, management, and monitoring methods; it has also been employed to evaluate the cost-effectiveness of differing approaches to diagnosis, screening, and management [72].

Therefore, the definition of EBM, which focuses on individual physicians and their decisions, is too limited and should be expanded to comprise not only evidence-based decision making by the individual physician, but also evidence-based systematic reviews, guidelines, and other types of policies, including the patient's choice.

This new approach is moving medical practices faster, more consistently, and more efficiently toward evidence than evidence-based individual decision making alone.

In summary, EBM is a set of principles and methods intended to ensure that, to the greatest extent possible, medical decisions, guidelines, and other types of policies are based on and consistent with good evidence of efficacy and benefit [27].

Patients are the primary beneficiary of EBM, since they receive the most advanced care, proven in the medical literature that offer them the best chance for survival. It has been shown that reducing the individual variability in care improves its quality by lowering propensity for errors.

National health systems can also benefit, because where systematic procedures have been instituted, cost control coupled with the highest quality of care seems to result. Therefore, EBM is a good practice for patients, physicians, and business, too.

The best information from the field shows that serving a patient well benefits the physician's practice. It is axiomatic that if patients are treated with the best standard of care their outcomes are optimal [23].

14.2 EBM and the Development of Clinical Practice Guidelines (CPGs)

Transferring existing research results into consistent patient-oriented strategies in the form of evidence reviews is a key step in the process of improving cancer care and patient outcomes [66].

Clinicians practicing EBM seek out the best available evidence on which to base their decisions in order to offer the individual patient the highest-quality and most effective care, and ultimately to improve outcome; [87] an EBM exercise can also identify areas in which evidence is lacking, and further studies are needed. A review of the available evidence is at the core of the clinical practice guideline (CPG) development process.

CPGs are a set of systematically developed statements to assist both practitioners and patients with the decision-making process concerning the most appropriate healthcare for one specific clinical circumstance; [31] they are also a useful mechanism to break down complex data sets into more manageable pieces, and ideally allow busy clinicians to effectively use them for individual patient care.

Several regulatory bodies and professional organizations such as the American Society of Clinical Oncology (ASCO) and the Cancer Care Ontario Practice Guideline Initiative (CCOPGI) in Canada have become heavily involved in the development of CPGs, and their potential impact can be estimated by understanding who is creating them, and who is using them and how. Also, in most European countries, numerous CPG development programs have been set up in various fields, including oncology [16].

Literature searching, critical appraisal, and synthesis of the evidence play a key role in CPG development and updating processes. Although some of them should give consistent results, cultural diversity among European countries (particularly in terms of healthcare structure and organization) can lead to legitimate variability in guideline recommendations

showing marked differences in cancer survival across Europe despite tangible improvements in diagnosis and treatment [30, 75].

Heterogeneity in several aspects of the guideline-development process is controversial. Therefore, it is pivotal to identify the predictors of high-quality care in oncology for CPGs to be developed and to inspire confidence in prospective users, and also to ensure that they have an influence on clinical practice [4].

Predictors of high-quality care for CPG in oncology were identified by Fervers et al. The quality scores for 32 oncology guidelines from 13 countries were determined by four independent appraisers using the Appraisal of Guidelines for Research and Evaluation (AGREE) instrument. The results showed that the availability of background information had the greatest impact on the guideline quality score.

Surprisingly, the absence of an exclusive focus on oncology programs was associated with significantly lower quality scores in the applicability domain. The guidelines generally failed to address issues such as barriers to implementation and cost implications, and did not include monitoring criteria; this may be explained in settings where links with regional cancer networks do exist since they incorporate CPGs into local implementation protocols [69].

Actually, no standard algorithm for producing CPGs is of proven superiority, the assessment parameters and methods to measure such superiority being poorly defined.

So far, no unique rating scale for evaluating the level of evidence/strength of recommendation has been adopted widely [65]. However, users of CPGs and other recommendations need to know how much confidence they can place on them.

A systematic and explicit approach to making judgments about the quality of evidence and the strength of recommendations can help to prevent errors, to facilitate critical appraisal of these judgments, and to improve communication.

14.3 Levels of Evidence from Healthcare Research

Clinical decision making incorporates collection of the best evidences to answer specific questions, and their subsequent critical evaluation in order to clarify validity, impact, and transferability into clinical practice. Different study designs on the same topic often answer rather different questions. It should also be kept in mind that there is a hierarchy of quality of evidence, and that it is essential to develop a methodology to assess the hierarchy of medical evidence and to grade healthcare recommendations about a specific clinical intervention [45].

Rules of evidence have been developed to help assess the validity of a given clinical finding to address and answer the ultimate questions: *Are the findings of this study believable? How close are they to the truth?* [24].

Central to the idea of applying EBM is the need for thorough review and appraisal of existing literature by the treatment provider. EBM stratifies the available evidence into discrete categories, placing more emphasis on those in which the sources of bias have been systematically minimized. In this respect, prospective, placebo-controlled, randomized clinical trials (RCTs) are top-ranked, whereas case reports are bottom-ranked [58].

Indeed, random allocation to a treatment or control group is the basis of all experimental designs, and it is the only way to isolate the effect of a single factor under study on a given outcome, thereby avoiding the distorting effects of confounding. Even though potential confounders still exist among study subjects, randomization is designed to distribute them evenly between the test and control groups to remove possible bias.

Based on the above considerations, a "5S" pyramid-like model has been proposed to rank evidence-based information: original *studies* are buried at the base, *syntheses* (that is, systematic reviews, such as Cochrane Reviews) sit at the next level, followed by *synopses* (very brief descriptions of the original papers and reviews, such as those appearing in evidence-based journals such as ACP Journal Club), *summaries* (succinct descriptions of an individual study or a systematic review), and *systems* (such as computerized decision support systems that link individual patient characteristics to pertinent evidence) at the top [48].

14.4 EBM and Quality of Evidence

EBM is based on a *quality-of-evidence* concept that indicates to what extent one can be confident that an estimate of effect is correct.

The *strength of a recommendation* indicates to what extent one can be confident that adherence will do more good than harm [3].

Pivotal to the idea of EBM is that there is a hierarchy of quality of evidence that is related to the design and conduct of the study or studies from which it is derived.

Moreover, it should be borne in mind that different study designs on the same topic often answer rather different questions. However, not all evidence is created equal, and certain findings are closer to the truth than others. There must exist some rational system to determine whether the results of one study are more reliable than those achieved by another trial.

The first stage of evidence-based decision making is to look closely at the information available.

Clinicians should consider four key elements: study design, study quality, consistency, and directness.

14.4.1 Study Design

Although there were usually no apparent differences between the results of observational studies and those attained by RCTs, this is not always the case.

An example of such a discrepancy is given by the differing results of observational studies that suggested that hormone replacement therapy would decrease the risk of coronary heart disease, and those achieved by subsequent RCTs showing no risk reduction but rather an increase. Unfortunately, it is not possible to know in advance whether observational studies can accurately predict the findings of subsequent randomized trials [50, 71].

As a result, most clinicians rightfully believe that evidence collected in RCTs and organized according to standard principles of study design and conduct is superior to that obtained from uncontrolled clinical experience.

On the other hand, we should keep in mind that MOPP or PVB combination chemotherapy regimens in the treatment of Hodgkin's disease or testicular cancer, respectively, have revolutionized modern clinical practice on the basis of case-series or single-arm prospective studies [24].

Another core (and related) tenet of scientific inquiry is the idea of comparison or control group. In clinical research, in the absence of a control group similar in every respect to the test group receiving the experimental treatment, it is impossible to discern how many subjects have benefited from the new therapy as opposed to those with spontaneous improvement of their conditions.

14.4.2 Study Quality

It refers to the basic study designs, i.e., observational studies and randomized trials. Whatever the case may be, a mistake to avoid absolutely is to regard any finding that is statistically significant as remarkable, as this is necessary, but not sufficient to guarantee importance.

A simple example is represented by a randomized phase III study by Moore et al. [61], that in an attempt to explore the effects of adding the HER1/EGFR-targeted agent erlotinib to gemcitabine in patients with unresectable, locally advanced, or metastatic pancreatic cancer demonstrated a statistically significant improvement in survival rates by combining any agent to gemcitabine.

Overall survival (OS) based on an intent-to-treat (ITT) analysis was significantly prolonged in the erlotinib/gemcitabine arm with a hazard ratio (HR) of 0.82 ($p>0.038$; adjusted for stratification factors; median 6.24 vs. 5.91 months). Therefore, the benefit was equal to an extended median survival time of less than 2 weeks.

Also progression-free survival (PFS) was significantly longer with an estimated HR of 0.77 ($p>0.004$, adjusted for stratification factors; median 3.75 vs. 3.55 months).

Out of 282 patients who had received erlotinib, 79 had no skin rash, 102 had grade 1 rash, and 101 had grade 2 or higher rash; altogether there was a higher incidence of some adverse events with erlotinib plus gemcitabine. The deep analysis of these data showed that in the study arm, there was considerable toxicity but no impact on the quality of life and survival.

Therefore, high-quality evidence does not necessarily imply strong recommendations, and strong recommendations can arise from low-quality evidence.

14.4.3 Consistency

It refers to the similarity of the estimates of effect across studies: broadly differing estimates suggest true differences in the underlying treatment effect [44]. Variability may arise from differences in populations, interventions, or outcomes. Should important unexplained inconsistency in the results be recorded, our confidence in the estimate of effect for that outcome would decrease. Moreover, should a compelling explanation for inconsistency be identified, separate estimates of the magnitude of effect for different subgroups should follow.

14.4.4 Directness

It is high when there is overlapping between the people of interest and those under study, and when studies use outcomes that are important to people and not surrogate outcomes, which require much more stringent criteria.

An important factor to consider when evaluating oncology research, particularly studies concerning new cancer treatments, is the selection of end-points, ranging from health outcomes (total mortality, cause-specific mortality, and quality of life) to indirect surrogates for any of them [3].

Total mortality: it is the proportion of the study population that died. It is frequently called death (or mortality) rate, and it is measured from a given point in time, such as the time of diagnosis or the time since treatment was initiated.

Cause-specific mortality: it is meant as death from a specified cause in the study population, for example, death from cancer vs. death from treatment side effects vs. death from other causes.

Quality of life: although it is very subjective, this endpoint is extremely important to patients. The strength of a quality-of-life assessment depends on the validity of the instruments (questionnaires, psychological tests, etc) used.

Indirect surrogates: they are measures that substitute for actual health outcomes, and they are subject to an investigator's interpretation.

Examples of surrogate end-points are disease-free survival (DFS) (length of time during which no cancer is detected after treatment), PFS (length of time during which disease is stable or does not worsen after treatment), or tumor response rate (TRR) (the proportion of patients whose disease responds to treatment, and the degree or extent to which the disease responds). Studies of surrogate end-points represent weaker, more indirect evidence; however, a clinician may rank studies differently depending on the patient's individual values.

Once the results of high-quality randomized trials are available, few people would argue for continuing to base recommendations on nonrandomized studies with discrepant results.

RCTs are not always feasible, and in some instances, observational studies may provide better evidence, as is generally the case for rare adverse effects. Moreover, their results may not always be applicable – for example, if the participants are highly selected and motivated as against the population of interest.

14.5 Grades of Recommendations

Recently, groups of experts have been asked to classify the levels of evidence by using informal processes, which means that the process integrity could be undermined by lack of transparency and methodology.

As a result, new and often expensive molecules have been introduced into clinical practice despite limited evidence of their efficacy and safety, and badly defined indications, leaving a potential for inappropriate use.

Two different strategies can obviate this problem, of which one applies a structured approach for collecting, analyzing, and summarizing evidences, and the other produces and grades evidence-based recommendations.

The strength of a recommendation reflects to what extent we can be confident that, across the range of patients for whom it is intended, the desirable effects of an intervention would outweigh the undesirable effects. Alternatively, in considering two or more possible management strategies, the strength of a recommendation represents our confidence that the net benefit clearly favors one alternative or the other [43].

Desirable effects of an intervention include decreased morbidity and mortality rates, improved quality of life, reduced burden of treatment (such as the inconvenience of having to take drugs or blood tests, or going to the doctor's office for check-ups), and lower costs. Undesirable consequences include adverse effects that may have a detrimental impact on morbidity, mortality, or quality of life, or increase resource consumption [43].

Several quality-rating scales have been published to evaluate the quality, quantity, rigor, and consistency of the evidence base, and hence to assess the level of evidence and strength of recommendations [26, 46].

Previous grading approaches have sometimes used complex systems of recommendations with up to nine categories of strength of recommendations [36].

14.6 The GRADE Approach

The grading of recommendations, assessment, development, and evaluation (GRADE) system has been developed in order to overcome the shortcomings of previous approaches. Since its appearance, it has been adopted extensively, and it is being used by 25 organizations, including the Cochrane Collaboration.

It is based on a sequential assessment of the quality of evidence followed by a benefit-risk analysis and subsequent evaluation of the strength of recommendations.

The study design remains critical to judgments about the quality of evidence. According to the GRADE approach, RCTs without important limitations are ranked as high-quality evidence, whereas observational studies without special strengths or important limitations are regarded as low-quality evidence. Limitations or special strengths can, however, have an impact on the quality of evidence. The quality of evidence is classified in four levels, namely high, moderate, low, and very low, but only in the first level, additional research does not change our confidence in the estimate of effect.

The GRADE approach identifies five factors than can lower the quality of evidence: study limitations (*including lack of allocation concealment, lack of blinding, a large loss of follow-up, failure to adhere to an intention-to-treat analysis, stopping early for benefit, or selective reporting of outcomes*) inconsistency of results (*due to variability arising from differences in populations, interventions, or outcomes*), indirectness of evidence (*randomized trials may allow indirect comparisons of the magnitude of effect of two drugs vs. placebo, but in addition to the evidence from indirect comparisons, substantial evidence from direct comparisons is required*), imprecision (*when the study includes relatively few patients and few events and thus has wide confidence intervals*), publication bias (*reporting studies that they have undertaken*), and three factors that might increase the quality of evidence (*large magnitude of effect, plausible confounding, which would reduce a demonstrated effect, and dose response gradient*) [3].

While the current US Food and Drug Administration (FDA) and European Medicine Agency (EMEA) regulations require as a prerequisite that a drug be found effective in well-conducted clinical trials before approval, the reality is that regulatory approval for a new drug is often based only on surrogate outcomes, with limited follow-up and sometimes using data obtained from phase II rather than phase III studies.

As an example of the practical exertion in oncology, De Palma et al. [22] describe the application of the GRADE approach to the development of CPGs for breast, colorectal, and lung cancer treatment.

In this study, 12 clinical questions on adjuvant treatment (namely three, four, and five for breast, colorectal, and lung cancer, respectively) were identified and discussed by a panel of 57 members (of which 16 were medical oncologists) on the basis of the following three criteria:

- The relative importance of treatment.
- The lack of conclusive recommendations in the existing guidelines.
- The interest of the local oncology community.

With regard to colorectal cancer, the four questions were as follows:

- In patients with stage II colon cancer is adjuvant chemotherapy recommended?
- In patients with stage III colon cancer should oxaliplatin be used in association with FU + folinic acid?
- In patients with stage III colon cancer is capecitabine recommended instead of FU + folinic acid?
- In patients with stage II and III rectal cancer is chemoradiotherapy recommended presurgery instead of postsurgery?

Overall, for breast and colon cancer there were one strong and five weak recommendations, and one instance in which the panel concluded that no recommendation could be formulated, underlying that in some cancers, evidences over some molecular target drugs are less powerful.

De Palma et al. [22] highlight several advantages of the GRADE method: first, it makes guideline developers focus on key methodological issues; second, it organizes the presentation of the evidentiary base on specific outcomes; and third, it provides guidance for balancing trade-offs among risks, benefits, and costs.

However, De Palma et al. document considerable variability among the participants in their assessments of evidence quality, risk-benefit trade-offs, and strength of recommendations suggesting that there are likely known, and perhaps some unknowable, factors that influence the way the participants will interpret data and apply them to their judgments [12].

In using GRADE, the most common classification of guideline recommendations one might expect in oncology is between "probably use it" or "probably do not use it," that is to say between strong or weak [12].

14.7 Implications of Recommendations

14.7.1 The Implications of a Strong Recommendation

For patients – most people in your situation would want the recommended course of action, and only a small proportion would not; request discussion if the intervention is not offered; for clinicians – most patients should receive the recommended course of action; for policy makers – the recommendation can be adopted as a policy in most situations.

14.7.2 The Implications of a Weak Recommendation

For patients – most people in your situation would want the recommended course of action, but many would not; for clinicians – you should recognize that different choices will be appropriate for different patients and that you must help each patient to arrive at a management decision consistent with her/his values and preferences; for policy makers – policy making will require substantial debate and involvement of many stakeholders [43].

However, the GRADE methodology leaves considerable room for individual interpretations. This is not surprising, because cancer care options are often linked with important risks, benefits are often incremental, and individual patient and societal values are not necessarily aligned as in the case of expensive drugs that yield arguably modest gains [12].

14.8 Colon Cancer

Early diagnosis of colorectal cancer significantly decreases morbidity and mortality rates. Five-year survival for patients diagnosed with Dukes A colorectal cancer is approximately 90%, which drops down to as little as 5% for patients with Dukes D, or metastatic, disease.

Staging provides essential prognostic information relevant for choosing adequate therapy, and it should also identify patients with resectable distant metastases.

Preoperative clinical staging consists of clinical examination, blood counts, liver and renal function tests, carcino-embryonic antigen (CEA), chest X-ray or CT scan, abdominal CT, and colonoscopy of the entire large bowel. Postoperative repeat colonoscopy is recommended if proximal parts of the colon were not accessible preoperatively.

Pathologic staging should be carried out according to the TNM 2002 system with optional listing of the modified Dukes stage [86].

14.8.1 Colon Cancer Adjuvant Setting

Adjuvant therapy has been recommended for stage III colon cancer patients because it decreases relapse and mortality rates by 30–40% when compared to observation alone after surgery [63]. Standard adjuvant treatment consists of fluoropyrimidine-based chemotherapy; 5-fluorouracil (5-FU), leucovorin (LV) plus oxaliplatin combination regimens significantly improve DFS and OS [1].

In contrast, ongoing controversy exists as to whether adjuvant therapy should also be advised for patients with stage II colon cancer.

For this reason, numerous clinical trials have been performed in this setting, but unfortunately their results are still inconclusive. Based on those considerations, ASCO entrusted an expert panel including professionals in clinical medicine, clinical research, and health services research with the development of guidelines to facilitate clinical decision making.

In order to determine if adjuvant therapy improves survival for stage II colon cancer patients as against surgery alone, papers were selected for inclusion in the CCO systematic review evidence-based on the following criteria: RCTs with appropriate control groups, or meta-analyses of RCTs comparing adjuvant therapy with observation in stage II colon cancer patients who had undergone curative surgery.

Stage II colon cancer was defined according to the American Joint Committee on Cancer (AJCC)-TNM system classification as any pT3N0M0 or pT4N0M0 tumor of the colon.

In this study, 37 RCTs and 11 meta-analyses of adjuvant chemotherapy or immunotherapy for colon cancer were identified. Overall, 20,317 patients (7,803 with colon cancer and 12,514 with colorectal cancers) were included. In the trials under review, the proportion of patients with stage II disease ranged from 23 to 100% (average 48%).

A literature-based meta-analysis of selected data from the trials identified demonstrated that adjuvant therapy was associated with a small absolute improvement in DFS (from 5 to 10%), but this did not translate into a statistically significant difference in OS [8].

A literature-based meta-analysis on a subset of 12 out of 37 RCTs selected on the basis of more stringent criteria requiring inclusion of a surgery-alone control arm and at least one FU-based chemotherapy arm came to the same conclusion: adjuvant chemotherapy does not improve survival significantly. Failure to document a statistically and clinically relevant benefit is largely due to the relatively good prognosis for stage II patients after surgery alone, and the resulting requirement to randomize thousands of patients to demonstrate a small margin of absolute improvement in survival with adequate statistical power [8].

Based on that, ASCO issued a guideline stating that direct evidence from RCTs does not support the routine use of adjuvant chemotherapy for stage II colon cancer patients.

However, the subset of stage II colon cancer patients includes subgroups with a high risk of relapse.

Patients for whom the number of sampled lymph nodes was very small can be considered as inadequately staged and at greater risk of having microscopic residual disease. As a result, patients with inadequately sampled nodes could be offered adjuvant chemotherapy.

Other patients with any of a number of poor prognostic features such as T4 lesion (defined as adherence to or invasion of local organs), perforation, or poorly differentiated histology might also be regarded as candidates for adjuvant chemotherapy [38, 76].

The question of whether or not to offer adjuvant chemotherapy to stage II patients at higher risk or with inadequately sampled nodes should be considered in the light of the available evidence.

Direct evidence from RCTs and meta-analyses of such trials does not demonstrate any survival benefit for adjuvant chemotherapy in high-risk stage II disease, yet, and there are toxic effects of treatment. On the other hand, in the high-risk setting, it is reasonable for oncologists and patients to invoke indirect evidence of benefit by generalizing from the positive results of adjuvant chemotherapy in stage III colon cancer patients.

The clinical decision should be based on a discussion with the patient about the nature of the direct evidence supporting treatment.

Both the quality of surgery and lymph node sampling have been evaluated extensively, and the latter has most often been implicated in assessing prognosis for high-risk colon cancer. Inherent in the accurate staging of a patient with stage II disease is the retrieval and examination of an adequate number of lymph nodes. In a series of 35,787 stage II colon cancer cases from the National Cancer Data Base (NCDB), the 5-year survival rate varied from 64%, if only one or two lymph nodes were examined, to 86% if over 25 lymph nodes were tested.

Although the precise number of lymph nodes to be examined is not known, the NCDB investigators concluded that at least 13 lymph nodes should be retrieved and declared pathologically negative for a patient to be labeled or treated as having stage II disease.

Therefore, it is important that the definition of stage II colon cancer be restricted to patients with at least 10–13 lymph nodes examined [6, 9], and to cases with T4 disease who received en bloc resection and did not have a perforated tumor. Otherwise, lax criteria for stage II disease may include patients at higher risk of undetected lymph node metastases or spillage of cancer cells in the peritoneal cavity at surgery. These and other potential prognostic factors have been described [47, 62].

Patients with resected colon cancer should be staged appropriately, and only those with no tumor involvement in at least 10–13 regional lymph nodes, real en bloc resection for T4 tumor, and no evidence of tumor perforation into the peritoneal cavity should be classified as stage II. They have excellent prognosis, and if over 60 years of age, they are unlikely to benefit from adjuvant therapy. Clinical adjuvant trials involving patients with stage II colon cancer must be restrictive in their definition of stage.

Two larger trials – namely, the MOSAIC (Multicenter International Study of Oxaliplatin/5-Fluorouracil/Leucovorin in the Adjuvant Treatment of Colon Cancer) trial [2] and NSABP (National Surgical Adjuvant Breast and Bowel Project) C-07 study [59] – have evaluated the introduction of oxaliplatin as adjuvant therapy for stage II or III colon cancer.

The MOSAIC trial is a large ($n > 2,246$), international, multicenter, phase III, randomized, open-label, active-controlled study comparing the efficacy and safety of oxaliplatin in combination with an infusional de Gramont schedule of 5-FU/LV (FOLFOX-4 regimen) or infusional 5-FU/LV alone (LF5FU2 regimen) for 6 months in patients with stage II (40%) or III (60%) colon cancer. The primary trial end-point was DFS; secondary end-points included toxicity and OS.

The NSABP C-07 study is a large ($n > 2,492$), international, multicenter, phase III, randomized, active-controlled trial comparing the efficacy and safety of oxaliplatin in combination with a bolus of 5-FU/LV (FLOX regimen) or bolus 5-FU/LV alone (Roswell Park Regimen) for 24 weeks in patients with stage II (29%) or III (71%) colon cancer. The primary and secondary trial end points were the same as in the MOSAIC trial.

In the MOSAIC trial, the probability of recurrence for the intention-to-treat (ITT) population was 73.3 and 67.4% for FOLFOX-4 and LV5FU2 groups, respectively (HR = 0.80; $p = 0.003$), which means a 20% reduction in the relapse risk in favor of FOLFOX-4.

In patients with stage III (any T, N1 or N2, M0) colon cancer, the probability of remaining disease-free at 5 years was 66.4 and 58.9% for FOLFOX-4 and LV5FU2 groups, respectively (HR = 0.78; $p = 0.005$).

However, among stage II patients, the probability of DFS events at 5 years was 83.7 and 79.9% in the FOLFOX-4 and LV5FU2 groups, respectively (HR = 0.84; $p = 0.258$), failing to demonstrate a significant improvement.

In the stage III subsetting, the probability of surviving at 6 years was 72.9 and 68.7%, respectively (HR = 0.80; $p = 0.023$), that is a 20% reduction in the death risk in favor of FOLFOX-4. In patients with stage II disease, the probability of surviving at 6 years was 86.9 and 86.8%, respectively (HR > 1.00; $p > 0.986$).

It can be inferred from the above that FOLFOX-4 is useful after surgery for patients undergoing curative treatment for stage III colon cancer, but a similar conclusion cannot be drawn for stage II disease as a whole.

However, the NSABP C-07 trial had already shown the same findings. The overall DFS rates at 4 years were 73.2% for FLOX and 67.3% for 5-FU/LV. The HR for FLOX vs. 5-FU/LV was 0.80 ($p = 0.0034$), corresponding to a 20% relative relapse risk reduction in favor of FLOX.

These data from two independent large controlled clinical trials establish unequivocally the efficacy of the oxaliplatin-FU-LV combination as postoperative adjuvant therapy for stage III disease. Despite that MOSAIC trial has found a trend toward improved DFS at 5 years in patients with high-risk stage II disease treated with FOLFOX-4 and the NSABP C-07 trial has not found significant interactions between stage and treatment, the role of adjuvant therapy for stage II colon cancer remains controversial. However, neither study was powered to detect improvement in patients with stage II disease.

Therefore, both FOLFOX-4 and FLOX are more effective as adjuvant therapy for colon cancer than the same regimens without oxaliplatin. In patients with node-positive colon cancer, the combination of FU, LV, and oxaliplatin unequivocally improves DFS and can be recommended in clinical practice. These studies do not rule out the benefits for stage II colon cancer patients, although their absolute magnitude is likely to be small in unselected patients [64].

The evidence to support the use of oral capecitabine as adjuvant treatment is shown in the large ($n > 1,987$), international, multicenter, phase III, randomized, open-label, active-controlled X-ACT study [84], which compared oral capecitabine with a bolus Mayo Clinic regimen of 5-FU/LV for a total of 24 weeks in patients with stage III (Dukes' C) colon cancer. The primary trial endpoint was at least equivalent in DFS.

Capecitabine therapy was shown to be at least equivalent to 5-FU/LV in that the primary endpoint (DFS) was met. The HR comparing DFS in the capecitabine group with that in the 5 FU-FV/LV group was 0.87 (95% CI 0.75–1.00). The upper limit of the confidence interval (1.0) was significantly lower than both preset values of 1.25 and 1.20, or at least equivalent ($p < 0.001$ for both comparisons), providing confidence that capecitabine is at least as effective as 5 FU-FV/LV.

The adverse events most commonly leading to dose modifications (including treatment interruption and dose reduction) were hand–foot syndrome (31%) and diarrhea (15%) in the capecitabine group, and stomatitis (23%) and diarrhea (19%) in the 5 FU-FV/LV group.

Patients receiving capecitabine experienced significantly less grade 3 or 4 stomatitis (2 vs. 14%; with 5-FU/LV $p < 0.001$) and alopecia (0 vs. <1%; $p < 0.02$) and grade 3 or 4 neutropenia requiring medical intervention (0.6 vs. 5% $p > 0.001$). Grade 3 hand–foot syndrome was significantly more common in the capecitabine arm (18 vs. 0.6% $p < 0.001$) [77].

As a result of toxicity, both the groups required dose modifications (42% of the patients receiving capecitabine vs. 44% of those treated with 5-FU/LV).

14.8.1.1 Colon Cancer Adjuvant Setting Recommendations

The ASCO has been providing clinical recommendations on different clinical entities for several years. As far as gastrointestinal cancer is concerned, there are three guidelines: the ASCO 2006 update and Recommendation for the use of tumor markers in gastrointestinal cancer; the Colorectal Cancer Surveillance: 2005 Update of the ASCO Practice Guideline; and the ASCO Recommendation on Adjuvant Chemotherapy for Stage II Colon Cancer published in 2003. An update of the latter guideline is in progress.

A recent Italian publication [22] adopting the GRADE approach has investigated also on the colon cancer adjuvant setting. The conclusion has been: "probably use it, weak positive" recommendation for stage III. Furthermore, the same recommendation has been produced with regard to the use of oxaliplatin in association with FU and folinic acid vs. FU and folinic acid, and the use of capecitabine instead of FU and folinic acid infusion. For stage II colon cancer, the suggested recommendation has been: "no recommendation." In fact, nowadays, only the so-called high-risk stage II colon cancer (inadequate number of analyzed lymph nodes, grade 3 tumors, perforation/occlusion, and age under 50) patients are included in the ongoing or recently closed RCTs.

14.8.2 Colorectal Metastatic Setting. First-Line Chemotherapy

Stage IIIC and IV advanced colorectal cancer (ACRC) is so locally diffuse that surgical resection is unlikely to be carried out with curative or metastatic intent. Out of those cases, around 50% will have liver metastases. Clearly, there is much interest in evaluating targeted monoclonal antibodies, and notable studies have explored the clinical effectiveness of bevacizumab and cetuximab as first-line treatment of metastatic colorectal cancer.

Three RCTs [51, 56, 57] were included in the assessment of bevacizumab, of which one compared bevacizumab plus irinotecan, fluorouracil, and leucovorin (IFLV) vs. IFLV alone, whereas the remaining two trials compared bevacizumab plus 5-FU/LV vs. 5-FU/LV alone. OS was the primary endpoint in all studies.

The addition of 5 mg/kg bevacizumab to IFLV resulted in a statistically significant increase in median OS by 4.7 months (HR = 0.66; $p < 0.001$), which means a 34% reduction in the death risk in the bevacizumab group, and in a statistically significant increase in median PFS by 4.4 months (HR = 0.54, $p < 0.001$).

As compared with IFL alone, the IFL plus bevacizumab regimen increased PFS from a median of 6.2 months to 10.6 months, the overall response rate from 34.8 to 44.8%, and the median response duration from 7.1 to 10.4 months.

Furthermore the clinical benefit was accompanied by a relatively modest increase in the treatment-related adverse events, which were easily managed. Only the incidence of hypertension was significantly increased in the bevacizumab plus IFLV group ($p < 0.01$), with all episodes being manageable with standard oral antihypertensive agents [51].

To evaluate the safety and efficacy of bevacizumab in metastatic colorectal cancer, Kabbinavar et al. [57] designed a trial in which 5 mg/kg bevacizumab were added to bolus 5-FU/LV as first-line therapy. Median survival was 16.6 and 12.9 months for the FU/LV/bevacizumab group and for the FU/LV/placebo patients, respectively, resulting in a non-significant increase in median OS by 3.7 months (HR = 0.79; $p = 0.16$). Also within this study, the addition of 5 mg/kg bevacizumab to 5-FU/LV resulted in a statistically significant increase in median PFS by 3.7 months (HR = 0.50; $p = 0.0002$).

Another study [56] investigated the safety and efficacy of adding 5 mg/kg bevacizumab to 5-FULV/FA, and found a non-significant increase in median OS by 7.7 months (HR = 0.63). This study did not report on PFS but on the time to disease progression (TTP), defined as the time from randomization up to objective tumor progression. TTP was used as a primary endpoint for this trial. The results showed that the addition of bevacizumab at 5 mg/kg produced a statistically

significant increase in TTP by 3.8 months as against FU/LV alone (9.0 vs. 5.2 months, $p = 0.005$).

The combined analysis of the above three studies reported a 26% reduction in the daily death risk with bevacizumab plus 5-FU/LV vs. 5-FU/LV or IFLV alone, with an HR of 0.74 ($p = 0.0008$) and a significant benefit in terms of median PFS in patients treated with FU/LV plus bevacizumab vs. FU/LV or IFLV (8.77 vs. 5.55 months, $p = 0.001$) [55].

The trials indicate that bevacizumab plus 5-FU/LV and bevacizumab plus IFLV are clinically effective in comparison with standard chemotherapy options for the first-line treatment of metastatic CRC.

Randomized phase II and III studies on metastatic colorectal cancer have demonstrated efficacy and tolerability of cetuximab as monotherapy or in combination with irinotecan after previous irinotecan and/or oxaliplatin-based chemotherapy regimens.

Two studies reported OS estimates for patients receiving cetuximab in combination with irinotecan. The BOND trial [19] randomly assigned 329 patients whose disease had progressed during or within 3 months after treatment with an irinotecan-based regimen to receive either cetuximab and irinotecan or cetuximab alone. The reported median OS was 8.6 and 6.9 months for patients receiving the combined cetuximab plus irinotecan regimen and cetuximab alone, respectively (HR = 0.91; $p = 0.48$). The HR for disease progression in the combination-therapy group was 0.54 ($p < 0.001$) indicating a 46% reduction in the disease progression risk as against the monotherapy group.

Cetuximab in combination with irinotecan had significantly more adverse events (any grade 3 or 4 adverse event) than cetuximab alone, 65.1 vs. 43.5% ($p < 0.001$). Key toxicities associated with cetuximab plus irinotecan were the presence of an acne-like rash (80% in each group), diarrhea, and neutropenia.

Based on scientific background, Saltz et al. [74] conducted a phase II study to formally evaluate the activity and safety of cetuximab plus irinotecan in patients with irinotecan-refractory colorectal cancer. Five patients achieved a partial response, whereas 21 additional patients had stable disease or minor responses. Median OS, meant as the time span from the beginning of treatment to death, for the 57 treated patients was 6.4 months, and the median time to progression was 2.9 months. Therefore, the evidence on TRRs suggests that cetuximab plus irinotecan has some clinical activity.

Furthermore, in the first-line setting, building on promising phase II data, the Crystal trial, a randomized phase III study of irinotecan and 5-FU/LV (FOLFIRI) with or without cetuximab as front-line therapy in 1,217 patients with metastatic colorectal cancer, found a significant increase in both response rates (46.9 vs. 38.7%; $p=0.005$) and the primary endpoint of PFS (8.9 vs. 8 months, $p=0.036$) in the cetuximab arm [85].

In the subgroup analysis, a quantitative PCR method in codons 12/13 was used to assess the K-RAS status in 587 patients whose tumor samples were available, and it showed a statistically significant difference in PFS (HR=0.68; $p=0.0167$) in favor of 346 patients with K-RAS wild-type genes who had received cetuximab, and the best overall response was 59.3% (cetuximab+FOLFIRI) vs. 43.2% (FOLFIRI) ($p=0.0025$). When the K-RAS mutation status was assessed for cetuximab and FOLFIRI vs. FOLFIRI alone, no significant differences in PFS (HR=1.07; $p=0.75$) or the best overall response ($p>0.46$) were observed. In the ITT population, there was no OS advantage in all patients who had received cetuximab vs. FOLFIRI alone (19.9 vs. 18.6 months; HR=0.931 p = 0.305).

In K-RAS wild-type patients, median OS was 24.9 months in those treated with cetuximab vs. 21 months in those who had been given FOLFIRI alone, but again the difference was not significant (HR=0.844; $p=0.217$). The lack of significance here was thought to be driven by high crossover for the placebo group and low statistical power.

The OPUS trial, a randomized phase III study of FOLFOX-4 regimen with or without cetuximab as first-line therapy in 338 patients with metastatic colorectal cancer, found that the overall response rate increased by 10% (46 vs. 36%) following addition of cetuximab to FOLFOX-4 vs. FOLFOX-4 alone. However, it was not possible to determine a statistically significant increase in the odds of response ($p=0.064$). The risk of disease progression was similar for both the ITT ($n>337$) (HR=0.93; $p=0.6170$) and K-RAS populations (DNA suitable for the K-RAS mutation analysis was extracted from the tumor samples of 233 patients) (HR=0.928; $p=0.6609$).

However, when retrospective efficacy analyses were carried out in the K-RAS group according to K-RAS mutation status, striking differences were seen. Patients whose tumors were K-RAS wild-type had a clinically relevant increase in the chance of response (61 vs. 37%; odds ratio 2.544; $p=0.011$), and

a just as significant decrease in the risk of disease progression (61 vs. 37%; HR=0.57; $p=0.0163$). On the contrary, patients whose tumors carried a K-RAS gene mutation were more likely to derive a trend for improved PFS time if treated with FOLFOX-4 alone rather than with cetuximab plus FOLFOX-4 (HR=1.830; $p=0.0192$) [11].

These data, like those from the CRYSTAL study, confirm the activity of cetuximab to be restricted to patients with K-RAS wild-type tumors.

Furthermore, given that in the CRYSTAL study subgroup analyzes by K-RAS mutation status for cetuximab and FOLFIRI vs. FOLFIRI alone demonstrate no difference in PFS between the treatment groups, the type of chemotherapy may be a factor in any possible interaction.

It is interesting to note that the phase III CAIRO2 trial, in which patients were randomized to receive CAPOX (capecitabine/oxaliplatin) and bevacizumab or the same combination regimen plus cetuximab, found that the addition of cetuximab to CAPOX plus bevacizumab did not have any impact on the overall response, median PFS, or OS rates. When patients were grouped according to their K-RAS status, patients with mutant K-RAS who received CAPOX with the dual biologic agents experienced a significant 4-month reduction in median PFS compared with CAPOX plus bevacizumab with excess toxicity, particularly skin toxicity and diarrhea [83]. The findings from this study demonstrate that the use of bevacizumab plus cetuximab in combination with CAPOX chemotherapy in the first-line setting did not provide any clinical benefit, and raised the possibility of a negative interaction between anti-EGFR antibodies and bevacizumab when combined with chemotherapy.

Another randomized phase III trial ($n>1,053$) evaluated panitumumab plus bevacizumab and (oxaliplatin – and irinotecan-based) chemotherapy as first-line treatment for metastatic colorectal cancer. Within each chemotherapy cohort, patients were randomly assigned to bevacizumab and chemotherapy with or without panitumumab. The primary endpoint was PFS within the oxaliplatin cohort, whereas the primary endpoint for irinotecan-based chemotherapy was to describe safety. PFS was significantly worse in the panitumumab arm within the oxaliplatin-based chemotherapy group (HR= 1.44; $p=0.004$). K-RAS analyzes showed adverse outcomes for the panitumumab arm in both wild-type and mutant groups. Therefore, the addition of panitumumab to bevacizumab and oxaliplatin or irinotecan-based chemotherapy resulted in increased toxicity and decreased PFS [49].

14.8.2.1 Metastatic Colon Cancer Setting Recommendations

In metastatic colon cancer care, there have been a very rapid progress of knowledge and a wealth of new data in recent years, which has no match in the adjuvant setting that necessitates a longer time period to obtain the results from RCTs.

This amount of information and data needs to be confirmed and classified before strong guidelines and recommendations can appear, and therefore in the short run, the correct application of the information derived from RCTs is the only way to pursue the interest of each single patient. Furthermore, the cost of such new treatments needs to be carefully balanced against potential advantages, which is up to regulatory entities and national governments.

Anyway, ASCO has recently published and introduced the "provisional clinical opinions (PCOs)" which are based on the expedited review of potentially practice-changing evidence. The first PCO was on the use of K-RAS to help select patients with advanced/metastatic colon cancer to be treated with the monoclonal antibody cetuximab or panitumumab.

14.9 Breast Cancer

Breast cancer is the most common malignancy in women worldwide with a higher prevalence in industrialized countries, and it is the leading cause of cancer-related mortality. Some patients with early breast cancer may be cured with loco-regional treatment alone, whereas the majority will have undetectable (micrometastatic) disease and require adjuvant systemic therapy. Both adjuvant hormonal therapy and chemotherapy together with the new targeted therapies like trastuzumab can improve DFS and OS rates in premenopausal and postmenopausal women. The decision on how to treat early stage breast cancer with a multidisciplinary approach is one of the most difficult, due to the large amount of clinical trials sometimes

having contradictory results. To help clinicians in the decision-making process, different tools have been made available including treatment guidelines developed by experts on the basis of evidences provided by clinical trials and transferred into applications for individual patient care (for example, the National Cancer Center Network Guidelines are updated yearly in line with new data appearing in the literature as well as with the American Society Clinical Oncology Guidelines).

Moreover, since 1978, experts' opinions are summarized in a consensus conference that takes place in St. Gallen every 2 years in order to define recommendations on how to select the best options for adjuvant systemic treatments in each specific subgroup of early breast cancer patients [39]. Established prognostic factors are age, nodal status, tumor size, and grade. The amount of estrogen and progesterone receptors define the so-called endocrine responsiveness that may be regarded as a prognostic and predictive factor, and may be used to classify tumors into three major categories: estrogen and progesterone-receptor-positive tumors, which may be considered as highly endocrine responsive, and for which the main (and eventually the only necessary) adjuvant therapy may be hormone therapy; estrogen and progesterone-receptor negative tumors, which may be regarded as endocrine nonresponsive, for which adjuvant chemotherapy is effective, and so far, the only evidence-based therapy, irrespective of menopausal status; and an intermediate category with tumors having a low level of receptors, for which both endocrine therapy and chemotherapy would be required. Another prognostic and predictive marker is human epidermal growth factor receptor 2 (HER-2), which is the target of the monoclonal antibody trastuzumab. Gene expressing profiles (the 21-gene assay Oncotype DX, and the 70-gene assay MammaPrint) are newer prognostic, and probably predictive, tests. Clinical trials are ongoing to validate these tools for the selection of the most adequate treatment.

As we know, EBM was created to make order in a jungle of data and to help young clinicians who have no personal experience with the interpretation of data, and to give them the ability to select important findings from anecdotic data, applying a scale of levels of evidence ranking from bottom to top as the one obtained from meta-analyses of RCTs. Some examples on the issue of early breast cancer treatment found in the literature are reported.

14.9.1 Adjuvant Endocrine Therapy

Hormonal treatment with ovariectomy was the first "target therapy" used as adjuvant endocrine treatment. More recently, hormonal agents including ovarian suppression with luteinizing hormone-releasing hormone (LHRH), the antiestrogen tamoxifen and aromatase inhibitors (AI), which are divided into nonsteroidal (e.g., anastrazole and letrozole) and steroidal (e.g., exemestane) were used. A level I of evidence was proven for tamoxifen as adjuvant treatment in stage I or stage II breast cancer patients. Actually, the benefit of tamoxifen was investigated by a meta-analysis published in 2005: the 15-year absolute reductions in recurrence and mortality rates with a 5-year administration were confined to women with ER-positive or ER-unknown tumors, irrespective of lymph node status, menopausal status, age, and use of chemotherapy [25]. Tamoxifen, taken for 5 years, reduces the annual odds of disease recurrence and death by 47 and 26%, respectively [25]. For this reason, tamoxifen has become the "gold standard" hormonal agent. Two randomized trials (NSABP-14 and the Scottish study), which compared 5 years vs. 10 years of adjuvant tamoxifen administration, failed to show any advantage for the continuation of therapy beyond 5 years. Both trials even demonstrated a trend toward a worse outcome associated with prolonged treatment mainly due to an excess risk of tamoxifen-induced endometrial cancer [32, 81]. The value of adjuvant tamoxifen after chemotherapy in premenopausal breast cancer women was assessed in numerous trials, including, for instance, the IBCSG 13–93 trial, in which 1,246 assessable premenopausal women with axillary node-positive, operable breast cancer received chemotherapy (cyclophosphamide plus either doxorubicin or epirubicin for four courses followed by immediate or delayed classical cyclophosphamide, methotrexate, and fluorouracil for three courses) followed by either tamoxifen (20 mg daily) for 5 years or no further treatment [14]. Tamoxifen improved DFS in the ER-positive cohort (HR for tamoxifen vs. no tamoxifen=0.59; 95%; CI, 0.46–0.75; $p<0.0001$) but not in the ER-negative cohort (HR=1.02; 95% CI, 0.77–1.35; $p=0.89$). In an unplanned exploratory analysis, tamoxifen showed a detrimental effect on patients with ER-absent disease vs. no tamoxifen (HR=2.10; 95% CI, 1.03–4.29; $p=0.04$). Patients with ER-positive tumors who had achieved chemotherapy-induced amenorrhea had a significantly improved outcome (HR for amenorrhea vs. no amenorrhea = 0.61; 95% CI, 0.44–0.86; $p=0.004$), regardless of whether they received or did not receive tamoxifen. Different RCTs were designed to compare tamoxifen plus chemotherapy vs. tamoxifen alone in postmenopausal women: the overall results of the available evidence suggest that the addition of chemotherapy to tamoxifen has a significant, albeit small impact on survival advantage [33–35]. It is difficult, however, to try and identify whether sufficient levels of evidence are available to spare chemotherapy in patients with a highly endocrine-responsive disease who are not expected to have an additional benefit from cytotoxic drugs, and also to identify the optimal treatment regimens to be combined with hormonal therapies.

In premenopausal women, a meta-analysis showed that ovarian ablation or suppression reduce the 15-year absolute risk of recurrence by 4.3% and the mortality risk by 3.2% [25]. The comparison between ovarian ablation and suppression with different chemotherapy regimens has been the object of several clinical trials, most of which found no difference in the OS and DFS rates between the treatment groups. However, the chemotherapy regimens did not include antracyclines and taxanes, which are more effective drugs in comparison to CMF regimen. Whether ovarian suppression may provide an alternative to chemotherapy and whether LHRH may induce any additional benefit when associated with tamoxifen or AI requires further investigation which is now ongoing in the SOFT trial.

AI have recently challenged tamoxifen as "gold standard" hormonal treatment for postmenopausal patients. They have been studied in prospective trials either as up-front therapy or sequential treatment after 2–3 years of tamoxifen administration. A large randomized trial (ATAC trial) compared tamoxifen vs. anastrazole vs. a combination of tamoxifen and anastrazole as adjuvant endocrine therapy in postmenopausal women with both node-negative and node-positive breast cancer [37]. The results of this study suggest an advantage in terms of DFS, time to recurrence, and contralateral breast cancer rate for the anastrazole arm as compared to the tamoxifen and the combination arms. The absolute benefit for time to recurrence has increased from 2.8% at 5 years to 4.8% at 100 months, showing a carry-over effect similar to that reported with tamoxifen and indicating that the benefit persists after discontinuation of the drug. No significant difference in the OS rates has been observed so far. Three randomized trials (ABCSG 8, ARNO 95, and ITA trials) were performed to evaluate the switch to anastrazole after 2–3 years of tamoxifen administration. The overall results suggest that switching to anastrazole improves DFS rates significantly as compared to continuing tamoxifen [10, 52]. A meta-analysis on upfront, switching, and sequencing anastrozole in the adjuvant treatment of early breast cancer was published in 2008 [5]. The combined hazard ratio of four trials for event-free survival (EFS) was 0.77 (95%CI: 0.70–0.85; $p < 0.0001$) for patients treated with anastrozole vs. tamoxifen. In the second analysis in which only ITA, ABCSG 8, and ARNO 95 trials were included and ATAC (up-front trial) was excluded, the combined hazard ratio for EFS was 0.64 (95%CI: 0.52–0.79; $p < 0.0001$). In the third analysis including the hazard ratio for recurrence-free survival (excluding nondisease related deaths) of estrogen receptor-positive patients for the ATAC trial and the hazard ratio for EFS of all patients for the remaining trials, the combined hazard ratio was 0.73 (95%CI: 0.65–0.81; $p < 0.0001$).

In conclusion, it seems that a level I of evidence was reached for AI, which are more effective than tamoxifen in the adjuvant hormonal treatment of early breast cancer. An analysis of the elderly population was performed in another four-arm double-blind randomized trial (BIG-1-98) that compared 5-year tamoxifen vs. 5-year letrozole vs. crossover to a sequence of both drugs at 2 years [18]. The results confirmed that the aromatase inhibitor letrozole was safe also in this group of patients. The updated study was presented at the last San Antonio Breast Cancer Symposium: at a median follow-up time of 71 months, the monotherapy update suggests improved survival for the letrozole group vs. the tamoxifen arm. The sequential treatments did not improve DFS as against letrozole alone. Trends support the initial use of letrozole in patients at higher risk of relapse as, for instance, those with a large number of positive nodes. Patients commenced on letrozole can be switched to tamoxifen if required. Until further clinical evidence comes up, AI should be the initial hormonal therapy in postmenopausal early breast cancer patients, and switching should be considered only for patients who are currently receiving tamoxifen. Distant DFS was taken as a surrogate endpoint for survival, due to the large amount of crossover treatment among patients that probably will obscure the survival benefit in the entire population.

Letrozole was evaluated also as extended therapy after 5 years of tamoxifen in a randomized, double-blind trial (MA-17) in a group of postmenopausal women already treated with tamoxifen [40]. The first interim analysis (median, 2.4 patient years) showed substantial benefits from letrozole in terms of DFS and distant DFS, and all patients were unblinded and offered the drug. An OS advantage was observed in the node-positive patient subgroup. Despite two thirds of the patients crossing over to letrozole, an ITT analysis at 54 months' follow-up continued to demonstrate the strong beneficial effect of extended adjuvant letrozole [40–42]. Furthermore, a significant benefit was demonstrated among patients who had been randomized to placebo but elected to take letrozole after a prolonged washout from previous tamoxifen (late extended adjuvant therapy).

In one randomized trial (Breast International Group-9702), the switch to exemestane after 2–3 years of treatment with tamoxifen was investigated. This study compared a 5-year tamoxifen administration vs. 2–3 years of tamoxifen followed by exemestane up to 5 years, and it demonstrated an advantage in terms of DFS, but not in terms of OS, for the switching arm [15].

On the basis of the DFS advantage, AI have become the new standard adjuvant therapy in postmenopausal women especially if at higher risks; however, because of lack of evidence of a clear benefit in terms of OS, tamoxifen remains a valid option as standard treatment, especially in lower-risk patients. Survival benefits must be balanced against long-term adverse events and costs.

14.9.2 Adjuvant Chemotherapy

A level I of evidence exists for adjuvant chemotherapy that improves disease-free and OS rates for early stage breast cancer patients, irrespective of nodal status. According to the National Comprehensive Cancer Network (NCCN) guidelines and St. Gallen recommendations, adjuvant chemotherapy is indicated for healthy patients with node-positive breast cancer or node-negative disease at high risk of relapse for the presence of other unfavorable prognostic factors, such as tumor size greater than 1 cm, younger age (<35 years), high tumor grade, and estrogen and progesterone-receptor negative status [39]. These data came from the EBCTCG meta-analysis, which summarized the results of about 80 randomized adjuvant trials initiated in 1995 [25]. An antracycline-based chemotherapy regimen is the first choice chemotherapy, but its benefits vary among patient groups. Generally, the benefit is probably greater in HER2 and topoisomerase II overexpressing tumors and younger patients, whereas it is smaller in hormonal receptor-positive patients, HER2-negative, and node-negative patients. Several RCTs explored the impact of adding taxane (paclitaxel and docetaxel) to an antracycline-based regimen: a meta-analysis of 13 trials has shown that inclusion of taxane improved both DFS and OS, with an absolute benefit of 5 and 3%, respectively [21]. More recently, a Cochrane review focusing on the role of taxanes in the adjuvant setting has examined the results of 12 out of 20 RCTs, and it has found out that adjuvant chemotherapy including a taxane drug lowers the cancer death risk and reduces the number of recurrences: the HR for DFS and OS was 0.81 (95% CI 0.77–0.86; $p<0.00001$) and 0.81 (95% CI 0.75–0.88; $p<0.00001$), respectively, which is in favor of taxane-containing regimens [29]. Further trials are needed to find the best way to use a taxane drug when it is given in combination with other nontaxane chemotherapy drugs. The Oncology Research Trial 9735 compared four courses of a nonantracycline-containing regimen (Docetaxel-Cyclophosphamide, DC regimen) vs. the standard adriamycin plus cyclophosphamide (AC) regimen : after a 7-year follow-up period, the DC regimen significantly improved DFS and OS as against the AC regimen, and the benefit was independent of HER2 status and age [54]. This study demonstrated for the first time an advantage of a nonantracycline containing regimen over antracycline-based chemotherapy in a subgroup of patients for whom a shorter length of therapy (four courses) may be adequate, such as intermediate or low risk patients (node-negative, one to three positive lymph nodes, ER-positive) or patients with cardiovascular disease or already treated with antracycline. Even if the subgroup analysis should be regarded only as "hypothesis-generating" and is not a valid tool for EBM, it is to be considered ,for instance, when evaluating a special patient population like the elderly. In this case, what is "evidence-based" for younger patients may not apply due to comorbidities typical of older age. For instance, even if the meta-analysis suggested the benefit of anthracycline containing regimens in

node-positive patients, this approach may be contraindicated in a woman who suffered a previous myocardial infarction. Moreover, an increased risk of heart failure following anthracycline administration is noted mainly in the subgroup of patients over 65 [82]. Furthermore, until recently, all RCTs have had an upper age limit of 65 years that prevented their results from being extended to the overall population of women aged 70 or more. On the other hand, only few trials started in this group of patients due to different and well-noted methodological problems [17].

14.9.3 Monoclonal Antibodies

HER2 receptor, which is overexpressed in about 20% of primary breast cancer, is the target of the recombinant humanized monoclonal antibody trastuzumab. This molecular therapy was proven to be one of the most successful rationally designed biological cancer therapies, contributing to a major achievement in the oncology field. The important role of the drug was first demonstrated in a work on metastatic breast cancer patients, but the survival advantage in this study was noted with a post-hoc analysis in the pivotal trial of the group of patients with IHC 3+ staining [79], which confirmed the assumption that not all HER 2-positive patients (as, for instance, those with 1+ or 2+ staining) derive the same survival advantage, but only a minority of them. On the other hand, we would have lost one of the most important drugs of the last decades if we had concentrated on the overall data and not on the real target group with HER 2 overexpression. Six RCTs have addressed the role of this drug in the adjuvant setting in combination or in sequence with chemotherapy: the NSABP B-31 study, the North Central Cancer Treatment Group (NCCTG) N9831 trial, the herceptin adjuvant (HERA) trial, the Breast Cancer International Research Group (BCIRG) 006 study, the Finland Herceptin (FinHER) study and the French and Belgian cooperative study programs d'Actions Concertees 04 (PACS-04) [70, 80]. Overall, the results of all available studies show with a level I of evidence that the addiction of trastuzumab to chemotherapy or its use after chemotherapy have a positive effect in early-stage HER2-positive breast cancer patients. The NCCN Guidelines recommend that adjuvant trastuzumab therapy be administered as a standard treatment in patients with node-negative, high risk, or node-positive early-stage breast cancer overexpressing HER2: trastuzumab improves disease-free, and probably overall, survival rates, irrespective of age, axillary node metastases, and estrogen and progesterone-receptor status. Direct comparison of these studies is difficult because they differed in design: in the NSABP B-31 and the NCCTG N9831 trial, trastuzumab was administered during and after a taxane regimen following four cycles of doxorubicin and cyclophosphamide; [70] the HERA trial explored 1 or 2 years of trastuzumab therapy after completion of adjuvant chemotherapy; [67] the BCIRG 006 trial assessed the use of trastuzumab in combination with platinum-based chemotherapy; [78] the FinHER trial tested a short course of trastuzumab administered concomitantly with adjuvant chemotherapy; [53] finally, the PACS-04 trial focused on a 1-year administration of trastuzumab after the end of chemotherapy in node-positive, HER2-positive breast cancer patients [80]. As a result of different trial designs, uncertainties remain about the ideal timing, optimum schedule, and preferable duration of treatment with trastuzumab as well as the optimal chemotherapy regimen it should be associated with. However, current data do not support the use of trastuzumab for longer than 1 year. Trastuzumab has an acceptable toxicity profile: the incidence of cardiac toxicity derived from chemotherapy associated with trastuzumab ranges from 0.5 to 4%. Other targeted therapies such as lapatinib and pertuzumab are going to be investigated in further investigational trials.

14.9.4 Neoadjuvant Therapy

Primary systemic chemotherapy (PSC) or neoadjuvant chemotherapy has been increasingly used in order to obtain tumor downstaging and consequently increase the rate of breast-conservation surgery, to evaluate the treatment effect in vivo, and possibly to improve outcomes. Early trials of primary systemic therapy compared the same schedule of chemotherapy before or after standard surgical treatment. The NSABP B-18 trial randomized patients to four courses of antracycline-based chemotherapy before and after surgery [88]. No difference in OS was observed, but the rate of breast-conservation surgery performed among patients receiving PSC was higher. Furthermore, patients with complete

pathological response to PSC had improved DFS and OS. Subsequent trials evaluated if different neoadjuvant regimens could improve outcome: the NSABP B-27 trial is a three-arm study comparing a preoperative antracycline-based regimen (AC) vs. an AC followed by four courses of docetaxel (T); the addition of T to AC did not have a significant impact on DFS or OS. Preoperative T added to AC significantly increased the proportion of patients with pathological complete responses (pCRs) over preoperative AC alone (26 vs. 13%, respectively; $p<0.0001$) [7]. An update of the NSABP Protocols B-18 and B-27 was published: in both studies, patients who had achieved pCR continued to have significantly better DFS and OS outcomes vs. patients who had not. B-18 and B-27 suggest that preoperative therapy is equivalent to adjuvant therapy. B-27 also shows that the addition of preoperative taxanes to AC improves response rates [68]. A first meta-analysis assessed the effectiveness of neoadjuvant chemotherapy on clinical outcome [60] by reviewing the results of fourteen RCTs comparing adjuvant and neoadjuvant chemotherapy. Overall, these trials included 5,500 patients with early breast cancer. Survival rate was equivalent in both groups; however, breast conservation surgery was offered more frequently to patients treated with neoadjuvant therapy without having an influence on the local recurrence rate and therefore giving more opportunities to women to conserve their breast. A second meta-analysis on the use of taxanes as primary chemotherapy for early breast cancer was performed by Cuppone et al. [20]. Seven RCTs were identified collecting 2,455 patients. Patients receiving taxane-containing regimens had a significantly higher rate of breast conservation surgery ($p=0.012$) and pCRs, but the differences were not statistically significant. Patients receiving taxanes as a sequential schedule had a significant higher probability to achieve pCR ($p=0.013$), whereas the use as a concomitant schedule gives the patients a significantly higher probability to achieve BCS ($p=0.027$). The complete response rate was significantly higher in the taxane arms, regardless of the adopted strategy. In conclusion, the combination of taxanes and anthracyclines as neoadjuvant chemotherapy for early breast cancer improves the chance of achieving both higher BCS and pCR rates. The role of trastuzumab in the neoadjuvant setting has been evaluated by several phase II trials. One phase III randomized trial showed a higher pCR rate in patients with HER2-positive breast cancer after concurrent administration of trastuzumab and paclitaxel followed by concurrent trastuzumab and 5-fluorouracil, epirubicin, and cyclophosphamide (FEC) preoperative chemotherapy: 42 patients were randomly assigned to either four cycles of paclitaxel followed by four cycles of FEC or to the same chemotherapy with simultaneous weekly trastuzumab for 24 weeks [13]. In the second cohort, the pathological CR rate was 54.5% (95% confidence interval, 32.2–75.6%), and the pathological CR rate among all patients treated with chemotherapy plus trastuzumab was 60% (95% CI, 44.3–74.3%). The safety data did not demonstrate any significant difference between the two treatment arms.

In conclusion, early breast cancer treatment is one of the oncology domains in which EBM is the leading condition to look at the enormous amount of published data. This methodology can help in the decision-making process. As already mentioned, we have now the opportunity to summarize the findings of similar trials in meta-analysis that can help when contrasting data are reported but, in spite of all that, many open questions remain to be clarified by future well-planned and well-conducted trials.

14.10 Closing Remarks

In modern medicine there is a growing need to define strategies, recommendations and guidelines, which support clinicians in their daily practice, and make patients much more confident that their best interest is being taken care of. In oncology, knowledge has evolved so rapidly, particularly in the last decade, and the quantity and quality of new therapeutic possibilities and strategies have changed so quickly that it is objectively difficult to keep oneself up-to-date and take account of new developments in order to make the right decision (to be updated for the right decision. One of the modern ways in the clinical decision-making process is to rely on evidence, follow guidelines and their recommendations.

However, the gap between the amount of information produced yearly and the time to get guidelines updated is increasing tremendously. Actually, ASCO produced the first guideline on the correct use of hematopoietic growth factors in 1994, published thereafter 25 additional guidelines, and as a rule intended to update them every 3 years. However, it is currently developing nine new guidelines and updating eleven old ones. Furthermore, ASCO has very recently introduced "PCOs," which are based on expedited review of potentially practice-changing evidence.

The first PCO has been published in the very recent past to help select patients with advanced/metastatic colon cancer for treatment with the monoclonal antibody cetuximab or panitumumab.

At the same time (November 2008) also the NCCN announced important updates of the Guidelines on Colon and Rectal Cancer. The recommendation is that a determination of the K-RAS gene status of either the primary tumor or a site of metastasis be part of the pretreatment work-up for all patients diagnosed with metastatic colorectal cancer. Consequently, the epidermal growth factor receptor (EGFR) inhibitors, cetuximab and panitumumab, either as single agents or, in the case of cetuximab, in combination with other agents, are now recommended only for patients with K-RAS wild-type tumors.

In the late '90 numerous organizations in Europe began to establish rules to improve the quality of medicine. In particular, within the Cochrane Collaboration several national organizations, like NICE in Great Britain, and the European Society for Medical Oncology (ESMO), were created to support the use of EBM.

In particular, ESMO has developed and disseminated clinical recommendations to all European and non-European oncologists to achieve high common standards of medical practice for patients all over Europe. The principles of the ESMO Clinical Recommendations are: "*to create a set of statements for an essential standard of care; to be disease or topic-oriented; to be evidence-based; to have an emphasis on medical oncology; and to be annually updated.*"

In this respect, by recognizing the continuous huge amount of new information deriving from the increasing number of clinical trials, the ESMO has made a big effort to produce up-to-date recommendations. The last publication in Annals of Oncology (Volume 20, Supplement 4, May 2009) deals with ten different topics and 54 different clinical recommendations.

The evolution in the area of EBM has been so rapid that from the early '90s a profound revision of terms and strategies occurred. ASCO and ESMO clinical recommendations still use the grading system divided into five levels of evidence (from I, the strongest, to V, the weakest) and four grades of recommendations (from A to D).

The evolution of this system is represented by the GRADE system, currently adopted worldwide by more than 25 health organizations. This approach provides a complete and transparent methodology for grading the level of evidence and strength of recommendations for patient management. The quality of evidence is classified in four levels, namely high, moderate, low and very low. In the process of grading evidence, an important role is played also by patient representatives.

References

1. André T, Boni C, Mounedji-Boudiaf L, Navarro M, Tabernero J, Hickish T, Topham C, Zaninelli M, Clingan P, Bridgewater J, Tabah-Fisch I, de Gramont A (2004) Multicenter international study of oxaliplatin/5-fluorouracil/leucovorin in the adjuvant treatment of colon cancer (MOSAIC) investigators. N Engl J Med 350:2343–2351

2. Andrè T, Boni C, Navarro M, Tabernero J, Hickish T, Topham C, Bonetti A, Clingan P, Bridgewater J, Rivera F, de Gramont A (2009) Improved overall survival with oxaliplatin, fluorouracil, and leucovorin as adjuvant treatment in stage II or III colon cancer in the MOSAIC trial. J Clin Oncol 27:1–8

3. Atkins D, Best D, Briss PA, Eccles M, Falck-Ytter Y, Flottorp S, Guyatt GH, Harbour RT, Haugh MC, Henry D, Hill S, Jaeschke R, Leng G, Liberati A, Magrini N, Mason J, Middleton P, Mrukowicz J, O'Connell D, Oxman AD, Phillips B, Schünemann HJ, Edejer TT, Varonen H, Vist GE, Williams JW Jr, Zaza S, GRADE Working Group (2004) Grading quality of evidence and strength of recommendations. BMJ 328:1490

4. Austoker J (2001) The potential and pitfalls for developing guidelines in oncology. Ann Oncol 12:1189–1190

5. Aydiner A, Tas F (2008) Meta-analysis of trials comparing anastrozole and tamoxifen for adjuvant treatment of postmenopausal women with early breast cancer. Trials 9:47

6. Baxter NN, Virnig DJ, Rothenberger DA, Morris AM, Jessurun J, Virnig BA (2005) Lymph node evaluation in colorectal cancer patients: a population-based study. J Natl Cancer Inst 97:219–225

7. Bear HD, Anderson S, Smith RE, Geyer CE Jr, Mamounas EP, Fisher B, Brown AM, Robidoux A, Margolese R, Kahlenberg MS, Paik S, Soran A, Wickerham DL, Wolmark N (2006) Sequential preoperative or postoperative docetaxel added to preoperative doxorubicin plus cyclophosphamide for operable breast cancer: National Surgical Adjuvant Breast and Bowel Project Protocol B-27. J Clin Oncol 24: 2019–2027

8. Benson AB 3rd, Schrag D, Somerfield MR, Cohen AM, Figueredo AT, Flynn PJ, Krzyzanowska MK, Maroun J, McAllister P, Van Cutsem E, Brouwers M, Charette M, Haller DG (2004) American Society of Clinical Oncology recommendations on adjuvant chemotherapy for stage II colon cancer. J Clin Oncol 22:3408–3419

9. Berger AC, Sigurdson ER, LeVoyer T, Hanlon A, Mayer RJ, Macdonald JS, Catalano PJ, Haller DG (2005) Colon cancer survival is associated with decreasing ratio of metastatic to examined lymph nodes. J Clin Oncol 23:8706–8712

10. Boccardo F, Rubagotti A, Guglielmini P, Fini A, Paladini G, Mesiti M, Rinaldini M, Scali S, Porpiglia M, Benedetto C, Restuccia N, Buzzi F, Franchi R, Massidda B, Distante V, Amadori D, Sismondi P (2006) Switching to anastrozole versus continued tamoxifen treatment of early breast cancer. Updated results of the Italian tamoxifen anastrozole (ITA) trial. Ann Oncol 17:vii10–vii14

11. Bokemeyer C, Bondarenko I, Makhson A, Hartmann JT, Aparicio J, de Braud F, Donea S, Ludwig H, Schuch G, Stroh C, Loos AH, Zubel A, Koralewski P (2009) Fluorouracil, leucovorin, and oxaliplatin with and without cetuximab in the first-line treatment of metastatic colorectal cancer J. Clin Oncol 27:663–671

12. Brouwers MC, Somerfield MR, Browman GP (2008) A for effort: learning from the application of the GRADE approach to cancer guideline development. J Clin Oncol 26:1033–1039

13. Buzdar AU, Valero V, Ibrahim NK, Francis D, Broglio KR, Theriault RL, Pusztai L, Green MC, Singletary SE, Hunt KK, Sahin AA, Esteva F, Symmans WF, Ewer MS, Buchholz TA, Hortobagyi GN (2007) Neoadjuvant therapy with paclitaxel followed by 5-fluorouracil, epirubicin, and cyclophosphamide chemotherapy and concurrent trastuzumab in human epidermal growth factor receptor 2-positive operable breast cancer: an update of the initial randomized study population and data of additional patients treated with the same regimen. Clin Cancer Res 13:228–233

14. Colleoni M, Gelber S, Goldhirsch A, Aebi S, Castiglione-Gertsch M, Price KN, Coates AS, Gelber RD, International Breast Cancer Study Group (2006) Tamoxifen after adjuvant chemotherapy for premenopausal women with lymph node-positive breast cancer: International Breast Cancer Study Group Trial 13-93. J Clin Oncol 24:1332–1341

15. Coombes RC, Hall E, Gibson LJ, Paridaens R, Jassem J, Delozier T, Jones SE, Alvarez I, Bertelli G, Ortmann O, Coates AS, Bajetta E, Dodwell D, Coleman RE, Fallowfield LJ, Mickiewicz E, Andersen J, Lønning PE, Cocconi G, Stewart A, Stuart N, Snowdon CF, Carpentieri M, Massimini G, Bliss JM, van de Velde C, Intergroup Exemestane Study (2004) A randomized trial of exemestane after two to three years of tamoxifen therapy in postmenopausal women with primary breast cancer. N Engl J Med 350:1081–1089

16. Courtè-Wienecke S, Engelbrecht R, v Eimeren W (1999) A survey on the current state of development, dissemination and implementation of guidelines of clinical practice in European countries. Report conducted in the text of the Telematics Application programme for Health Care in the European Union. Medis Institute of Medical Informatics and Health Services Research, Neuherberg

17. Crivellari D, Aapro M, Leonard R, von Minckwitz G, Brain E, Goldhirsch A, Veronesi A, Muss H (2007) Breast cancer in the elderly. J Clin Oncol 25:1882–1890

18. Crivellari D, Sun Z, Coates AS, Price KN, Thürlimann B, Mouridsen H, Mauriac L, Forbes JF, Paridaens RJ, Castiglione-Gertsch M, Gelber RD, Colleoni M, Láng I, Del Mastro L, Gladieff L, Rabaglio M, Smith IE, Chirgwin JH, Goldhirsch A (2008) Letrozole compared with tamoxifen for elderly patients with endocrine-responsive early breast cancer: the BIG 1-98 trial. J Clin Oncol 26:1972–1979

19. Cunningham D, Humblet Y, Siena S, Khayat D, Bleiberg H, Santoro A, Bets D, Mueser M, Harstrick A, Verslype C, Chau I, Van Cutsem E (2004) Cetuximab monotherapy and

cetuximab plus irinotecan in irinotecan-refractory metastatic colorectal cancer. N Engl J Med 351:337–345

20. Cuppone F, Bria E, Carlini P, Milella M, Felici A, Sperduti I, Nisticò C, Terzoli E, Cognetti F, Giannarelli D (2008) Taxanes as primary chemotherapy for early breast cancer: meta-analysis of randomized trials. Cancer 113:238–246

21. De Laurentiis M, Cancello G, D'Agostino D, Giuliano M, Giordano A, Montagna E, Lauria R, Forestieri V, Esposito A, Silvestro L, Pennacchio R, Criscitiello C, Montanino A, Limite G, Bianco AR, De Placido S (2008) Taxane-based combinations as adjuvant chemotherapy of early breast cancer: a meta-analysis of randomized trials. J Clin Oncol 26:44–53

22. De Palma R, Liberati A, Ciccone G, Bandieri E, Belfiglio M, Ceccarelli M, Leoni M, Longo G, Magrini N, Marangolo M, Roila F, Programma Ricerca e Innovazione Emilia Romagna Oncology Research Group (2008) Developing clinical recommendations for breast, colorectal, and lung cancer adjuvant treatments using the GRADE system: a study from the Programma Ricercae Innovazione Emilia Romagna Oncology Research Group. J Clin Oncol 26:1033–1039

23. Deguara C, Dozier N (2007) Evidence-based medicine: setting the standard for high quality patient care. US Oncol (2)

24. Djulbegovic B, Lyman G, Ruckdeschel JC (2000) Why evidence-based oncology? Evid Based Oncol I:2–5

25. Early Breast Cancer Trialists' Collaborative Group (EBCTCG) (2005) Effects of chemotherapy and hormonal therapy for early breast cancer on recurrence and 15-year survival: an overview of the randomised trials. Lancet 365:1687–1717

26. Ebell MH, Siwek J, Weiss BD, Woolf SH, Susman J, Ewigman B, Bowman M (2004) Strength of Recommendation Taxonomy (SORT): a patient-centered approach to grading evidence in the medical literature. J Am Board Fam Pract 17:59–67

27. Eddy DM (2005) Evidence–based medicine: a unified approach. Health Aff 24:9–17

28. Evidence-Based Medicine Working Group (1992) Evidence-based medicine: a new approach to teaching the practice of medicine. JAMA 268:2420–2425

29. Ferguson T, Wilcken N, Vagg R, Ghersi D, Nowak AK (2009) Taxanes for adjuvant treatment of early breast cancer (Review). Cochrane Database Syst Rev (2)

30. Fervers B, Burgers JS, Haugh MC, Brouwers M, Browman G, Cluzeau F, Philip T (2005) Predictors of high quality clinical practice guidelines: examples in oncology. Int J Qual Health Care 17:123–132

31. Field MJ, Lohr KN (1990) Clinical practice guidelines. Institute of Medicine, National Academy, Washington, DC

32. Fisher B, Dignam J, Bryant J, Wolmark N (2001) Five versus more than five years of tamoxifen for lymph node-negative breast cancer: updated findings from the National Surgical Adjuvant Breast and Bowel Project B-14 randomized trial. J Natl Cancer Inst 93:684–690

33. Fisher B, Dignam J, Wolmark N, DeCillis A, Emir B, Wickerham DL, Bryant J, Dimitrov NV, Abramson N, Atkins JN, Shibata H, Deschenes L, Margolese RG (1997) Tamoxifen and chemotherapy for lymph node-negative, estrogen receptor-positive breast cancer. J Natl Cancer Inst 89:1673–1682

34. Fisher B, Jeong JH, Bryant J, Anderson S, Dignam J, Fisher ER, Wolmark N (2004) National Surgical Adjuvant Breast and Bowel Project randomised clinical trials. Treatment of lymph-node-negative, oestrogen-receptor-positive breast cancer: long-term findings from National Surgical Adjuvant Breast and Bowel Project randomised clinical trials. Lancet 364:858–868

35. Fisher B, Redmond C, Legault-Poisson S, Dimitrov NV, Brown AM, Wickerham DL, Wolmark N, Margolese RG, Bowman D, Glass AG (1990) Postoperative chemotherapy and tamoxifen compared with tamoxifen alone in the treatment of positive-node breast cancer patients aged 50 years and older with tumors responsive to tamoxifen: results from the National Surgical Adjuvant Breast and Bowel Project B-16. J Clin Oncol 8:1005–1018

36. Fleisher LA, Bass EB, McKeown P (2005) Methodological approach: American College of Chest Physicians guidelines for the prevention and management of postoperative atrial fibrillation after cardiac surgery. Chest 128:17S–23S

37. Forbes JF, Cuzick J, Buzdar A, Howell A, Tobias JS, Baum M, Arimidex, Tamoxifen, Alone or in Combination (ATAC) Trialists' Group (2008) Effect of anastrozole and tamoxifen as adjuvant treatment for early-stage breast cancer: 100-month analysis of the ATAC trial. Lancet Oncol 9:45–53

38. Gill S, Loprinzi C, Sargent D, Thomé SD, Alberts SR, Haller DG, Benedetti J, Francini G, Shepherd LE, Francois Seitz J, Labianca R, Chen W, Cha SS, Heldebrant MP, Goldberg RM (2004) Pooled analysis of fluorouracil-based adjuvant therapy for stage II and III colon cancer: who benefits and by how much? J Clin Oncol 22:1797–1806

39. Goldhirsch A, Wood WC, Gelber RD, Coates AS, Thürlimann B, Senn HJ (2007) 10th St. Gallen conference Progress and promise: highlights of the international expert consensus on the primary therapy of early breast cancer. Ann Oncol 18:1917

40. Goss PE, Ingle JN, Martino S, Robert NJ, Muss HB, Piccart MJ, Castiglione M, Tu D, Shepherd LE, Pritchard KI, Livingston RB, Davidson NE, Norton L, Perez EA, Abrams JS, Cameron DA, Palmer MJ, Pater JL (2005) Randomized trial of letrozole following tamoxifen as extended adjuvant therapy in receptor-positive breast cancer: updated findings from NCIC CTG MA.17. J Natl Cancer Inst 97:1262–1271

41. Goss PE, Ingle JN, Pater JL, Martino S, Robert NJ, Muss HB, Piccart MJ, Castiglione M, Shepherd LE, Pritchard KI, Livingston RB, Davidson NE, Norton L, Perez EA, Abrams JS, Cameron DA, Palmer MJ, Tu D (2008) Late extended adjuvant treatment with letrozole improves outcome in women with early-stage breast cancer who complete 5 years of tamoxifen. J Clin Oncol 26:1948–1955

42. Goss PE, Muss HB, Ingle JN, Whelan TJ, Wu M (2008) Extended adjuvant endocrine therapy in breast cancer: current status and future directions. Clin Breast Cancer 8:411–417

43. Guyatt GH, Oxman AD, Kunz R, Falck-Ytter Y, Vist GE, Liberati A, Schünemann HJ, GRADE Working Group (2008) Going from evidence to recommendations. BMJ 336:1049–1051

44. Guyatt GH, Oxman AD, Kunz R, Vist GE, Falck-Ytter Y, Schünemann HJ, GRADE Working Group (2008) What is "quality of evidence" and why is it important to clinicians? BMJ 336:995–998

45. Guyatt GH, Sackett DL, Sinclair JC, Hayward R, Cook DJ, Cook RJ (1995) Users guides to the medical literature. IX. A method for grading health care recommendations. JAMA 274:1880–1884

46. Harris RP, Helfand M, Woolf SH, Lohr KN, Mulrow CD, Teutsch SM, Atkins D, Methods Work Group, Third US Preventive Services Task Force (2001) Current methods of the US Preventive Services Task Force: a review of the process. Am J Prev Med 20:21–35

47. Hase K, Ueno H, Kuranaga N, Utsunomiya K, Kanabe S, Mochizuki H (1998) Intraperitoneal exfoliated cancer cells in patients with colorectal cancer. Dis Colon Rectum 41:1134–1140

48. Haynes RB (2006) Of studies, syntheses, synopses, summaries, and systems: the "5S" evolution of information services for evidence-based health care decisions. Evid Based Med 11:162–164

49. Hecht JR, Mitchell E, Chidiac T, Scroggin C, Hagenstad C, Spigel D, Marshall J, Cohn A, McCollum D, Stella P, Deeter R, Shahin S, Amado RG (2009) A randomized phase IIIB trial of chemotherapy, bevacizumab, and panitumumab compared with chemotherapy and bevacizumab alone for metastatic colorectal cancer. J Clin Oncol 27:672–680

50. Hulley S, Grady D, Bush T, Furberg C, Herrington D, Riggs B, Vittinghoff E (1998) Randomized trial of estrogen plus progestin for secondary prevention of coronary heart disease in postmenopausal women. JAMA 280:605–613

51. Hurwitz H, Fehrenbacher L, Novotny W, Cartwright T, Hainsworth J, Heim W, Berlin J, Baron A, Griffing S, Holmgren E, Ferrara N, Fyfe G, Rogers B, Ross R, Kabbinavar F (2004) Bevacizumab plus irinotecan, fluorouracil, and leucovorin for metastatic colorectal cancer. N Engl J Med 350:2335–2342

52. Jakesz R, Jonat W, Gnant M, Mittlboeck M, Greil R, Tausch C, Hilfrich J, Kwasny W, Menzel C, Samonigg H, Seifert M, Gademann G, Kaufmann M, Wolfgang J, ABCSG and the GABG (2005) Switching of postmenopausal women with endocrine-responsive early breast cancer to anastrozole after 2 years' adjuvant tamoxifen: combined results of ABCSG trial 8 and ARNO 95 trial. Lancet 366:455–462

53. Joensuu H, Kellokumpu-Lehtinen PL, Bono P, Alanko T, Kataja V, Asola R, Utriainen T, Kokko R, Hemminki A, Tarkkanen M, Turpeenniemi-Hujanen T, Jyrkkiö S, Flander M, Helle L, Ingalsuo S, Johansson K, Jääskeläinen AS, Pajunen M, Rauhala M, Kaleva-Kerola J, Salminen T, Leinonen M, Elomaa I, Isola J, FinHer Study Investigators (2006) Adjuvant docetaxel or vinorelvine with or without trastuzumab for breast cancer. N Engl J Med 23:809–820

54. Jones S, Holmes FA, O'Shaughnessy J, Blum JL, Vukelja SJ, McIntyre KJ, Pippen JE, Bordelon JH, Kirby RL, Sandbach J, Hyman WJ, Richards DA, Mennel RG, Boehm KA, Meyer WG, Asmar L, Mackey D, Riedel S, Muss H, Savin MA (2009) Docetaxel with cyclophosphamide is associated with an overall survival benefit compared with doxorubicin and cyclophosphamide: 7-year follow-up of US Oncology Research Trial 9735. J Clin Oncol 27:1177–1183

55. Kabbinavar F, Hambleton J, Mass RD, Hurwitz HI, Bergsland E, Sarkar S (2005) Combined analysis of efficacy: the addition of bevacizumab to fluorouracil/leucovorin improves survival for patients with metastatic colorectal cancer. J Clin Oncol 23:3706–3712

56. Kabbinavar F, Hurwitz HI, Fehrenbacher L, Meropol NJ, Novotny WF, Lieberman G, Griffing S, Bergsland E (2003) Phase II, randomized trial comparing bevacizumab plus fluorouracil (FU)/leucovorin (LV) with FU/LV alone in patients with metastatic colorectal cancer. J Clin Oncol 21:60–65

57. Kabbinavar F, Schulz J, McCleod M, Patel T, Hamm JT, Hecht JR, Mass R, Perrou B, Nelson B, Novotny WF (2005) Addition of bevacizumab to bolus fluorouracil and leucovorin in first-line metastatic colorectal cancer: results of a randomized Phase II trial. J Clin Oncol 23:3697–3705

58. Kruer MC, Steiner RD (2008) The role of evidence-based medicine and clinical trials in rare genetics disorders. Clin Genet 74:197–207

59. Kuebler JP, Wieand HS, O'Connel MJ, Smith RE, Colangelo LH, Yothers G, Petrelli NJ, Findlay MP, Seay TE, Atkins JN, Zapas JL, Goodwin JW, Fehrenbacher L, Ramanathan RK, Conley BA, Flynn PJ, Soori G, Colman LK, Levine EA, Lanier KS, Wolmark N (2007) Oxaliplatin combined with weekly bolus fluorouracil and leucovorin as surgical adjuvant chemotherapy for stage II and III colon cancer: results from NSABP C-07. J Clin Oncol 25:2198–2204

60. Mieog JS, van der Hage JA, van de Velde CJ (2007) Neoadjuvant chemotherapy for operable breast cancer. Br J Surg 94:1189–1200

61. Moore MJ, Goldstein D, Hamm J, Figer A, Hecht JR, Gallinger S, Au HJ, Murawa P, Walde D, Wolff RA, Campos D, Lim R, Ding K, Clark G, Voskoglou-Nomikos T, Ptasynski M, Parulekar W, National Cancer Institute of Canada Clinical Trials Group (2007) Erlotinib plus gemcitabine compared with gemcitabine alone in patients with advanced pancreatic cancer: a phase III trial of the National Cancer Institute of Canada Clinical Trials Group. J Clin Oncol 25:1960–1966

62. Nathanson SD (1994) Is there a role for clinical prognostic factors in staging patients with colorectal cancer? Semin Surg Oncol 10:176–182

63. NIH consensus conference (1990) Adjuvant therapy for patients with colon and rectal cancer. JAMA 264:1444–1450

64. O'Connell MJ (2009) Oxaliplatin or irinotecan as adjuvant therapy for colon cancer: the results are in. J Clin Oncol 27:1–3

65. Pentheroudakis G, Stahel R, Hansen H, Pavlidis N (2008) Heterogeneity in cancer guidelines: should we eradicate or tolerate? Ann Oncol 19:2067–2078

66. Philip T, Fervers B, Haugh M, Otter R, Browman G (2003) European cooperation for clinical practice guidelines in cancer. Br J Cancer 89:SI–S3

67. Piccart-Gebhart MJ, Procter M, Leyland-Jones B, Goldhirsch A, Untch M, Smith I, Gianni L, Baselga J, Bell R, Jackisch C, Cameron D, Dowsett M, Barrios CH, Steger G, Huang CS, Andersson M, Inbar M, Lichinitser M, Láng I, Nitz U, Iwata H, Thomssen C, Lohrisch C, Suter TM, Rüschoff J, Suto T, Greatorex V, Ward C, Straehle C, McFadden E, Dolci MS, Gelber RD (2005) Herceptin Adjuvant (HERA) Trial Study Team Trastuzumab after adjuvant chemotherapyin HER2-positive breast cancer. N Engl J Med 20:1659–1672

68. Rastogi P, Anderson SJ, Bear HD, Geyer CE, Kahlenberg MS, Robidoux A, Margolese RG, Hoehn JL, Vogel VG, Dakhil SR, Tamkus D, King KM, Pajon ER, Wright MJ, Robert J, Paik S, Mamounas EP, Wolmark N (2008) Preoperative chemotherapy: updates of National Surgical Adjuvant Breast and Bowel Project Protocols B-18 and B-27. J Clin Oncol 26:778–785

69. Ray-Coquard I, Philip T, Lehmann M, Fervers B, Farsi F, Chauvin F (1997) Impact of a clinical guidelines program for breast and colon cancer in a French cancer center. JAMA 278:1591–1595

70. Romond EH, Perez EA, Bryant J, Suman VJ, Geyer CE Jr, Davidson NE, Tan-Chiu E, Martino S, Paik S, Kaufman PA, Swain SM, Pisansky TM, Fehrenbacher L, Kutteh LA, Vogel VG, Visscher DW, Yothers G, Jenkins RB, Brown AM, Dakhil SR, Mamounas EP, Lingle WL, Klein PM, Ingle JN, Wolmark N (2005) Trastuzumab chemotherapy for operable HER2-positive breast cancer. N Engl J Med 20:1673–1684

71. Rossouw JE, Anderson GL, Prentice RL, LaCroix AZ, Kooperberg C, Stefanick ML, Jackson RD, Beresford SA, Howard BV, Johnson KC, Kotchen JM, Ockene J, Writing Group for the Women's Health Initiative Investigators (2002) Risks and benefits of estrogen plus progestin in healthy post-menopausal women. Principal results from the women's health initiative randomized controlled trial. JAMA 288:321–333

72. Rubenstein JH, Inadomi JM (2006) Evidence based medicine (EBM) in practice: applying results of cost-effectiveness analyses. Am J Gastroenerol 6:1169–1171

73. Sackett DL, Rosenberg WM, Gray JA, Haynes RB, Richardson WS (1996) Evidence based medicine: what it is and what it isn't. BMJ 312:71–72

74. Saltz LB, Meropol NJ, Loehrer PJ Sr, Needle MN, Kopit J, Mayer RJ (2004) Phase II trial of cetuximab in patients with refractory colorectal cancer that expresses the epidermal growth factor receptor. J Clin Oncol 22:1201–1208

75. Sant M, Capocaccia R, Coleman MP, Berrino F, Gatta G, Micheli A, Verdecchia A, Faivre J, Hakulinen T, Coebergh JW, Martinez-Garcia C, Forman D, Zappone A (2001) EUROCARE Working Group Cancer survival increases in Europe, but international differences remain wide. Eur J Cancer 37:1659–1667

76. Sargent DJ, Goldberg RM, Jacobson SD, Macdonald JS, Labianca R, Haller DG, Shepherd LE, Seitz JF, Francini G (2001) A pooled analysis of adjuvant chemotherapy for resected colon cancer in elderly patients. N Engl J Med 345:1091–1097

77. Scheithauer W, McKendrick J, Begbic S, Borner M, Burns WI, Burris HA, Cassidy J, Jodrell D, Koralewski P, Levine EL, Marschner N, Maroun J, Garcia-Alfonso P, Tujakowski J, Van Hazel G, Wong A, Zaluski J, Twelves C, X-ACT Study Group (2003) Oral capecitabine as an alternative to i.v. 5-fluorouracil-based adjuvant therapy for colon cancer: safety results of a randomized, phase III trial. Ann Oncol 14:1735–1743

78. Slamon D, Eiermann W, Robert N, Pienkowski T, Martin M, Pawlicki M, Chan A, Smylie M, Liu M, Falkson C, Pinter T, Fornander T, Shiftan T, Valero V, Mackey J, Tabah-Fisch I, Buyse M, Lindsay M, Riva A, Bee V, Pegram M, Press M, Crown J (2006) BCIRG 006: 2nd interim analysis Phase III randomized trial comparing doxorubicin and cyclophosphamide followed by docetaxel and trastuzumab (AC>T) with docetaxel, carboplatin and trastuzumab (TCH) in HER2/neu positive early breast cancer patients. Breast Cancer Res Treat 106:52a

79. Slamon DJ, Leyland-Jones B, Shak S, Fuchs H, Paton V, Bajamonde A, Fleming T, Eiermann W, Wolter J, Pegram M, Baselga J, Norton L (2001) Use of chemotherapy plus a monoclonal antibody against HER2 for metastatic breast cancer that over expresses HER2. N Engl J Med 344:783–792

80. Spielmann M, Roché H, Humblet Y, Delozier T, Bourgeois H, Serin D, Romieu G, Canon JL, Monnier A, Piot G, Maerevoet M, Orfeuvre H, Extra JM, Hardy AC, Martin AL, Kramar A, Geneve J (2007) 3-year follow-up of trastuzumab following adjuvant chemotherapy in node-positive HER2-positive breast cancer patients: results of the PACS-04 trial. Breast Cancer Res Treat 106:S72

81. Stewart HJ, Forrest AP, Everington D, McDonald CC, Dewar JA, Hawkins RA, Prescott RJ, George WD (1996) Randomised comparison of 5 years of adjuvant tamoxifen with continuous therapy for operable breast cancer. The Scottish Cancer Trials Breast Group. Br J Cancer 74:297–299

82. Swain SM, Whaley FS, Ewer MS (2003) Congestive heart failure in patients treated with doxorubicin: a retrospective analysis of three trials. Cancer 97:2869–2879

83. Tol J, Koopman M, Rodenburg CJ, Cats A, Creemers GJ, Schrama JG, Erdkamp FL, Vos AH, Mol L, Antonini NF, Punt CJ (2008) A randomised phase III study on capecitabine, oxaliplatin and bevacizumab with or without cetuximab in first-line advanced colorectal cancer, the CAIRO2 study of the Dutch Colrorectal Cancer Group (DCCG). An interim analysis of toxicity. Ann Oncol 19:734–738

84. Twelves C, Wong A, Nowacki MP, Abt M, Burris H 3rd, Carrato A, Cassidy J, Cervantes A, Fagerberg J, Georgoulias V, Husseini F, Jodrell D, Koralewski P, Kröning H, Maroun J, Marschner N, McKendrick J, Pawlicki M, Rosso R, Schüller J, Seitz JF, Stabuc B, Tujakowski J, Van Hazel G, Zaluski J, Scheithauer W (2005) Capecitabine as adjuvant treatment for stage III colon cancer. N Engl J Med 352:2696–2704

85. Van Cutsem E, Nowacki M, Lang I, Cascinu S, Shchepotin I, Maurel J, Rougier P, Cunningham D, Nippgen J, Köhne C (2007) Randomized Phase III study of irinotecan and 5-FU/FA with or without cetuximab in the first-line treatment of patients with metastatic colorectal cancer (mCRC): the CRYSTAL trial. ASCO Annual Meeting Proceedings Part I. J Clin Oncol 25:18S

86. van Cutsem EJ, Oliveira J (2008) Colon cancer: ESMO clinical recommendations for diagnosis, adjuvant treatment and follow-up. Ann Oncol 19:ii29–ii30

87. Wolff CA, Desch CE (2005) Clinical practice guidelines in oncology: translating evidence in to practice (and back). J Oncol Pract 4:160–161

88. Wolmark N, Wang J, Mamounas E, Bryant J, Fisher B (2001) Preoperative chemotherapy in patients with operable breast cancer: nine-year results from National Surgical Adjuvant Breast and Bowel Project B-18. J Natl Cancer Inst Monogr 30:96–102

Francesco Chiappelli

Core Message

> This book presented a state-of-the-art compilation of chapters by several experts in the field of research synthesis and evidence-based decision making in the clinical setting. This collection of work, taken together, not only sets the present state of knowledge in the field, but also points to *lacunae*, which will be addressed and resolved in the next one or two decades.

15.1 Comparative Effectiveness

This work did not focus on comparative effectiveness, because it will be considered in a separate series. It is, nevertheless, necessary to stress that evidence-based treatment and comparative effectiveness analysis of treatments are two sides of the same coin. Both together would provide a strong scientific foundation in formulating evidence-based policies thereby improving the quality, efficiency, effectiveness, long-term consistency, and sustainability of the health care system. These evidence-based policies would be equated to the standard of care, which would have a higher bar in courts. The preceding chapters have clearly made the point that clinical evidence-based decisions are driven by a clinical question that either the clinician poses, or (and) the patient may pose as well. Hence, from that starting point, a research synthesis question is developed, which is framed within the constraints of the patient characteristics, the interventions under consideration, and the clinical outcome sought – hence the acronym, PICO.

The PICO question is so stated as to provide the keywords necessary to gain access to the entire body of published reports on the question of interest, the *available* bibliome corpus. Several fully validated instruments are then utilized to establish the *best* research evidence. Having obtained the best available evidence, the research synthesis investigator then obtains a consensus statement, which the clinician integrates in the process of clinical decision making for treatment intervention. These decisions incorporate on an equal footing the best available evidence, and the patients' needs/wants, medical and clinical history, and insurance coverage (or means for private payment). The process is grounded on the logic model, which, as discussed in earlier chapters, permits careful formative and summative evaluation by means of fully validated instruments (e.g., AMSTAR, AGREE, GRADE).

Typically, an evidence-based provider would approach the patient with a statement such as: *the best available evidence for your condition recommends this or that treatment intervention. Now, in your case, with your history, etc., these are my clinical recommendations.*

In other words, the best available evidence is an adjuvant for optimal treatment care for every individual patient. Clinical evidence-based decision making is *par excellence* personalized health care.

F. Chiappelli
Divisions of Oral Biology and Medicine, and Associated Clinical Specialties (Joint), University of California at Los Angeles, School of Dentistry, CHS 63-090, Los Angeles, CA 90095-1668, USA
e-mail: fchiappelli@dentistry.ucla.edu

F. Chiappelli et al. (eds.), *Evidence-Based Practice: Toward Optimizing Clinical Outcomes*,
DOI: 10.1007/978-3-642-05025-1_15, © Springer-Verlag Berlin Heidelberg 2010

Comparative effectiveness research[1] (or analysis) also rests on the best available evidence, which it obtains by means of exactly the same research synthesis process: a PICO question is formulated, in which the outcome, O, focuses on cost– and risk–benefit relationships. Differences arise at the tail-end of the process, where decisions are grounded on a probabilistic model (cf., earlier chapters), akin to the Markov decision tree. Clinical decisions that rest on comparative effectiveness analysis are oriented toward societal benefits (i.e., financial, risk-minimizing).

It is fair to say, as has already been proposed in the pertinent research literature, that comparative effectiveness analysis is the other side of the same coin as evidence-based treatment interventions [5, 6]. One focuses on effectiveness issues from the viewpoint of societal benefit and reducing overall costs, the other is directed at individualized health care. One cannot be considered without consideration of the other.

Future research in the field will increasingly establish the intertwined nature of the relationship between comparative effectiveness research and analysis on one hand, and evidence-based clinical decisions for optimal treatment on the other.

Moreover, cognizant of the fact that both these elements rely on the entire body of available information about a given patient population ("P" in PICO), future research will increasingly recognize the urgency of the need for human information technology (HIT) in this sector. It is urgent, timely, and critical that we develop databases of patient histories, so that as the product of research synthesis becomes available, they may be integrated with these HIT repositories, and probabilistic (comparative effectiveness) or logic model (evidence-based treatment) decisions obtained by computerized algorithms.

Finally, and perhaps most importantly, because both comparative effectiveness analysis and evidence-based intervention depend upon the systematic

---

[1]Comparative effectiveness research (or analysis) in health care is best defined as the process of generation and synthesis of scientific evidence that compares the benefits and harms of alternative methods to prevent, diagnose, treat, and monitor clinical conditions, or to improve the delivery of care, in a concerted effort to assist patients, clinicians, purchasers, and policy makers to make informed decisions that will improve health care at both the individual and the population levels. (from the Committee on Comparative Effectiveness Research, Institute of Medicine, 2009).

evaluation of the best available research evidence (i.e., research synthesis), future research in the field of research synthesis must reach novel and improved frontiers in the next decade.

15.2 Research Synthesis: Where Do We Need To Go in the Next Decade?

15.2.1 Level of the Evidence vs. Quality of the Evidence

Currently, most systematic reviews present an assessment of the "level of the evidence," as was discussed in several chapters. This is typically obtained based on the pyramid schematic representation of research. The pyramid, which places systematic reviews and clinical trials at the top, and animal and bench research at the very bottom, was constructed with an effort to provide some guidance for grading the usefulness of research reports in the context of immediate use in the clinical context [2, 6]. Although by its mere structure, it implies that clinical trials are "better than" fundamental mechanistic research, the pyramid was not really meant to proffer such a (destructive and blatantly wrong) message. It is clear in the minds of most clinicians that basic experiments involving genomic or proteomic endpoints, or cells in culture or animals can, and do, provide novel and critical knowledge, which is indispensable for developing sound clinical trials. In fact, in the absence of solid fundamental studies, randomized clinical trials could never see the light of day, they would be impossible to run if they did, and if they were run, they could never be interpreted.

So, really, the pyramid – if that is what we want to use – should be inverted.

Another issue that disqualifies the pyramid of the level of evidence as presently used is that it places cohort studies at a mediocre "level of evidence." However, researchers know well that, before a clinical trial can be effectively designed, observational studies, such as cohort studies, will provide critical data. Moreover, in several clinical situations, randomization is not possible, and control group would be unethical: thus, negating the possibility of running a clinical trial, and of obtaining a "high level of evidence" study.

So, in fact, the pyramid should be done away with!

Last but not the least, the pyramid, in addition to providing a loose assessment of what is now being called "level of evidence" – although that too could be argued to be a gross misnomer: what the pyramid does is to provide an artificial ranking list of study designs supposedly pertinent to the clinical realm – not at all a "level" of the "evidence" – has engendered a situation that is proven to be increasingly detrimental to the field. By, in effect, closing in on certain study designs to the exclusion of others, it has emarginated certain areas of research with critical relevance for patient well-being. For instance, by artificially pushing down the value of experimental designs that serve to test new materials in dental and medical care (e.g., prostheses), it de facto excludes the possibility of performing evidence-based decision making (or comparative effectiveness analysis) on materials. The same is true for diagnostic studies, which frankly are not all represented in the pyramid.

In brief, whereas the pyramid concept was useful to get us started in the field in the past 2–3 decades, it is now time to get rid of it, or at least to reassess seriously what it is meant to do, what its limitations are, and what information it really provides. Projections are that continuing development in research synthesis in the next decade will yield to a new position with respect to the concept of the level of evidence.

The same can be said about the concept of the quality of the evidence. In fact, level and quality of the evidence are two intertwined constructs, which must be carefully redefined and reassessed so that novel and better tools may be developed in the near future [2]. The salient issues with the level of evidence concept were discussed in the preceding section. With respect to the quality of the evidence, we presently have several tools that are based on widely accepted criteria and standards for adequate-to-good research. Case in point, the Consolidated Standards of Randomized Trials (CONSORT), and the QUORUM and PRISMA criteria for assessing the quality of meta-analyses ([3]; cf., Chap. 1). Nevertheless, two issues are salient: (1) the assessment of the quality of the evidence is not as widely used in research synthesis as it ought to be, and (2) instruments that are all-encompassing of recognized criteria of excellence for research methodology (e.g., sampling issues, measurements issues), design, and statistical handling of the data are rare. It is often the case that research synthesis reports will attempt an evaluation of the quality of the evidence based on this

trilogy of criteria, but when that is done it often suffers from the fact that the instrument used is an in-house and ad-hoc-made tool with no or little validation data.

To counter this problem, we reported elsewhere the full psychometric characterization of reliability, coefficient of agreement and validity of a simple instrument that rigorously assesses the quality of the evidence gathered in clinical trials, observational studies, fundamental experimental research, materials research, and any such related investigation [7]. Instruments such as these are, and remain, however, few and far between.

It will behoove the field of research synthesis, and its applications and implications to both comparative effectiveness analysis and evidence-based clinical decision making to establish further the criteria of good and acceptable research, and, based upon those, novel or improved instruments for evaluating systematically the quality of the evidence.

To make a mundane example: the level of the evidence relates to what was done, such as what did you have for dinner last night. We rank clinical trials at the top and observational studies as less desirable, as we may rank sirloin at the top and chicken as a less desirable dish. Quality of the evidence describes how the study was done: if the sirloin was burnt, it certainly was not a pleasant dinner! In the same fashion, a top level of evidence (clinical trial) does not ensure that the trial was in fact conducted well. If it was not, its outcomes ought not to be applied to patient care: better we rely on a well done observational study.

This brings us to another point of systematic research synthesis that will see increased activity in the next decade. We need to refine our analyses so that we can red flag studies that are less than acceptable, based on quantifiable measures of the quality of the evidence. We ought to discuss and come to an agreement as to whether we should incorporate in meta-analyses all the reports obtained in the systematic search (*all* available evidence), or only those reports that are determined to be acceptable based on acceptable sampling analysis (*best* available evidence).

From a statistical theoretical viewpoint, one might argue that in a Bayesian view on evidence-based decision making, which was proposed and discussed elsewhere [1, 2], the true population of the outcome of interest will be best approximated by incorporating all the available evidence, whether or not it meets acceptable criteria. A mundane example, however, points us to the fallacy of this argument: if I use all the oranges

I have in my fruit salad, unripe oranges, ripe oranges, and unacceptably over-ripe (read: rotten) oranges, the fruit salad is bound to be unpalatable. Should we then be surprised if, when we use acceptable and unacceptably deficient reports (based on established criteria of research methodology, design, and statistical analysis of the data), we obtain less than convincing meta-analysis results.

In brief, the principle of acceptable sampling is to assess systematically what paper is acceptable based on commonly held criteria of research excellence, and to include only those in meta-analyses, and to use these assessments of the *best available evidence* in evidence-based decision making [2, 4, 6]. The next decade will see, expectations are, substantial developments in acceptable sampling analysis, and refinements in fixed and random model meta-analyses.

15.2.2 Quality of Systematic Reviews

The last two decades have witnessed an explosion in our ability to generate systematic reviews of the literature. The procedure and protocols have been, and continue to be refined. We have generated systematic reviews that most of us recognize to be superb, and other reviews that most of us have no hesitation in finding wanting. As a field, we have been able to outline a set of simple criteria of what makes a "good" systematic review. We generally agree that following the Cochrane Group protocol ensures pursuance of a high quality systematic review – even though that too is not full proof, and some Cochrane reviews are much better than others. Be that as it may, based on widely shared criteria of adequate-to-excellent systematic reviews, the field has generated a number of instruments that are designed to assess the quality of systematic reviews [2, 6]. A good example of that is the AMSTAR ([6], cf., Chap. 1).

Research efforts in the next decade must converge on transforming the qualitative nature of the AMSTAR, and related instruments for the assessment of the quality of systematic reviews, into tools of measurements that permit full quantification of these outcomes. These revised tools must then be fully validated psychometrically to ensure reliability and validity of the assessments.

These transformations must be actualized with the AMSTAR, the GRADE, the SORT, the CASP, the AGREE and all the assessments tools currently in use,

and with any new ones in development. Ongoing work by our own research group, which will be published shortly, demonstrates the feasibility of this enterprise with the publication of the Revised AMSTAR, which permits full quantification of the assessment of systematic review quality.

15.2.3 Quantifying Clinical Relevance

Today, even under the best of circumstances when the meta-analysis is convincingly demonstrating statistically significant trends, systematic reviews generally produce a statement of clinical relevance that is bland and often misleading. We label the overall evidence as good or limited, but hardly any of us would not be hard pressed to explain in detail to the clinician what we mean, exactly.

Here again, research in the forthcoming decades will advance our field by providing clearer and better evaluations of clinical relevance. Our research group, again in a publication to be soon disseminated, has developed a simple algorithm by which valid and reliable scores are obtained, pooled, and expressed in quartiles. In this fashion, the upper quartile can be labeled with a letter grade, say A; the upper middle quartile might be represented by a B, the middle lower quartile might be given a C; and the lowest quartile might be valued as a D. In this simple representation of the final product of the systematic evaluation of the literature, including systematic reviews, the reader will have an immediate sense of the quality and clinical relevance of the overall *best available* evidence: an A evidence being better than a B evidence, better than C evidence and so on – a bit like, if I am permitted to return to a mundane example, the consumer is immediately alerted of the quality of restaurant by the rating, A, B, or C, that hangs from the window.

15.2.4 Toward Complex Systematic Reviews and Meta-Meta-Analyses for Evidence-Based Policies

As we stated above, the field of research synthesis that we use in comparative effectiveness analysis and in evidence-based research has exploded in the last decade.

Systematic reviews will continue to multiply, and the bibliome for any given PICO question can be expected to consist increasingly of multiple systematic reviews, in addition to multiple primary research papers.

That is to say, evidence is becoming increasingly more complex: it used to be the case when evidence was to be found in one or in several trials or observational studies. Now, evidence is to be found not only in primary research, but also in several systematic reviews, often published only a few months apart. Expectations are that evidence, increasingly, will have to be obtained as systematic reviews of systematic reviews – that is to say, "complex" systematic reviews, or "meta-systematic reviews" [2, 3, 6].

It is unclear at this point how these gargantuan systematic analyses of the best available research evidence will be conducted, reported, and evaluated. It is also unclear as to how the data of the meta-analyses from each of the systematic reviews incorporated in a meta-systematic review can be pooled into a *meta*-meta-analysis. There are serious conceptual as well as statistical problems that need to be carefully addressed and confronted.

It is fair to say that, of all the topics of future research in the field, this latter point is the issue of major concern. We are driven toward it, and yet we know little how to face it, what to expect once we will have faced it, and where the caveats will trip us. Yet, it is crucial that we do so within the next decade, lest we fail to serve our patient with the *best available* evidence.

15.3 Conclusion

It must be understood that the future of research synthesis in health care depends not only upon the topics the authors of this *opus* so eruditely discussed, but also on the few points outlined above. The future of the field depends as well upon two fundamental principles:

- First, research synthesis for evidence-based decision making and comparative effectiveness research must aim at utilizing the *best available* evidence for sustainable solutions [3].
- Second, research synthesis for evidence-based decision making and comparative effectiveness research

must be grounded on a solid pedagogy. Students must be educated not only on *how we do* research synthesis, and *why we must do it*, but also on *how we interpret it* and *why such interpretation is beneficial* for the individual (cf., logic model, evidence-based health care) or for the society (cf., probabilistic model or the Markov decision tree for comparative effectiveness analysis). Education[2] in the principles, fundamentals, and applications of research synthesis in comparative effectiveness and evidence-based decisions is both crucial and critical for the survival of the society and the quality of life of all of us, at a local and a global level (cf., ifebdcer.org).

References

1. Bauer JG, Spackman S, Chiappelli F, Prolo P, Stevenson RG (2006) Making clinical decisions using a clinical practice guideline. Calif Dent Assoc J 34:519–528
2. Chiappelli F (2008) The science of research synthesis: a manual of evidence-based research for the health sciences – implications and applications in dentistry. NovaScience, Hauppauge, NY
3. Chiappelli F (2010) Sustainable evidence-based decision-making. Monograph. NovaScience, Hauppauge
4. Chiappelli F, Cajulis OS (2009) The logic model in evidence-based clinical decision-making in dental practice. J Evid Based Dent Pract 9(4):206–210
5. Chiappelli F, Cajulis O, Newman M (2009) Comparative effectiveness research in evidence based dental practice. J Evid Based Dent Pract 9:57–58
6. Chiappelli F, Cajulis OC, Oluwadara O, Ramchandani MH (2009) Evidence-based based decision making – implications for dental care. In Columbus F (ed) Dental care: diagnostic, preventive, and restorative services. NovaScience, Hauppauge, NY
7. Chiappelli F, Navarro AM, Moradi DR, Manfrini E, Prolo P (2006) Evidence-based research in complementary and alternative medicine III: treatment of patients with Alzheimer's disease. Evid Based Compl Alt Med 3:411–424

---

[2]In this context, the concepts of "hard" vs. "soft" knowledge cited in the introductory chapter as arising from the academic domain of knowledge management, clearly signal a novel domain of teaching/learning of the tenets proposed in this book, and which will, we predict, see increased exploration, implications, and application in the field of evidence-based decision-making in health care.

Index

Printing and Binding: Stürtz GmbH, Würzburg